A SYNOPSIS OF
CONTEMPORARY PSYCHIATRY

A SYNOPSIS OF
CONTEMPORARY
PSYCHIATRY

GEORGE A. ULETT, A.B., M.S., M.D., Ph.D.

Professor and Chairman, Missouri Institute of Psychiatry (St. Louis),
University of Missouri School of Medicine;
Visiting Professor of Psychiatry, University of Istanbul, Istanbul, Turkey;
Director, Division of Mental Health for the State of Missouri,
Jefferson City, Missouri

FIFTH EDITION

THE C. V. MOSBY COMPANY

SAINT LOUIS 1972

VH/VH/B   9   8   7   6   5   4   3   2

Preface

What a challenge is presented by contemporary psychiatry! New discoveries in the brain sciences continually bring us closer to the causes of mental illnesses. Psychopharmacological agents and behavioral techniques offer hope for recovery where previously there was none. Serious limitations in budgets and mental health manpower are real obstacles to delivery of optimal mental health care to all, even with computer assistance. United States Public Health Service statistics estimate 17% of the population have some form of mental illness, and some recent studies show up to 80% of persons with troublesome psychiatric symptoms. While psychotropic drugs continue to reduce overcrowding in state hospitals, a steady rise in admissions and readmissions increases the work load. As the length of hospital stay becomes ever shorter, more patients are followed or receive initial care in psychiatric units in general hospitals, community mental health centers, burgeoning outpatient clinics, partial hospitals (day care/night care), emergency services, rehabilitation services, halfway houses, foster homes, and even foster communities.

Today patient care moves steadily into the community, while at the same time admissions to hospital inpatient services continue to rise. Ever greater numbers of persons are becoming involved in the treatment and rehabilitation of the mentally ill. Thus, more than ever before, there is need for a brief eclectic textbook to present the facts about mental illness simply and to serve as an introduction to this complex field for the beginning medical student, nurse, or mental health worker. Previous editions of this small book have also found use as a review for professional examinations and as a concise pocket compendium for busy general physicians.

George A. Ulett

v

Contents

A SYNOPSIS OF
CONTEMPORARY PSYCHIATRY

1
Introduction

The beginning student of psychiatry is confronted by a confusion of different diagnostic terminologies of the several schools within this medical specialty. He may be perplexed as he attempts to define the limits of a psychiatry which now ranges from the microbiology of individual cells through anatomy, biochemistry, genetics, neurophysiology, clinical medicine and neurology, psychology, and sociology to include pronouncements in law, foreign relations, and religion. Psychiatry even includes an involvement in practical politics at the community level as groups of people seek fulfillment of the promises of a better society through the application of forces and facilities at the community level in their search for solutions to local public mental health problems.

In the present handbook our scope is less broad. The actual number of factually supportable observations in the field of psychiatry is readily encompassed between the covers of this small volume. Despite some regional differences in classification of mental illness, there is considerable agreement on broad groupings of the major clinical entities and their management which we will present as standard fare. In view of current limitations of knowledge it is obviously unwise for one who seeks for his patients the best treatment method that is available to settle for either the dogma of psychoanalysis or the latest puffery of some chemotherapeutic agent as the single answer to the complex psycho-bio-social problems of psychiatric sickness. It is hoped, as a result of an increasingly rigorous application of research and statistical fact gathering to the methods and outcome of decision making in psychiatry, that treatment procedures for the mentally ill will become ever more based on reality. In the interim period an increase in popular knowledge about the problems of mental illness and a more ready availability of existing treatment methods will be promoted through legislative and public action such as has produced the current community mental health center movement.

As much as possible, this book will be organized as are other medical synopses to serve as a convenient, easy reference. It is divided into three sections: *diagnostic procedures, major disease entities,* and *therapeutics.* The topic headings of the *Diagnostic and Statistical Manual of Mental Disorders** (second edition) will be used. Where knowledge exists, the histological, physiological, or chemical pathology of the brain will be described. Little attempt will be made to present theoretical formulations of etiology except where they are widely used as a basis for a therapy of some demonstrated efficacy. Added evidence from the important research of recent years gives rise to the belief that the future of psychiatry may be more scientifically productive than its past.

Despite the promising advances of the past 50 years in our understanding of human brain function, personality development, and various therapeutic techniques, psychiatric disorders are today as abundantly with us as ever and constitute a major public health problem. Although since 1955 the overcrowded populations in state mental hospitals have been steadily decreasing, the number of persons seeking treatment for mental illness has been increasing at a rate of over 5% per year. Obviously this is one of medicine's most challenging frontiers.

Because of the many gaping holes in our knowledge about the relationships between biological factors and psychosocial forces, practical therapeutic measures tend to have an either-or quality at present. The beginning student will soon encounter a great variety of operating psychiatric philosophies. It may be helpful to mention a few of these. For example, some hope that when detailed knowledge of intracellular and intercellular biochemical processes is available, answers to mental illness will appear. Others are intrigued with the need for clarifica-

---

*Washington, D. C., 1968, American Psychiatric Association.

tion of the neurophysiological connections between large groups of neurons which constitute complex functional systems. Still others tend to view the brain more as a necessary substrate for psychological functioning but one having little differential effect on personality. The latter look for concepts which will clarify the effects of life experience upon an individual's patterns of behavior, feeling, and thinking. Since no scientific body of knowledge exists which to any appreciable extent unifies the above complex of possibly relevant etiological factors, each researcher, teacher, or practitioner tends to base his own particular diagnostic-therapeutic system somewhat upon his personal experience with patients.

We would like to emphasize the great need for application of the scientific method to collection and analysis of psychiatric data—to correct a failure which is almost universal in reports in the field of clinical psychiatry and which fills our literature with much confusing misinformation. It is our belief that an answer to many problems in this field can be found through well-planned comprehensive studies of human behavior, utilizing a multidimensional approach which includes observations by neurophysiologists, biochemists, geneticists, anthropologists, psychiatrists, sociologists, and a host of other workers. Evaluation of treatment procedures should include the use of adequate controls, statistical validation, and methods of handling data which will permit a ready acceptance of psychological observations into the general body of scientific knowledge.

In view of the above, it is with considerable trepidation that one writes a text in this field—especially a brief text—where lack of space for giving alternate theories forces a somewhat dogmatic presentation. We feel, however, with the current trend toward detailed encyclopedic compilations which attempt to cover the total mushrooming field of psychiatric schools, philosophies, and theories, that the need is now greater than ever before for a brief, factual and eclectic introduction to the increasingly complex field of psychiatry.

SUGGESTED READINGS

Throughout this book reference is made to writings of particular interest or historical importance. Many good books and articles are omitted, since selection must be made from the vast literature in this field.

Arieti, S.: American handbook of psychiatry, New York, 1967, Basic Books, Inc., Publishers, vols. 1 to 3.

Berelson, B., and Stiner, G. A.: Human behavior, New York, 1964, Harcourt, Brace & World, Inc.

Cumming, J., and Cumming, E.: Ego and milieu, New York, 1966, Atherton Press.

Franks, C. M.: Conditioning techniques in clinical practice and research, New York, 1964, Springer Publishing Co., Inc.

Freedman, A. M., and Kaplan, H. I.: Comprehensive textbook of psychiatry, Baltimore, 1967, The Williams & Wilkins Co.

Mayer-Gross, W., Slater, E., and Roth, M.: Clinical psychiatry, ed. 3, London, 1969, Bailliere, Tindall & Cassell, Ltd.

Menninger, K., and Devereux, G.: A guide to psychiatric books with a suggested basic reading list, ed. 2, New York, 1956, Grune & Stratton, Inc.

Redlich, F. C., and Freedman, D. X.: Theory and practice of psychiatry, New York, 1966, Basic Books, Inc., Publishers.

Satir, V.: Conjoint family therapy, Palo Alto, Calif., 1964, Science & Behavior Books, Inc.

VonderBerg, J. H.: The phenomenological approach to psychiatry, Springfield, Ill., 1955, Charles C Thomas, Publisher.

2
History of psychiatric thought

Man has always feared mental illness, and the tendency to ascribe its phenomena to supernatural causes is even yet extant. Progress in banishing these beliefs has been slow despite the fact that long before the Christian era enlightened Greeks treated their mentally sick by baths, music, exercise, drugs, venesection, and the surroundings of beautiful gardens. *Hippocrates* promulgated the concept of mental disease resulting from natural causes and included among his many keen descriptions the syndromes of mania, melancholia, and dementia. For 700 years, beginning with Hippocrates and ending with the death of *Galen,* A.D. 200, patients with mental diseases were treated with some degree of humanitarianism. Then, with the fall of the Roman Empire and disintegration of classical civilizations, 15 centuries of primitive attitudes of fear ensued, attitudes which were typified by the Inquisition with its accusation and persecution of the mentally ill as witches.

Philippe Pinel of France in 1792 started the era of "the moral treatment of the insane" by striking off the chains of patients in the Bicêtre. In England a similar role was played by *William Tuke,* representing the Quakers in the founding of the York Retreat. At this time in Philadelphia an energetic pioneer physician and signer of the Declaration of Independence, *Benjamin Rush,* was protesting against conditions and punishment of mental patients in the Pennsylvania Hospital.

During the early nineteenth century, *Jean-Etienne Esquirol,* a pupil of Pinel, applied statistical methods to his clinical studies. In Germany *Wilhelm Griesinger* advocated nonrestraint, while other Germans created the first modern description of mental disease (*Hecker*—hebephrenia; *Kahlbaum*—catatonia and cyclothymia). In America in the years following 1824 numerous state hospitals were developed and men such as *Pliny Earle, Isaac Ray, Luther Bell, Amariah Brigham, John Butler,* and *Thomas Kirkbride* were prominent in plans, construction, and administration. *Samuel Woodward* was the first president (1844) of the Association of Medical Superintendents of American Institutions for the Insane—later to become the American Psychiatric Association. In 1841 *Dorothea Lynde Dix* began her courageous crusade to remove mental patients from the jails and almshouses into mental hospitals.

Early unsuccessful attempts to classify personality disorders in terms of will, emotions, and intellect were resolved by the classification of *Paul Moebius,* which divided the mental diseases into exogenous and endogenous types, and by *Emil Kraepelin* (1855-1926) whose work established the basis for the present clinical classification. Using concepts which originated with *Morel* in 1860, Kraepelin established the general form of both dementia praecox and manic-depressive psychosis. He believed that the outcome of mental disease is predetermined and laid great stress on the physical causation of these disorders. About this time an attempt was made by *Ernst Kretschmer* to relate manic-depressive disease and dementia praecox to bodily types, an effort which represented a further outgrowth of German psychiatry. Finally *Eugen Bleuler* (1857-1939), revising the Kraepelinian concept of dementia praecox, introduced the term "schizophrenia"; he conceived of schizophrenia not as a progressive deteriorative mental disease but rather as a group of psychotic reactions characterized by a basic disturbance in associative thought processes, accompanied by emotional irritability, indifference, and autistic symptoms. A foreshadowing of today's wide research interest in physiological-psychological correlates occurred with *William Falconer's* book entitled *The Influence of the Passions Upon the Disorders of the Body* (1796) and with *Johann Heinroth's* discussion of the psychosomatic determinants of insomnia (1818).

Paralleling this development of descriptive psychiatry, an increasing understanding of psychological mechanisms developed. Pursuing a path shown earlier by *Franz Anton Mesmer* (1734-1815) in France and later by *James Braid* (1795-1850) in England, *August Liebault* and *Hippolyte-Marie Bernheim* (Nancy school) revived an interest in the use of hypnosis and treatment by suggestion. These methods flourished under the influence of such men as *Emil Coué* (new Nancy school), *Jean-Martin Charcot* (Salpêtrière school), and *Josef Babinski.* It was in this atmosphere that *Pierre Janet,* a pupil of Charcot, studied and defined hysteria, described various automatisms, fixed ideas, and a syndrome characterized by obsessions, doubts, and phobias which he named psychasthenia. He also introduced (1889) the concepts of dissociation, the subconscious, and psychological tension.

Sigmund Freud (1856-1939) early studied with Charcot and Bernheim and then returned to Vienna to collaborate with *Joseph Breuer* in 1893 in the publication of a new method of investigation and treatment of hysteria. This technique of releasing repressed ideas and their associated affect (i.e., catharsis) led later to the development of techniques of free association and dream analysis, the hypothesis of the unconscious, studies of the stages of psychosexual development, studies of the psychopathology of everyday life, and the analysis of transference reactions. These concepts form the historical basis for modern psychotherapy. Additional significant contributions to psychiatric thought were made by several of Freud's collaborators who later diverged from the main stream of analytic thought. *Carl Gustav Jung* (1875-1961) of Zurich, who earlier headed the psychoanalytic movement, made significant contributions to the study of word association techniques, schizophrenic processes, and personality types (introvert-extrovert); in addition, he wrote extensively of psychological aspects of man's religious and cultural strivings (the collective unconscious). *Alfred Adler,* an early supporter of Freud, later separated to form his own school which promulgated the theories of "individual psychology," including notably a theory of aggression (power instinct) producing neurotic symptoms and resulting from organ inferiority. His simple formulations, such as overcompensation, masculine protest, and inferiority complex, and the use of organ jargon ("pain in the neck," etc.) had great popular appeal. Another early collaborator of Freud's, *Otto Rank,* believed the cause of all neurosis lay in the individual's attempt to overcome the trauma of birth with its associated "primary" anxiety. His method (will therapy) involved a reexperiencing of separation from the mother figure (therapist) in an effort to strengthen the will.

Karl Abraham (1877-1925), a productive contributor to analytic theory, helped clarify the relation of the pregenital stages of personality development to character disorders. He observed a similarity between obsessive-compulsive neurotics and manic-depressive patients who are in remission. He contributed to the dynamic theories of depression by pointing out the basic ambivalence and increased oral eroticism. He gave clinical support to Freud's interpretation of the internalized struggle which results in the self-punishing desires and self-destructive behavior of depressed patients.

Wilhelm Reich published an outstanding paper entitled "On Character Analysis" (1933), presenting the theory of character defenses ("armor"), which he conceived of as habitual attitudes and ways of behavior that mask inner feelings and basic conflicts. He contributed to analytic technique by pointing out the necessity for dealing with such resistances early in the course of therapy. In her book *The Ego and Mechanisms of Defense* (1946), *Anna Freud* further described man's ways of making psychological adaptation to inner conflict.

Sandor Ferenczi's major contributions were in the realm of psychoanalytic technique and psychopathology. He early advocated active therapy as a way to heighten the emotions produced during the analytic hour but later, with an emphasis on the analyst's personality as the instrument of cure, he recommended an attitude of friendly acceptance on the part of the therapist.

Coincident with the development of psychoanalysis, other contributions to dynamic psychiatry appeared. Hysterical dissociative states were studied and described by *Morton Prince,* who used the method of hypnosis. A few years later the Dean of American psychiatry, *Adolph Meyer* (1866-1950), introduced the broad concepts of psychobiology (ergasiology). He focused the psychiatrist's attention upon the total context of social, emotional, and physical bases of personality. He introduced the life chart and distributive analysis. *Paul Schilder,*

History of psychiatric thought

German neuropsychiatrist and later student of Meyer, is well known for his formulation of "body image" concepts. *Harry Stack Sullivan* taught that personality develops in response to family patterns of social interaction and that anxiety is most basically an aspect of a relationship rather than of an individual. The therapist's role as a participant-observer in the patient's system of disturbed relationships was stressed. Along with *Paul Federn, Frieda Fromm-Reichmann,* and others, Sullivan promoted the use of psychotherapy in the treatment of the psychoses. His concepts of interpersonal relations, like those of *Karen Horney,* have formed a basis for relating the social sciences to psychiatry.

The study of the developmental origins of personality began with *A. Kussmaul's* observations of the neonatal period (1859) and with *Charles Darwin's* biographical sketch of an infant (1877). A landmark in child development was the report by *Wilhelm Preyer* in 1882 of growth in his son over the first 4 years. *G. Stanley Hall's* research on childhood and on adolescence (1893) was followed by *Alfred Binet* and *J. Simon's* elaborate studies of the development of intelligence (1916). Measurements of infant and preschool development were stimulated by *Arnold Gesell's* standard scheme (1923) for classifying the phasic achievement of simple sensorimotor and locomotor skills. Of historic importance have been the voluminous and careful studies of the development of cognitive capacities carried out since 1929 by *Jean Piaget.*

The neurophysiological processes underlying behavior are yet to find their proper place in relation to these dynamic psychiatric concepts. Early work by *Ivan Pavlov* (1849-1936) in Russia focused on the potentialities of this approach and gave us the concept of the conditioned reflex. Behaviorism, an extension of this theoretical framework in the field of psychology, was developed by *John B. Watson* in the United States and forms the foundation for certain modern concepts of brief psychotherapy. Various physical methods of altering neurophysiological processes, and hence behavior, have been useful. *Julius Wagner von Jauregg* in Vienna in 1918 initiated the method of malarial fever therapy in the treatment of general paresis. *Manfred Sakel* in Vienna in 1937 introduced insulin coma therapy for schizophrenia. *Von Meduna* (1935) popularized Metrazol shock therapy. In 1938 *Ugo Cerletti* and *Bini* in Italy first systematically described the successful use of electroshock treatments in mental disorders (although a case report of electroconvulsive treatment had been published by Babinski in 1903 and electrical stimulation therapy had begun in the eighteenth century). Subsequent to this, modified forms of electrocerebral therapy were introduced in France by *P. Delmas-Marsolet,* who used continuous stimulation, and in the United States by *Friedman, Paul Wilcox,* and *Vladimir Liberson,* who used unidirectional currents.

The surgical treatment of mental disorders probably began with primitive man, skulls being trephined for the treatment of those who were "possessed." Knowledge of the function of the frontal lobes had been gleaned mostly from cases of accidental destruction as in *Harlow's* report (1868) of Phineas Gage, an efficient and capable railroad foreman who became profane, irreverent, capricious, and obstinate following destruction of the frontal lobes by an iron, dynamite-tamping rod. *Burkhardt,* a Swiss, resected portions of the left hemisphere in 1888 for the relief of vivid hallucinations. In 1935 *C. F. Jacobsen* in the United States demonstrated that frustrated, anxious, and restless chimpanzees became calm and docile following lobectomy, and in the same year *Egaz Moniz* of Lisbon, Portugal, persuaded *Almeida Lima* to perform the first prefrontal lobotomies upon agitated patients refractory to other treatment. *Walter Freeman* and *J. W. Watts* popularized the method in the United States, and it is estimated that by 1955 more than 25,000 patients had been treated by this method.

The discovery of the behavioral effects of chlorpromazine by *Courvoisier* and associates and, from this, the development of important clinical studies by *Delay* and *Deniker* ushered in the new age of psychopharmacology. The availability and widespread use of potent psychotropic agents have resulted (since 1955) in a marked reduction of the chronic population of large public mental hospitals. This has been coupled with an increased emphasis upon rehabilitative techniques, which, according to *Maxwell Jones* (England), *Leighton, Caplan* (U. S. A.), and others, include the concepts of open ward, patient government, therapeutic milieu, and social and community aspects of psychiatry. In the United States the report of the Joint Commission on Mental Illness and Health, *Action for Mental Health* (1961), with ensuing community mental health center legislation (1963), represents attempts by an alerted public through legislative action to shift the emphasis from custodial care to active treatment. Although exciting and effective, these developments but presage the major attack which will be based upon research findings on the basic etiology of mental illnesses that must yet occur if we are ultimately to solve this grave and costly public health problem.

SUGGESTED READINGS

Ackerknecht, E.: Short history of psychiatry, New York, 1959, Hafner Publishing Co., Inc.

Alexander, F., and Selesnick, S.: The history of psychiatry, New York, 1966, Harper & Row, Publishers.

American Psychiatric Association: One hundred years of American psychiatry, New York, 1944, Columbia University Press.

Astrup, C.: Pavlovian psychiatry, Springfield, Ill., 1965, Charles C Thomas, Publisher.

Barton, W. E.: Prospects and perspectives: implications of social change for psychiatry, Amer. J. Psychiat. 125:147, 1968.

Bockoven, V. S.: Moral treatment in American psychiatry, New York, 1963, Springer Publishing Co., Inc.

Burnham, J. C.: Psychoanalysis and American medicine, New York, 1968, International Universities Press, Inc. In Psychol. Issues monograph no. 20.

Caldwell, A.: Psychopharmaca—a bibliography of psychopharmacology, 1952-1957, Washington, D. C., 1958, U. S. Government Printing Office.

Carlson, E. T., and Dain, N.: The psychotherapy that was moral treatment, Amer. J. Psychiat. 117:519, 1960.

Delay, J., Deniker, P., Ropert, R., and Wiart, C.: Les indications des cures neuroleptiques prolongées dans le traitement des psychoses chroniques, Arch. Psicol. Neurol. 17:401, 1956.

Deutsch, A.: The mentally ill in America, ed. 2, New York, 1949, Columbia University Press.

Freud, S.: The ego and the id, London, 1947, Hogarth Press, Ltd.

Freud, S.: The origins of psycho-analysis (letter to Wilhelm Fliess, drafts and notes, 1887-1902), edited by M. Bonaparte, A. Freud, and E. Kris, New York, 1954, Basic Books, Inc., Publishers.

Gesell, A. L., and Amatruda, C. S.: Developmental diagnosis, New York, 1941, Paul B. Hoeber, Inc.

Greenblatt, M., Sharaf, M. R., and Stone, E.: Dynamics of institutional change: the hospital in transition, Pittsburgh, 1971, University of Pittsburgh Press.

Hunter, R., and Macalpine, I.: Three hundred years of psychiatry 1535-1860, New York, 1963, Oxford University Press, Inc.

12   *A synopsis of contemporary psychiatry*

Janet, P.: Psychological healing, New York, 1925, The Macmillan Co., vols. 1 and 2.

Joint Commission on Mental Illness and Health: Action for mental health, New York, 1961, Basic Books, Inc., Publishers.

Jones, E.: The life and work of Sigmund Freud, New York, 1953 to 1957, Basic Books, Inc., Publishers, vols. 1 to 3.

Kraepelin, E.: One hundred years of psychiatry, New York, 1962, Citadel Press, Inc.

Leigh, D.: The historical development of British psychiatry, New York, 1961, Pergamon Press, Inc.

Lief, A.: The commonsense psychiatry of Dr. Adolph Meyer, New York, 1949, McGraw-Hill Book Co.

McKown, R.: Pioneers in mental health, New York, 1961, Dodd, Mead & Co., Inc.

Mora, G.: The history of psychiatry: a cultural and bibliographical survey, Psychoanal. Rev. 52:298, 1965.

Mullahay, P.: The contributions of Harry Stack Sullivan, New York, 1952, Hermitage House, Inc.

Piaget, J.: The construction of reality in the child, New York, 1954, Basic Books, Inc., Publishers.

Rank, O.: Will therapy and truth and reality, New York, 1945, Alfred A. Knopf, Inc.

Robach, A. A.: History of psychology and psychiatry, New York, 1962, Citadel Press, Inc.

Rome, H. P.: Prospects for a psi-net: the fourth quantum advance in psychiatry, Compr. Psychiat. 8:450, 1967.

Schneck, J. M.: A history of psychiatry, Springfield, Ill., 1960, Charles C Thomas, Publisher.

Soukes, T. L.: Biochemistry of mental disease, New York, 1962, Harper & Row, Publishers.

Stainbrook, E.: Psychosomatic medicine in the nineteenth century, Psychosom. Med. 14:211, 1952.

Tyhurst, J. S., et al.: More for the mind, a study of psychiatric services in Canada, Toronto, 1963, Canadian Mental Health Association.

Ulett, G. A., and Sletten, I. W.: Statewide electronic data-processing system, Hosp. Community Psychiat. 20:74, 1969.

Zillboorg, G.: Psychosomatic medicine—a historical perspective, Psychosom. Med. 6:3, 1944.

Zillboorg, G., and Henry, G. W.: A history of medical psychology, New York, 1941, W. W. Norton & Co., Inc.

1

HISTORY TAKING AND DIAGNOSTIC PROCEDURES

3

Examination of the psychiatric patient

It has long been traditional in psychiatry that to obtain a *mental status* is synonymous with making a psychiatric examination. With the advent of a psychiatry more interested in the study of etiological factors, more emphasis is now placed on the *longitudinal case history* in order to assess personality development as it relates to current symptoms. The psychiatrist should learn to use the mental status (behavioral status) and case history in a complete and orderly fashion to gain an initial diagnostic impression and to formulate tentative plans for treatment. Repeating the behavioral examination at regular intervals can lead to *progress notes* which will contribute to an objective basis for judging personality changes.

In his appraisal of the patient, the psychiatrist is aided by the instruments of the psychologist and neurologist. Through *intelligence tests* the psychologist furnishes a measure of present intellectual functioning as well as unrealized or damaged potentialities; by the use of *projective techniques* (which see behind the patient's psychological defenses) the psychologist forms an impression of habitual personality and areas of conflict.

It should not be forgotten that mentation and behavior are related to brain function and, although such theoretical concepts as id, superego, and ego may almost assume the proportions of tangible reality in some psychiatric formulations, it remains for the neurophysiologist and the biochemist to relate specific aspects of personality functioning to the topography of the neuraxis. At the present time, nevertheless, a clinical estimation of brain function obtained from neurological examination can give some useful clues to understanding the pathology of behavior. Psychiatric diseases such as pellagra, general paresis, and the senile psychoses have a recognized neuropathology; therefore, in these and in other mental diseases a careful *neurological examination* aided by the *electroencephalogram, spinal fluid studies,* and *roentgenography* can be of assistance to the psychiatrist.

INITIAL PSYCHIATRIC INTERVIEW

In psychiatry, therapy and history taking go hand in hand. Diagnosis and plans for treatment depend upon the results of appraisal of the *psychological functioning* of the patient. Initial immediate planning, working diagnoses, hospital orders, and instructions to aides and nurses must often be formulated after brief contact with the patient. This initial examination is also known as the mental or the behavioral status. To obtain significant diagnostic material, the patient's confidence must be won, and it should be remembered that the psychiatric patient is often initially less cooperative than are many medical patients. He may be frightened, anxious, hostile, agitated, or mute. He resents the implication that he is crazy and is brought to a mental hospital, or he fears that you may discover evidence to prove correct his apprehension that he is losing his mind.

The history-taking process may be expedited by a minute or two spent in getting acquainted, by discussing the patient's home town, occupation, or topics of some current interest. It is helpful to identify yourself and the purpose of the examination. Proceed slowly and ask questions about the mental state within as neutral a frame as possible—along with questions regarding other illness or habits of living, e.g.: "When you get 'nervous,' does it interfere with your thinking?" "Can you, for example, tell me the year you were born?" "Today's date?" Introduce the subject of delusions and hallucinations with care, e.g.: "Do you consider yourself a religious person?" "Some people say they have actually heard God's voice; has this happened to you?" "Do you hear other voices when no one is around?" "Have you ever felt that you are different from other people?" "In what way?" "Are others aware of this?" "Have they looked at you more than is usual?" "Do you believe in mental telepathy?" "Can others read your mind?" Approach with initial caution those areas about which many persons are reticent: suicide, sex, and hostile feelings. Always see the patient in private; his revelations may be embarrassing to him. Try to keep in tune with the patient's mood. Encourage him and let him know you are on his side by your warm understanding manner and nods of acknowledgement.

Initial examination of behavior (behavioral or mental status)

General appearance and attitudes. We should observe the patient's behavior in the presence of the examiner. His ability to participate appropriately and the peculiarities of his physical appearance, facial expression, amount of activity, mannerisms, posture, dress, gait, and voice may suggest characteristic attitudes such as denial, suspicion, irritability, fearfulness, and self-blame.

Speech activity. An accurate description of the patient's speech activity is important for an understanding of underlying thought processes. One should note the rapidity, pauses, blocking, flight of associations, distractibility, relevance of associations, rhyming, punning, neologisms, circumstantiality, confabulation, tone, slurring, and stuttering, as well as the extent of vocabulary and peculiar usage of words. The particular topics which are accompanied by increased speech disturbance should be noted for future investigation.

Emotional reactions. We should note whether the patient's predominant affect is depressed, euphoric, anxious, apathetic, hostile, or negativistic and the extent to which the mood is appropriate to the thought content.

Pathological thought content and adjustive techniques. In this section we describe such symptoms as delusions, false beliefs ("How are you treated? Do you feel that your troubles are the result of actions being taken against you by others?"), ideas of reference ("Do people talk about you? Do you feel that items in the newspaper refer to you?"), illusions (misperception of objects), hallucinations (hearing voices, seeing visions, etc.), obsessions (ideas or notions that persist despite conscious attempts to remove them), compulsions (acts committed against the conscious will of the individual), and phobias (obsessive, unreasonable fears). Feelings of unreality, of uncanniness, of being controlled by others, or of previously having experienced the present (déjà vu) should be noted.

If possible, relate the occurrence of pathological behavior or thought content to the preceding situation. Try to answer this question about each symptom: *In response to what sort of interpersonal situation does his symptom appear or become aggravated?*

Intellectual functions. An estimation of memory function is easily obtained both as to remote events and as to recent events. (Can he tell you what he has had for breakfast? Can he remember the names of several objects for a period of two minutes?) Impression of the patient's judgment should be formed. (What would he do in a theater if someone called out "fire"? What would he do if he found a stamped, addressed envelope on the street?) General information (names of rivers, presidents, states, etc.) should be sampled. Attention and concentration powers can be tested by asking the patient to make change or to subtract sevens serially, and his capacity for abstract concepts by obtaining his interpretation of simple proverbs. Orientation for time (exact date, place, name of hospital and person) should be determined, with careful attention being paid to differentiation between experiential confusion and true organic impairment. It should be determined how much insight the patient has into his illness, what he feels is wrong, and what he feels the etiological factors may be.

COMPLETE CASE STUDY

The psychiatric case study is completed not from one but from several interviews. In fact, psychotherapeutic interviews extending over many months' time are, at least in part, elaboration and addition to the patient's history. Over the course of such interviews, we seek to characterize the patient in terms of finding repetitive patterns of behavior which frequently associate with significant life events. The stress precipitating a symptom may be in the present or lie in the past. We are not concerned with how statistically abnormal a trait is in the population at large but rather with how much it bothers or affects *this* individual patient.

The history obtained from the patient may be unreliable

or lacking in detail. Relatives (who should be identified in the chart) may contribute additional history. Friends, employers, school records, etc. can all serve to round out the picture.

The following outline presents a form to follow in writing the complete history. Always remember that hospital records are public property and that even your notes may be subpoenaed; so state the problem in simple and safe terms. For example, the statement "difficulties in marital sexual adjustment" is adequate for the clinical record although it is of less interest to the curious than a story of sexual liberties which indiscreetly names the parties involved. Brevity, legibility, and good grammatical form mark the history written by a well-trained clinician. Longer, detailed psychotherapeutic notes may be kept in a separate research file for teaching or similar purposes. The complete psychiatric case study should include such data as the following.

Identifying data

This is the *(first, second, etc.)* hospital admission of this *(age)* year old *(race)* *(religion)* *(sex)* *(occupation or civil status, such as escapee, prisoner, parolee)* of *(residence)*, who was brought to the hospital by *(relatives, police, self)*.

Informants

Name, address, telephone, relationship, length of time they have known patient, frankness and reliability, attitude toward patient's illness ("can snap out of it," "just putting on," "a disgrace") and his admission to the hospital (concerned about patient's welfare, glad to be rid of him, overly solicitous, not understanding admission at this particular time).

Chief complaint

Chief symptoms (quote the patient if possible) and duration; circumstances surrounding admission.

Present illness

Patient was well until (chronological account of development of *symptoms*). Was *onset* sudden or gradual? Is the illness episodic? Was there a *precipitating factor* (death, separation, loss, frightening experience, domestic trouble)? When did patient quit *work* or begin neglecting housework? What time of day do symptoms get better or worse? Have *physiological functions* changed (eating, sleeping, elimination, menses, potency)? Any loss of weight? Changes in memory, mood, or judgment? Behavior changes suggesting *hallucinations? Suicidal* or *homicidal* tendencies? Any ideas of sin, persecution, infidelity, or jealousy?

Family, social, and cultural background

Family history of disease. Mental illness (relation, symptoms, age at which breakdown occurred, length of hospitalization, treatment used), alcoholism, eccentricity, suicides, epilepsy, mental retardation, delinquency, syphilis, glandular disorders.

Family constellation. Father, mother, siblings, spouse, children, stepparents, or foster parents. Whether raised in an institution. Give sketch of each member—name, maiden name of mother, age, marital status, children, health, occupation, residence, personality characteristics, attitudes toward patient.

Socioeconomic background. Housing conditions, number of rooms, plumbing, neighborhood; debts, whether breadwinner is steady worker or ill, hospitalization, insurance; race, minority group, community attitudes and values; religion, sect, regular attendance, scrupulousness, conversion experiences.

Past medical history

In chronological order—*operations, illnesses, injuries,* with duration, severity, sequelae. Inquire specifically about *syphilis* (lumbar puncture?—how treated) *encephalitis, convulsions* (how controlled), *head injury* (how long unconscious, sequelae). Inquire as to all chronic diseases, allergies, neurotic symptoms, etc. List previous attacks of *mental illness* (symptoms, duration, treatment, where hospitalized, degree of health between episodes, suicidal or homicidal attempts). Ask about drugs, especially narcotics, barbiturates, bromides, patent medicines. Amount and kind of alcoholic intake. Occupational *poisoning* (lead, arsenic, mercury).

School and occupational history

Grade completed and *age* when patient stopped and why, ability to read and write, whether failed or especially bright, relationships with teachers and classmates; whether *behavior problem,* hyperaggressive (truancy, cruelty, stealing, lying) or withdrawn. *Jobs,* how long, reason for changing, idle periods, how got along with boss and fellow workers, reasons for getting fired, is job commensurate with ability. *Time spent in the service,* duties, kind of discharge, any time spent in guardhouse or hospital. Juvenile court, reformatory, welfare, or police records.

Sexual and marital history

Some care should be exercised in pursuing this material in order not to create too much anxiety. With some patients, if information is requested in a matter-of-fact manner, much can be learned in the first interview; with others, information is obtained only after a positive relationship is formed with the therapist. The *experiences* and *attitudes* centering around the patient's early feeding and toilet-training situations, the degree of adolescent anxiety concerning sexual functions and the present sexual habits are desirable to know. Important homosexual or heterosexual experiences in the past should be noted, with the patient's feelings about them.

Age *menses* began, how prepared for it by parents (gives idea of family attitude toward sex), whether frightened. Whether menopausal? Age, number and duration of marriages, with age of spouse, sexual adjustment, and length of courtship. Use of contraceptives and whether pregnancies were wanted or planned. Guilt over extramarital affairs, abortions, illegitimate children, masturbation, perversions (sodomy, homosexuality, child molestation, fellatio, rape).

Developmental history
Rejected child, overindulged, birth injury, breast-fed, colic, bowel and bladder training, enuresis, temper tantrums, stuttering, tics, excessive thumbsucking, phobias, night terrors, sleep-walking, rituals, whether ever ran away from home. Age of sitting, walking, talking, coordination. Eating habits, weight curve, fainting spells, convulsions. Handicap such as crippling or blindness. Which parent seemed concerned, and in what manner, with development at different ages?

Personality traits
Kinds of activities enjoyed, whether solitary or group, active or passive, whether leader or follower. Aggressive or sub-assertive toward authority. Inclined to blame others or self. Demonstrative or reserved. Sense of humor. Mood fluctuations.

Adjustive techniques
It is well to describe briefly the behavior of a patient with the physician, particularly as related to emotionally laden material brought out in the interviews. Patient's facial expression, appearance, affect, verbal content, motor and autonomic reactions should be noted, with specific examples given. The therapist should attempt to understand in what ways the patient's behavior toward him is related to his behavior toward other important figures in life.

Impression
Use a phrase which fits the official psychiatric nomenclature and which indicates succinctly the principal types of pathology.

Recommendations
Diagnostic. For example—"further history from spouse by social worker, lumbar puncture, EEG, and skull films."

Therapeutic. These include *medical treatment,* current *milieu therapy,* and *rehabilitation planning.* For example—"hydrotherapy, electroshock, supportive psychotherapy; stay on locked ward, simple activities, no visiting; introduce vocational counselor for later planning when patient improves," or "intensive psychotherapy; hospital privileges, give patient ward jobs, family visit any time, encourage to occupational therapy; social worker to see wife."

Prognosis
Results to be expected and just how many months' hospitalization will be required. Whether patient will likely be able to return to old job, and

living arrangements to be made. Note any important factors likely to be crucial in determining outcome.

SUGGESTED READINGS

Burdock, E. I., and Hardesty, A. S.: Structured clinical interview manual, New York, 1969, Springer Publishing Co., Inc.

Deutsch, F., and Murphy, W. F.: The clinical interview, New York, 1954, International Universities Press, Inc.

Finesinger, J. E.: Psychiatric interviewing: some principles and procedures in insight therapy, Amer. J. Psychiat. 105:187, 1949.

Gill, M., Newman, R., and Redlich, F. C.: The initial interview in psychiatric practice, New York, 1954, International Universities Press, Inc.

Gregory, I.: Psychiatry: biological and social, Philadelphia, 1961, W. B. Saunders Co.

Menninger, K. A.: A manual for psychiatric case study, ed. 2, New York, 1962, Grune & Stratton, Inc.

Saslow, G., and Chapple, E. D.: A new life history form with instructions for its use, Appl. Anthropol. 4:1, 1945.

Stevenson, I.: Medical history-taking, New York, 1960, Paul B. Hoeber, Inc., Medical Book Department of Harper & Bros.

Sullivan, H. S.: The psychiatric interview, New York, 1954, W. W. Norton & Co., Inc.

Tarachow, S.: Initial interview conference, J. Hillside Hosp. 11:127, 1962.

Weiss, J. M. A.: Psychiatric emergencies. In Stephenson, H. E., editor: Emergency care and first aid, Boston, 1962, Little, Brown & Co.

Whitehorn, J. C.: Guide to interviewing and clinical personality study, Arch. Neurol. Psychiat. 52:197, 1944.

4
General physical and neurological examination

The physical examination of the psychiatric patient is no less important than of any other sick person. In one third of unselected psychiatric hospital admissions physical morbidity has been observed. Also, it is of special importance to remember that certain conditions, such as carcinoma of the pancreas, etc., may masquerade as psychiatric disorders, and that patients with surgically treatable brain tumors have died in mental hospitals with their pathology unsuspected. The medical examination of the patient is one of the contractual duties and responsibilities of the psychiatric physician. And the firsthand assurance of physical good health is often a strong initial step in the treatment of persons with anxiety reaction and other psychiatric disturbance. The technique will not be described here, as it is known to every physician and does not differ for psychiatric patients except that in very disturbed individuals some portions of it may, of necessity, be postponed. Particular attention should be paid to adequate chaperoning during rectal and vaginal examinations. A neurological examination is a necessary part of every complete psychiatric work-up because, after all, the symptoms of mental disease are mediated through the central nervous system. As elsewhere in physical diagnosis, the most common sins are those of omission. To interpret correctly the findings of the neurological examination requires the skill of specialized neurological training, but to suspect brain pathology requires only that the neurological examination be complete. "The neurologist differs from other physicians in that he tests *all* the cranial nerves." To aid in the performance of a complete neurological examination, the following outline is included.

EXAMINATION OF THE NERVOUS SYSTEM
GENERAL OBSERVATIONS
Position of body, head, extremities
Shape, tenderness, percussion of head
Tenderness and rigidity of neck

CRANIAL NERVES
I. **Olfactory**
   a. Subjective
      (1) Hallucinations of smell, loss or impairment of function
   b. Objective
      (1) Response to test odors

II. **Optic**
   a. Subjective
      (1) Failing vision, limitation of fields, hallucinations of light
   b. Objective
      (1) Visual acuity, perimetry. Fundi—shape, size, color of disc, lamina cribrosa, physiological cupping, engorged or tortuous veins, constriction or streaking of arteries, exudate, hemorrhage, choking

III. **Oculomotor**
IV. **Trochlear**
VI. **Abducens**
   a. Subjective
      (1) Diplopia
   b. Objective
      (1) External ocular movements, nystagmus, ptosis, palpebral fissures. Pupils—size, equality, regularity, reaction to light, accommodation

V. **Trigeminus**
   a. Subjective
      (1) Pain, paresthesia, numbness
   b. Objective
      (1) Sensory—anesthesia, hypesthesia, hyperesthesia, corneal reflex
      (2) Motor—deviation of jaw, paralysis of temporal and masseter muscles

VII. **Facial**
   a. Subjective
      (1) Hyperacusis, taste disturbance, spasmodic contractions of facial muscles, disturbance of lacrimal and salivary secretions, asymmetry of face
   b. Objective
      (1) Motor—facial expression, nasolabial folds, inability to retract corner of mouth, to close eye completely, to wrinkle forehead
      (2) Sensory—taste on anterior two thirds of tongue
      (3) Secretory—lacrimal and salivary secretions

VIII. **Acoustic**
    A. Cochlear
        a. Subjective
           (1) Impairment of auditory acuity, tinnitus
        b. Objective
           (1) Tick of watch
           (2) Tuning fork test—Rinné or Weber
           (3) Otoscopic examination
    B. Vestibular
        a. Subjective
           (1) Dizziness, unsteadiness of gait
        b. Objective
           (1) Bárány test
           (2) Items listed under cerebellum

 IX. **Glossopharyngeal**
        a. Subjective
           (1) Dysphagia
        b. Objective
           (1) Taste on posterior one third of tongue, pharyngeal reflex

  X. **Vagus**
        a. Subjective
           (1) Regurgitation of fluids, difficulty of speech, projectile vomiting
        b. Objective
           (1) Deviation of soft palate, pulse, laryngeal paralysis

 XI. **Spinal accessory**
    Paralysis of sternocleidomastoid and trapezius muscles

XII. **Hypoglossal**
    Paralysis of tongue

CORPUS STRIATUM

Muscular rigidity, tremors, slowness of voluntary movements, change of emotional expression

CEREBELLUM

Station, Romberg sign, gait, hypotonicity, nystagmus, dysarthria

Finger-to-finger ⎤
Finger-to-thumb ⎥
Finger-to-nose ⎥ Ataxia, asynergy
Heel-to-knee ⎥
Past-pointing ⎥
Adiadokokinesis ⎦

SPINAL CORD AND BODY SEGMENTAL REPRESENTATION OF SENSORY AND MOTOR FUNCTIONS—REFLEXES

Proceed in this examination so that neck, shoulders, upper extremities, trunk, abdomen, and finally lower extremities are covered in systematic manner.
a. Subjective

    (1) **Muscular weakness** (local or general), difficulty in walking, dragging toe of shoe, stumbling or falling, sphincteric disturbances
    (2) **Changes in sensation** (local or general), pain (fixed or radiating)
    (3) **Abnormal sweating**
  b. Objective
    (1) Motor—range of muscular movement, contractures, atrophy, strength of muscles against resistance, tremors
    (2) Sensory—segmental sensory level: pain, temperature, light touch, tactile discrimination, deep sensation (muscle, bone, joint, and vibratory sense)
    (3) Reflexes, superficial—abdominal, cremasteric, Babinski, Chaddock, Oppenheim, Gordon
    (4) Reflexes, deep—biceps, triceps, knee and ankle jerks, radial, periosteal, ankle clonus (indicate strength and equality by means of x's as on chart below)

NEUROLOGICAL SUMMARY

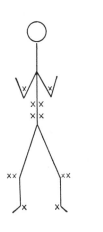

Cranial nerves	Done	Abnormality
I	√	———
II	√	———
III, IV, VI	√	———
V	√	———
VII	√	———
VIII	√	———
IX	√	———
X	√	———
XI	√	———
XII	√	———
Motor	√	———
Sensory	√	———
Gait	√	———
Other	√	———

SUGGESTED READINGS

Baker, A. B.: Clinical neurology, New York, 1962, Hoeber Medical Division, Harper & Row, Publishers.

Bickerstaff, E. R.: Neurological examination in clinical practice, Philadelphia, 1963, F. A. Davis Co.

Blackwood, W., Dodds, T. C., and Sommerville, J. C.: Atlas of neuropathology, ed. 2, Baltimore, 1965, The Williams & Wilkins Co.

Brain, W. R.: Recent advances in neurology and neuro-psychiatry, ed. 7, Boston, 1962, Little, Brown & Co.

Burr, H. S.: Classics in neurology, Springfield, Ill., 1963, Charles C Thomas, Publisher.

Gardner, E.: Fundamentals of neurology, ed. 4, Philadelphia, 1963, W. B. Saunders Co.

Haymaker, W., and Schiller, R.: The founders of neurology: one hundred and forty-six biographical sketches by eighty-nine authors, Springfield, Ill., 1970, Charles C Thomas, Publisher.

Maguire, G. P., and Granville-Grossman, K. L.: Physical illness in psychiatric patients, Brit. J. Psychiat. 114:1365, 1968.

Matthews, W. B.: Practical neurology, Philadelphia, 1963, F. A. Davis Co.

Merritt, H.: A textbook of neurology, ed. 4, Philadelphia, 1967, Lea & Febiger.

Monrad-Krohn, G. H.: The clinical examination of the nervous system, ed. 12, New York, 1964, Paul B. Hoeber, Inc.

Renfrew, S.: Introduction to diagnostic neurology, Baltimore, vol. 1, 1962; vol. 3, 1965, The Williams & Wilkins Co.

Spurling, R. G.: Practical neurological diagnosis, ed. 6, Springfield, Ill., 1960, Charles C Thomas, Publisher.

5
Examining for agnosia, apraxia, and aphasia

The current state of knowledge about the anatomy and physiology of thinking should command the attention of every serious student of psychiatry. Ultimately all psychological theory must be tested for its compatibility with the facts of cortical and subcortical functioning. The study of language disorder, in its broadest concept, should furnish the psychiatric researcher some help in his search for a model of thinking disorder. The careful clinician will consider aphasia in his differential diagnosis of the thought disorder seen in a variety of psychiatric conditions. A minimal brain lesion lying posterior to the motor area may produce only jargon aphasia and a clinical picture without other neurological signs, which could well be mistaken for schizophrenia with "word salad."

Although the physical basis of mind has puzzled thinkers from Hippocrates to Descartes, there has in the last quarter century appeared new and exciting information from biochemistry and neurophysiology. Evidence from histological studies of cell structure, from the chemistry of the synapse, and from brain stimulation in the intact, awake human patient continues to strengthen the belief that the basis of all memory, the permanent patterning of thoughts, must be located at the synapse. Here, where the branches of one nerve cell join the body of another, some physical-chemical alteration is produced by the passing stream of electrical potentials subsequent to sensory stimulation. Of such stuff are formed thinking and memory—the elusive engram pattern. The mechanism of recall has been succinctly described by Penfield. He suggests that the patient, upon seeing an old friend after many years, recognizes him through a memory flashback record of the past. By such a cerebral mechanism he is able to compare the present sensory picture with the old memory image, which is so vivid that small changes in the friend's mien are detectable. In order to produce such an experiential response a ganglionic record is activated. This engram is stored not in the cortex but rather, more likely, in the hippocampus. Such ganglionic patterns clearly formed by single exposures in earlier life, even when they have been forgotten for many years, can be immediately elicited by focal electrical stimulation or sometimes by hypnosis or by the free associational methods of psychoanalysis.

Attempts to localize language functions in the brain by *post hoc* case reconstructions of autopsy specimens have produced a voluminous, confused, and controversial literature. At best it appears that language function in most individuals resides in a dominant left hemisphere. This is regardless of handedness. Cerebral injuries early in life can reverse such dominance. Evidence from the work of Penfield and his collaborators at the Montreal Neurological Institute indicates clearly that the speech mechanism must function as a whole and is not, as the early phrenologists believed, divided into discrete areas of functioning. Man in his thinking may utilize several sets of neuronal patterns in his ideational speech mechanism, but the foci are only regions of a total network and not discrete localizations. On the sensory side, neuronal patterns are concerned with the sound of the word in listening and the visual units of the word in reading. On the motor side, the verbal units of speech and manual units for writing all contribute to language formulation. Three basic cortical areas have been outlined as utilized in the ideational elaboration of speech: (1) a large area in the posterior temporal and the posteroinferior parietal regions, (2) a small area in the posterior part of the third frontal convolution, and (3) part of the supplementary motor area within the midsagittal fissure. Motor mechanisms of speech, including voice control, articulating movements, and vocalization, and the mechanism for writing lie in the supplementary motor areas of either side. These areas are situated close to and between the principal areas for ideational speech. (See Figure 1.)

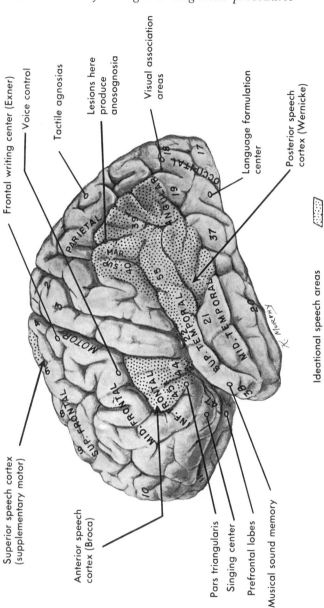

Figure 1. The human cerebral cortex, illustrating major anatomical divisions, important physiologically delineated areas, and regions designated as important for language function. (Adapted from Penfield, W., and Roberts, L.: Speech and brain mechanisms, Princeton, N. J., 1959, Princeton University Press.)

The functions of the cortical speech areas in man are coordinated by projections of the thalamus. It is obvious that the unilateral cortical speech mechanism must be integrated into the functional mechanisms of the whole brain. It has been hypothesized that nonspecific connections are made through a coordinating mechanism of the centrencephalic system.

Language is a function of human life that results from the dynamic interplay of several brain areas. It is concerned with more than just sensory (receiving) and motor (expressing) functions. Direct contact of sensory and motor neurons would result only in stereotyped, automatic, or mechanical responses. The richness of human speech, thought, and imagination is a resultant of the rich neural association network which intervenes. Recollection (reminiscence), which includes the recall both of experiential (detailed memory) and of conceptual (generalizing) images, is part of the stream of consciousness whose level of activity is controlled by the centrencephalon and inflow of the total reticular activating system.

The very complexity of this dynamic organization makes it highly unlikely that pure types of aphasia exist. When, however, the pathway is broken at any of several points, but the rest of the dominant hemisphere and its subcortical connections are intact, the subject is no longer able to find words though he knows what he wishes to say.

Rarely if ever is the aphasic patient perfect in any department of speech. However, his defect may be predominantly more in one area than another. If his difficulty appears greatest in understanding spoken language, he is said to be suffering from *sensory aphasia;* if, on the other hand, his difficulty is in expressing thoughts, it has been called *motor aphasia;* if in reading, *alexia;* or if in writing, *agraphia.*

The closer the lesion is to Broca's area (posterior part of third frontal convolution) and the adjacent precentral face area, the more the motor components of speech are involved. The nearer the lesion is to the junction of the parietal, temporal, and occipital lobes, the more are reading and writing affected; and the more the posterosuperior temporal region is involved, the greater is the difficulty in the comprehension of spoken words.

The patient-centered concepts of Wepman, which focus on aphasia testing as a means for planning therapy, are an important addition to the older writings in this field. Until the final clear answer becomes known, theories must guide the development of further knowledge. Admittedly such terms as "agnosia" and "aphasia" have their limitations, but their wide usage makes necessary some acquaintance with their commonly accepted definitions.

AGNOSIA

The term "agnosia" refers to loss of function through failure of recognition resulting from an organic cerebral lesion. Distinction must be made as to the sensory modality concerned, and merely to say visual agnosia is not enough. The type of visual agnosia can be further specified as the loss can be specific for animate or for inanimate objects, for their color, for distance, etc. Lesions may produce visual agnosia for various parts of the body (anosognosia, visual finger agnosia) or for the whole body (autotopagnosia).

Lesions causing agnosias in the sphere of language are more complex, but in general the area of cortex essential to visual recognition of letters, syllables, words, and musical notes is the angular gyrus. The terms "cortical" and "subcortical" were used to designate types of language agnosia occurring with lesions of the angular gyrus. "Cortical" was used by some to indicate the occurrence of agraphia in conjunction with the visual defect, whereas when agraphia was absent the term "subcortical" was applied.

Auditory agnosia occurs with involvement of the temporal lobe, and the patient may show paraphasia or senseless repetition of sounds heard (imperfect performance of the minor side).

Tactile agnosia (astereognosis) may result with parietal lesions. Such lesions, involving the gyri of Gratiolet, can produce disturbance in the tactile recognitions of one's own body.

Examining for agnosia. Test the patient's position sense, light touch, vibration sense, two-point discrimination, tactile recognition of objects, recognition of digits written on the palm by a dull instrument, and general visual, olfactory, and auditory recognition.

APRAXIA

The term "apraxia" refers to motor disturbances and therefore need not concern language function at all. However, "apractic (motor) aphasia" concerns disturbance of motor speech patterns as, for example, those located in the convolution of Broca. Similarly, apraxia of the cortical motor patterns used in writing may produce agraphia. Thus apraxia is a disturbance in which a patient without dementia, incoordination, or paralysis is nevertheless, because of a motor incapacity affecting association neurons, unable to apply his voluntary motor powers for parts of the body which are involved in a given purposive movement.

Examining for dyspraxia. A simple test routine might include such commands as "Show me how you would use these objects (pair of scissors, comb, or toothbrush—give each object to the patient), how you would light a cigarette, make a fist, clap hands, put out your tongue, put out tongue and scratch head at the same time, wink, blow a kiss, pretend to knock on a door, count money," etc.

It is important to ascertain whether the patient may be capable of executing a given movement spontaneously but will fail to carry out the same movement in response to a command. Failures may be due to inability to comprehend the command when there is sensory aphasia or when the movement involves manipulation of an object not recognized (dysgnosia). Perseveration may cause the patient to carry out a movement appropriate to a previous command. The patient's powers of imitation as well as response may be tested. Check for confusion. Check history of various motor incapacities and the patient's awareness of them and of the complexities of tasks involved.

APHASIA

Aphasia consists of an organic disease of the cerebral memory engrams for language (i.e., embraces those agnosias and apraxias that have to do with language). The term "aphasia" means loss of power to associate the sensory images of speech with the motor speech functions. Formulation aphasia (paraphasia, jargon aphasia) is the inability to formulate language.

When the power to determine the significance of the symbol

is lost as well, the adjective *semantic* is added. Thus one might recognize and repeat a word but be totally unaware of its significance. As pointed out by Head, an element of semantic aphasia (i.e., a quantitative reduction in speech comprehension or capacity) can occur with many types of diffuse brain damage, as well as with a focal lesion to speech centers. No portion of brain can be impaired functionally without affecting the function of the brain as a whole.

Examining for aphasia. Test the ability of the patient to pay attention, to see, to hear, and to act. If there is confusion, it is difficult to decide whether the amount present is sufficient to account for the aphasia observed. These patients fatigue easily, so examine for only 15 to 20 minutes at a time. Gain rapport, explain procedures, and gloss over failures with sympathy and encouragement. If patient can write well, he probably does not have aphasia of any kind. (Writing one's own name is not an adequate test for aphasia.) It is worth knowing how well the patient could formerly speak, read, and write. Follow the testing with logical thinking on your own part. "If the patient cannot recognize an object by sight (visual-occipital), can he by feel (touch-parietal)?" "If he cannot get the words by vision or sound, can he recognize them by feeling wooden letters?" A simple test routine includes measures of (1) the ability to understand spoken words, such as "close your eyes, touch your right ear with your left hand," (2) the ability to understand written words, (3) the ability to express oneself in speech (note defective grammar and syntax), (4) the ability to express oneself in writing, (5) the ability to name objects (the patient is asked to name a series of common objects shown to him, such as a penny, a button, a fountain pen, etc.—for tactile agnosia) to see if he can recognize objects in hand with the eyes closed, and (6) the ability to read aloud.

SUGGESTED READINGS

Agranowitz, A., and McKeown, M. R.: Aphasia handbook, Springfield, Ill., 1969, Charles C Thomas, Publisher.

Brain, W. R.: Speech disorders: aphasia, apraxia, and agnosia, Washington, D. C., 1961, Butterworth, Inc.

Decker, F.: Progressive lessons for language retraining, New York, 1960, Harper & Row, Publishers, books 1 to 4.

deHirsch, K., Jansky, J., and Langford, W.: Predicting reading failure, New York, 1966, Harper & Row, Publishers.

Forrest, D. V.: New words and neologisms, Psychiatry **32:**44, 1969.

Freud, S.: On aphasia, a critical study, 1891 (translated by E. Stengel), New York, 1953, International Universities Press, Inc.

Goldstein, K.: Language and language disturbances, New York, 1948, Grune & Stratton, Inc.

Goodglass, H., and Quadfasel, F. A.: Phrase length and the type and severity of aphasia, Cortex **1:**133, 1964.

Halstead, W. C., and Wepman, J. M.: The Halstead-Wepman aphasia screening test, J. Speech Hearing Dis. **14:**9, 1949.

Head, H.: Aphasia and kindred disorders of speech, London, 1926, Cambridge University Press, vol. 2.

Kleist, K.: Sensory aphasia and amusia, New York, 1962, Pergamon Press, Inc.

Linn, L., and Stein, M.: Sodium amytal in treatment of aphasia. A preliminary report, Bull. U. S. Army Med. Dept. **5:**705, 1946.

Martin, B. R.: Communicative aids for the adult aphasic, Springfield, Ill., 1962, Charles C Thomas, Publisher.

Nielsen, J. M.: Agnosia, apraxia, aphasia, ed. 2, New York, 1962, Hafner Publishing Co., Inc.

Osgood, C. E., and Murray, M. S., editors: Approaches to the study of aphasia, Urbana, 1962, University of Illinois Press.

Pavy, D.: Verbal behavior in schizophrenia: a review of recent studies, Psychol. Bull. **70:**164, 1968.

Penfield, W., and Robert, R.: Speech and brain mechanisms, Princeton, N. J., 1959, Princeton University Press.

Russell, W. R., and Espir, L. E.: Traumatic aphasia, New York, 1961, Oxford University Press, Inc.

Schilder, P.: The image and appearance of the human body, New York, 1951, International Universities Press, Inc.

Schuell, H., Jenkins, J., and Jimenez-Pabon, E.: Aphasia in adults: diagnosis, prognosis, and treatment, New York, 1964, Harper & Row, Publishers.

Taylor, M., and Marks, M.: Aphasia rehabilitation manual and therapy kit, New York, 1959, McGraw-Hill Book Co., Inc.

Wepman, J. M.: Aphasia and the "whole-person" concept, Amer. Arch. Rehab. Ther. **6:**1, 1958.

6
Electroencephalographic examination

The electroencephalogram (EEG) is a recording of the electrical activity of the brain. Unlike the EKG, which periodically repeats a characteristic cycle accompanying the activity of the heart, the EEG records brain waves, which are continually varying in form, frequency, and amplitude. The overall tracing, however, may demonstrate a pattern that is quite characteristic for a given individual. Different anatomical regions of the brain produce somewhat different patterns of resting activity. Thus, for example, the resting alpha rhythm of normal individuals is seen most clearly from parieto-occipital leads when the subject is at rest with eyes closed. Electroencephalograms are altered by attention, sensory stimulation, sleep or other disturbances of consciousness, central nervous system disease, and toxic and metabolic changes in the brain cells. Therefore similar EEG changes may be seen with morphological (anatomical) injury and with physiological (biochemical) insult.

By means of small silver or gold disks or needles attached to the scalp, the brain potentials (measured in millionths of a volt) are led by wires to a powerful amplifier. The brain patterns are then permanently recorded on moving paper by an ink-writing oscillograph. With proper spacing, a few pairs of electrodes provide a sampling of the activity from representative anatomical divisions of the brain and permit a comparison of homologous areas (left and right) which should show similar activity. The array of electrodes on the scalp may vary from one laboratory to another; however, the international (ten-twenty) electrode placement, or some modification, is becoming extensively used here as it is abroad. The brain wave activity from each electrode pair is fed into a separate amplifier and activates its own pen writer. Each such unit is called a channel. Modern machines with eight or more channels permit the simultaneous recording of many separate brain areas at one time. The pens write upon paper which moves at the rate of 3 cm./sec. Such paper is commonly ruled into 1-second and $\frac{1}{5}$-second divisions for ease in determining the frequency of waves in cycles per second. The average amplitude of normal activity is 20 to 75 microvolts, and calibration markings on the graph indicate the value in microvolts of the amount of pen deflection (usually 6 to 7 mm. $= 50\mu v$).

The brain waves as conventionally recorded vary from 1 to 50 cycles per second (c.p.s.) or hertz (Hz), although frequencies above and below this range exist. The most conspicuous activity in a normal recording is the *alpha* pattern, 8 through 13 c.p.s. (Figure 2), seen predominantly in the occipital region in about 75% of a control population either as occasional bursts or as a continuous pattern of varying amplitude. The alpha rhythm tends to disappear when the eyes are opened and when the subject is tense and, in many persons, with mental activity, attention, or anxiety. In about 10% of a control population no recognizable alpha is seen and the low-voltage background activity that predominates is called low-voltage fast (LVF). This is usually considered normal, although it frequently indicates some tension in the subject. Similar low-voltage fast activity is usual in the frontal and temporal areas of the head and in the occipital area when the eyes are open.

A moderate amount of activity below 8 c.p.s. is seen in some 10% to 15% of a control population. Activity in the range of 4 through 7 c.p.s. is called *theta* activity, and records containing it in any significant amount are considered to show a borderline disorder. In the Gibbs classification these are termed "S_1" records, the term "S_2" being reserved for records containing a large amount of slow or *delta* activity (under 4 c.p.s.). S_2 records are considered disordered or pathological and are seen in only 1% to 2% of a control population. Disordered records containing fast or *beta* activity (above 13 c.p.s.) are termed "F_1" or "F_2" records, depending upon the amount and voltage of the fast activity present.

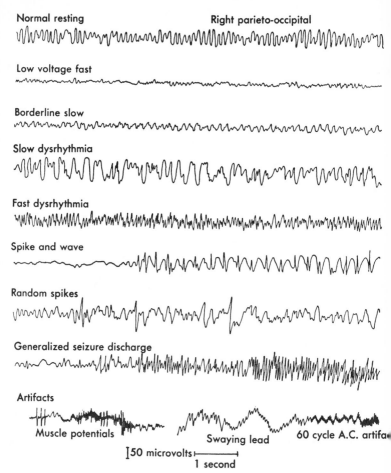

Figure 2. Representative samples of tracings taken from electroencephalographic recordings.

In an epileptic population 50% show diagnostically severe abnormality (Figure 2). Many of these records are paroxysmal in nature (i.e., have sudden bursts of high-voltage disordered activity differing in character from the background rhythm). Thirty percent of the remainder of the records show borderline disorder. The pattern of the EEG may even suggest the type of seizure (e.g., the 3/sec. spike and wave as seen with petit mal). Variants of this pattern occur in akinetic and myoclonic seizures. Although rapid activity (F_2) occurs with grand mal seizures, the interseizure records of persons with such disorder may show a paroxysmal slow dysrhythmia or even be entirely normal. A spike pattern or other paroxysmal abnormality occurring from a single pair of electrodes points to the location of abnormal brain tissue responsible for a focal seizure (e.g., temporal lobe spike of psychomotor epilepsy). In a similar fashion, a slow wave focus of 2 to 3/sec. activity may either lateralize or localize a brain tumor, abscess, or other focal encephalopathy.

As with other laboratory procedures, the EEG is to be interpreted in the light of clinical data. Its diagnostic suggestions are more often presumptive than positive. A single EEG tracing is of less worth than a series of tracings, which permits better evaluation of possible artifacts, the patient's state of apprehension, and his drowsiness. The series should include such techniques as hyperventilation and sleep recording.

It has been stated that the EEG is of little value in psychiatry. It is, however, becoming increasingly evident that disordered brain patterns occur in psychiatric disease and that with psychiatric screening of a control group the amount of electroencephalographic disorder found decreases. Abnormal EEG activity in an otherwise normal subject may well be evidence of some disturbance involving the central nervous system. Investigations using depth electrodes have demonstrated EEG abnormality not seen from scalp electrodes during strong emotion and in schizophrenics and other psychotic patients.

In the broad category of psychoneurosis, one third of patients show definite disorder and an almost equal number show borderline records. The abnormalities seen are usually of mild degree, such as 4 to 7/sec. activity or an increase in activity at fast frequencies. Mild slowing has been found in some obsessive-compulsive neurotics, whereas poor alpha organization and rapid activity are reported in patients with symptoms of anxiety.

Studies of intercorrelations between the EEG and personality type are of considerable interest, but as yet the findings are inconclusive.

For patients in hysterical trance states and under hypnosis the EEG is reported as but little altered, and arrest of alpha upon opening the eyes has been used as a test for hysterical blindness.

There is no relationship between the EEG and intelligence, although of course brain damage or anomalies that are associated with mental deficiency will account for some EEG disorder.

In neurosyphilis, as with other infectious diseases of the nervous system, the EEG abnormality may follow the course of the disease. In early untreated cases an increase in fast and slow activity is seen. High-voltage slow activity occurs in patients showing confusion, disorientation, and profound memory loss. Fast rhythms are seen in patients with mood change or thought disorder without mental confusion. The clinical improvement of paresis by treatment with penicillin is paralleled by improvement in the EEG. The EEG may be useful in evaluation and diagnosis of psychosis with epilepsy, or with drug or toxic encephalopathy, and corresponds in abnormality to the underlying pathology in organic psychoses. Abnormal EEG findings in children of patients with Huntington's chorea may identify carriers of the dominant mutant gene and indicate which offspring are more than likely to have the disease in at least incomplete expression.

Studies of the EEG in cases of psychopathic personality have been made difficult by a lack of accepted criteria for the clinical diagnosis of this condition. A review of studies in this field reported that nearly 50% of the subjects showed disorder, with the most characteristic finding being an increase of activity in the 5 to 7/sec. range. These EEG changes are nonspecific, neither focal or paroxysmal. The more severe the clinical disorder, the greater the percentage of EEG abnormality. In general these are viewed as signs of immaturity.

EEG studies of the major psychoses have been disappointing. No consistent diagnostic patterns have been described for manic-depressive disorder or schizophrenia. In the latter condition, however, the brain activity may be poorly organized with diffuse slow activity, and occasional paroxysmal rhythms have been reported in the catatonic phase.

To increase the diagnostic usefulness of the EEG, a number of activation techniques have been introduced. Such methods include hyperventilation, the intravenous introduction of repeated small doses of Metrazol or Megimide, exposure to a light flashing at different frequencies (photic stimulation), and the use of such photic stimulation in conjunction with Metrazol (pho-mac), hexazole, or other convulsant drugs.

These methods occasionally are successful in producing transient seizure discharges in the EEG. Such abnormal rhythms are often evoked more readily in the epileptic than in the non-epileptic, but there is such an overlap of the two groups that unless the findings are specific and focal the procedure may have little clinical value. Other activation techniques include intracarotid Amytal injection, carotid compression, and over-hydration from antidiuretic. Sodium Amytal injection is helpful in determining the location of a primary epileptogenic focus and also the side of cerebral dominance. Bilateral epileptic activity is reduced or stopped with injection on the side of the focus and ipsilaterally abolished when there is a contra-lateral focus. Diffuse slow activity may be brought about when there is significant occlusion of the opposite carotid artery and the normal one is compressed.

The use of sleep, both natural and induced, has served as an activation method of particular value in detecting focal temporal lobe pathology in patients with psychomotor seizures. Considerable attention has been given to the occurrence of positive spikes in the general frequency ranges of 14 and 6 c.p.s. appearing maximally over the posterior temporal area during light sleep. This pattern has been reported to relate to recurrent autonomic symptoms and to aggressive behavior but is also seen in the records of many apparently normal persons. Almost continuous high-voltage spindles have been found in the sleep records of some mentally retarded children.

In summary it can be stated that, at the present time, neither studies of the resting EEG pattern nor studies of records taken with activation techniques have presented substantial evidence of specific EEG patterns that relate to psychiatric diagnostic classifications. EEG findings of focal disturbances in temporal and diencephalic areas reported in patients previously classified as neurotic, behavior disorder, etc. may point to an overlap between diagnoses formerly considered purely psychiatric and certain of the seizure disorders. The interpretation of the EEG's of psychiatric patients is becoming increasingly complicated because the majority of such patients are now on psychotropic drugs, and these, almost without exception, can produce marked alterations in the EEG which may persist for weeks after medication has been withdrawn.

SUGGESTED READINGS

American Journal of EEG Technology, vols. 1 to 11, Cleveland, 1961-1971, American Society of EEG Technicians, Inc.

Anderson, P.: Physiological basis of alpha rhythm, New York, 1968, Appleton-Century-Crofts.

Berger, H.: The electroencephalogram of man, Amsterdam, 1969, Elsevier Publishing Co.

Brazier, M. A. B., editor: Bibliography of electroencephalography 1875-1948, New York, 1950, American Elsevier Publishing Co., Inc.

Brazier, M. A. B.: A history of the electrical activity of the brain, New York, 1961, The Macmillan Co.

Clinical EEG, vols. 1 and 2, Chicago, 1970-1971, The American Medical EEG Association.

Electroencephalography and clinical neurophysiology, vols. 1 to 30, Amsterdam, 1949 to 1971, Elsevier Publishing Co.

Fink, M., et al.: Bibliography of electroencephalography and human psychopharmacology 1951 to 1961, New York, 1963, American Elsevier Publishing Co., Inc.

Fois, A.: The electroencephalogram of the normal child (translated by N. L. Low), Springfield, Ill., 1961, Charles C Thomas, Publisher.

Fois, A.: Clinical EEG in epilepsy and related conditions in children, Springfield, Ill., 1963, Charles C Thomas, Publisher.

Gibbs, F. A., and Gibbs, E. L.: Atlas of electroencephalography, ed. 2, Reading, Mass., 1950, 1952, 1964, Addison-Wesley Publishing Co., Inc., vols. 1 to 3.

Gibbs, F. A., and Gibbs, E. L.: Fourteen and six per second positive spikes, Electroenceph. Clin. Neurophysiol. 15:553, 1963.

Gibbs, F. A., and Gibbs, E. L.: Medical electroencephalography, Reading, Mass., 1967, Addison-Wesley Publishing Co., Inc.

Glaser, G., editor: EEG and behavior, New York, 1963, Basic Books, Inc., Publishers.

Hill, D., and Parr, G.: Electroencephalography, New York, 1962, The Macmillan Co.

Hughes, R. R.: Introduction to clinical electroencephalography, Baltimore, 1961, The Williams & Wilkins Co.

Kiloh, L. G., and Osselton, J. W.: Clinical electroencephalography, ed. 2, London, 1966, Butterworth & Co., Ltd.

Kugler, J.: Electroencephalography in hospital and general consulting practice, New York, 1964, American Elsevier Publishing Co., Inc.

Laidlaw, J., and Stanton, J. B.: The EEG in clinical practice, Edinburgh, 1966, E. & S. Livingstone, Ltd.

Magoun, H. W.: The waking brain, Springfield, Ill., 1963, Charles C Thomas, Publisher.

Milnarich, R. F., and Potts, F.: A manual for EEG technicians, Boston, 1958, Little, Brown & Co.

Schwab, R. S.: Electroencephalography in clinical practice, Philadelphia, 1951, W. B. Saunders Co.

Stewart, L. F.: Introduction to the principles of electroencephalography, Springfield, Ill., 1962, Charles C Thomas, Publisher.

Ulett, G. A., Heusler, A., and Word, V.: The effect of psychotropic drugs on the EEG of the chronic psychotic patient. In Wilson, W., editor: Applications of electroencephalography in psychiatry: a symposium, Durham, N. C., 1965, Duke University Press.

Walter, W. G.: The living brain, New York, 1953, W. W. Norton & Co., Inc.

Wiener, N.: Cybernetics, ed. 2, Cambridge, 1961, Massachusetts Institute of Technology.

Williams, D.: Cerebral basis of temperament and personality, Lancet **2:**1, 1954.

Wilson, W. P., and Johnson, P. E.: Thyroid hormone and brain function, Electroenceph. Clin. Neurophysiol. **16:**321, 1964.

7
Psychological examination

On the psychiatric team the psychologist often functions as an expert on research design, a psychological theoretician, or even as a therapist. Originally his unique contribution to clinical psychiatry was in the realm of diagnostic testing. In those situations where prolonged observation of the patient is not feasible or where it is desirable quickly to pick up clues to covert symptomatology, the psychological test battery can be of great value.

The psychologist gathers his data from the patient's test responses and from observations of the patient functioning within the framework of a standardized test situation. His battery of psychological tests is carefully planned with a series of specific questions in mind intended to assess the patient's assets, conflicts, major defenses against anxiety, and amenability to various forms of treatment. The report of psychological findings usually includes a descriptive summary of the patient's personality problems. In order to obtain the greatest value from the psychologist's report, however, the psychiatrist should have some familiarity with the test instruments used. The following tests are commonly included in the diagnostic psychological battery. They are discussed briefly in this chapter and some mention is made of their component parts and scoring scales, but for further details the reader is referred to the list of suggested readings.

TESTS OF INTELLECTUAL FUNCTIONS
Tests of general intelligence
Wechsler Adult Intelligence Scale (WAIS)
Revised Stanford-Binet Scale

Wechsler Intelligence Scale for Children (WISC)
Bayley Infant Scales of Development
Tests of specific areas of function
Bender Visual-Motor Gestalt Test
Tests of abstract and concrete thinking
PROJECTIVE TESTS
Thematic Apperception Test (TAT)
Rorschach Psychodiagnostic Technique
Sentence Completion Test
Draw-A-Person Test
Word Association Test
Rosenzweig Picture-Frustration Test
INVENTORIES
General personality scales
Minnesota Multiphasic Personality Inventory (MMPI)
Guilford-Martin Temperament Profile
Symptom check lists
Saslow Screening Test
Cornell Index
Behavior rating scales
Evaluation of development or social performance
Vineland Social Maturity Scale, Revised
BRIEF TESTS
Proverbs
Comprehension and Similarities
Subtracting Serial Sevens
General Information
Memory for Digits
Kent E-G-Y Test

TESTS OF INTELLECTUAL FUNCTIONS
Tests of general intelligence

The oldest and most carefully standardized portion of the psychological examination is the assessment of intelligence. In these testing situations a number of perceptual, conceptual, memory, and performance abilities are judged. Although the results of these tests are quite easily interpreted and fairly consistent under standard conditions, the tests are affected by cultural and personality variables. Furthermore, it is now known that a large number of individuals vary from 15 to 30 points in functioning at different stages of maturity. Corrections must be made in scoring to account for the decline in intellectual function occurring in the senium.

Wechsler Adult Intelligence Scale (WAIS). Most commonly utilized by psychologists to measure adult intellectual functioning is the Wechsler Adult Intelligence Test. From scores obtained on 11 subtests (vocabulary, comprehension, information, similarities, digit span, arithmetic, picture arrangement, picture completion, object assembly, block design, and digit symbol) the intelligence quotient (I.Q.) is computed. On the basis of the I.Q. the population has been divided into seven groups: defective (69 and below, 2.2%), borderline (70 to 79, 6.7%), dull normal (80 to 90, 16.1%), average (90 to 109, 50.0%), bright normal (110 to 119, 16.1%), superior (120 to 129, 6.7%), and very superior (130 and over 2.2%). Although all subtests within this scale reflect certain aspects of intellectual functioning, there are interesting differences in the subtests, which are useful clinically.

The *Information* and *Vocabulary* subtests measure the subject's general intelligence, learning ability, and alertness to the world around him. In defining words a person tells much about his personality as well as his cultural background. Wechsler states that vocabulary scores decline least with age. *Comprehension* may be called a test of common sense and ability to evaluate past experience. Responses to this portion reveal much about personality or may provide clues to diagnosis of psychopathic personality or schizophrenia. The *Arithmetical Reasoning* subtest, while influenced by education, age, anxiety, and lapses of attention, seems to correlate reasonably well with intellectual capacity. The *Memory Span for Digits* subtest measures retentiveness. Decrease in memory span for digits, particularly in repeating digits backward, often reflects defects in attention and concentration and may be a sign of organic impairment. However, a low digit span score can also reflect marked manifest anxiety.

The *Similarities* subtest throws light upon the way a person reasons and his capacity for abstraction. The *Picture Arrangement* subtest measures an individual's grasp of a situation, his ability to size up what is going on socially; it seems to reflect general intelligence as applied in social situations. *Picture Completion* is useful for testing lower levels of intelligence and taps the ability to distinguish unessential from essential details. *Block Design* enables the examiner to observe how a person goes about discovering patterns and analyzing form. Success depends upon the ability to perceive the relations of the whole to its parts. It is a useful indicator of organic defect. On the *Digit Symbol* test the subject must speedily associate certain symbols with other symbols. Although this performance subtest measures intelligence, it is adversely affected by poor schooling as well as by the associative rigidity or the difficulty in concentration common in emotionally unstable patients. Another chance to observe a patient's intellectual approach to an unfamiliar task is provided by *Object Assembly,* which seems to reflect creative, mechanical, and conceptual abilities.

Revised Stanford-Binet Scale. For a number of years the Stanford-Binet has been widely applied in assessing the intellectual development of children from preschool years to adulthood. Unlike the Wechsler-Bellevue, the same items are not administered to and scored for all subjects; each age level is defined by a series of items which measure various intellectual capacities. The score is expressed in terms of both I.Q. and the mental age attained over all the test items.

Wechsler Intelligence Scale for Children (WISC). Popular with clinicians since its publication in 1949, the Wechsler Intelligence Scale for Children is constructed similarly to the WAIS and expresses the position of a child 5 through 15 years old in relation to others within his own age group.

Bayley Infant Scales of Development. In recent years reliable tests of mental, motor, and behavior development have been developed for ages 6 months to 3 years. These items have been standardized for infants from different cultures and ethnic groups. The relationship of these scales to later intelligence measurement begins to appear after the age of 15 months.

Tests of specific areas of function

Bender-Gestalt Test. This test consists of nine designs which the subject is asked to copy. The manner employed in reproducing this series of perceptual tasks reflects the patient's habitual ways of dealing with outer realities. For example, extreme embellishments of the original design may suggest a manic condition; overaccuracy can indicate compulsive trends. This test is often used to detect organic deficit, arrests, and regressions, shown through impairment of visual-motor function.

Tests of abstract and concrete thinking. A group of tests have been designed to explore the ways a patient has of seeing relationships between objects in the environment. Can he relate things only by their appearance in a very concrete way (as in organic brain damage)? Can he see different types of relationships in terms of function, connotation, etc.? The *Goldstein-Scheerer Tests of Abstract and Concrete Thinking* may be mentioned as well as the *Concept Formation Test* (by Hanfmann and Kasanin).

PROJECTIVE TESTS

Thematic Apperception Test (TAT). This test, developed by Morgan and Murray, is typical of the group. From 10 to 20 of a series of 30 pictures are shown. These are designed to permit identification with persons of both sexes and of different age levels; in some the details are quite indefinite and ambiguous. The subject projects his personality into the situation by building stories about each picture. The interpretation of the test depends upon the figures with which the subject seems to identify, the characteristic mood prevalent in the stories, endings, formal features, topical generalizations, and other dynamic clues. More so than many projective devices, the TAT reveals the content of the patient's fantasies.

Rorschach Test. The Rorschach is the best known of the projective techniques. Introduced by the Swiss psychiatrist Hermann Rorschach (1884-1922), it has been complexly elaborated. The test consists of a standard series of 10 ink blots, some in black and white and some colored. These are shown, one at a time, to a subject who is instructed to state what the blot looks like to him or of what it reminds him. Responses are recorded verbatim.

When all cards have been presented, the examiner scores the test, using a system of symbols (Table 1). Each response is examined with the following questions in mind: (1) Where on the blot area was the response object seen? *(Location.)* (2) What was seen? *(Content.)* (3) What characteristic of the blot suggested the response or why was it seen? *(Determinant.)* (4) How well did the response correspond to the contour of the blot area used? *(Form-level.)* (5) How commonly is this response given by other persons? *(Originality.)* The appro-

Table 1. Some typical Rorschach scoring symbols and their meaning

Location (where it is seen)		*Determinant* (how or why it is seen)	
W	Use of whole blot	Form	
Z	Organization toward whole	F	Responses on the basis of contour or form alone
D.	Usual detail of blot	Movement	
Dd	Rare or unusual area	M	Human-like action
S	White space	FM	Animal-like action
DW and Do Abnormal responses		m	Inanimate movement or force
Content (what is seen)		Color	
H	Living human being	FC	Colored object with form
Hd	Detail of human figure	CF	Color with indefinite form
A	Animal	C	Color only, form disregarded
Ad	Detail of animal	Shading and surface	
At	Anatomy (x-rays, surgical specimens, etc.)	FK	Shading suggesting three dimensions or vista
Obj	Objects	K	Shading as diffusion (smoke, clouds, etc.)
N	Nature (landscape, trees, etc.)	Fc	Surface shading (hairy, fur rug, etc.)
T	Topical (fire, blood, sex, etc.)	c	Shading as texture (furry shiny, etc.)
Form-Level (how well it is seen)		C′	White or black as a color
+	Superior form		
−	Poor form		
Originality (how commonly it is seen by others)			
P	Popular, seen by 1 of 5 persons		
O+	Good original responses (1 of 100 records)		
O−	Poor original response		

priate answer to each of these questions with reference to the subject's response is the Rorschach scoring category that best describes the perceptual processes used. For example, if the subject's reaction to the whole of a large butterfly-shaped ink blot is the popular response "flying bat," the scoring would be W, A, FM, +, P (i.e., whole blot, animal, moving animal, good form, and popular response).

The most difficult step in Rorschach technique is the interpretation of personality characteristics from the assembled

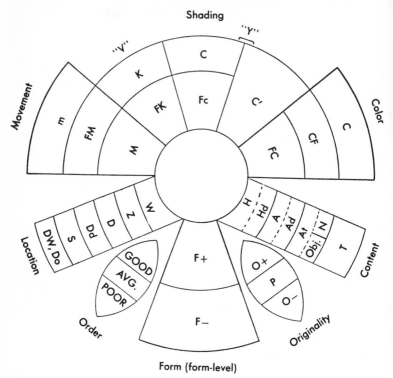

Figure 3A. Rorschach scoring symbol categories. (From Ulett, G.: Northwest Med. 48:545, Aug. 1949.)

totals of scoring symbols and analysis of content. An extremely oversimplified approach to this is seen in Figure 3A, in which the scoring symbol categories are arranged in a circle so that their logical relationships to one another may be readily discerned. The second circle in the diagram (Figure 3B), which may be superimposed upon the first, will serve here to suggest the various facets of personality that are related to the scoring categories. One cannot, however, make interpretative statements by simply noting that a subject's responses fall in certain scoring areas which in turn have some correspondence to a given characteristic of personality. The amount of scor-

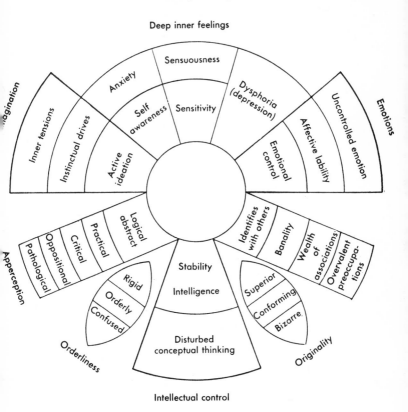

Figure 3B. Various personality facets relatable to Rorschach categories. (From Ulett, G.: Northwest Med. **48**:545, Aug. 1949.)

ing in any area of the diagram must be interpreted in the light of the total number of replies given by the subject, in terms of accepted norms for each symbol category, and with modification by interrelationships among several separate categories.

In the diagram of Figure 3*A* the sectors for *form, color,* and *movement* scoring become the three important interacting spheres of personality determination: *intellect, affect,* and *creative imagination,* as shown by the corresponding portions of Figure 3*B*. Other symbol categories are listed in similar manner. These are not just arbitrary descriptions but arise from a consideration of the ink blot material as follows:

Form answers suggested by the contour of the blot area used are most frequently given. Such answers result from associative and reasoning processes that select or recall previously laid down "engram" patterns in the brain; hence these may be considered to give some measure of intellectual processes. The form level (+ or −) relates to the quality of such associative processes.

The ink blots do not move. Therefore, to see *movement,* as in "bat flying" implies the use of creative imagination.

Color has long been known to portray emotion in everyday life. The color on the cards seems to stimulate the subject. Some patients completely block on colored cards, with great show of emotion. Others use the color in a productive artistic way, indicating good constructive control of the emotions.

Shading responses to the black and white cards have, for want of a better term, been labeled "deep inner feelings." Such responses can indicate anxiety, oversensitiveness, or dysphoric feelings of depression. *Fc* and *c* responses seem to indicate sensitivity and desire for affection. The subject may actually run his hand across the design in giving a response such as "hairy." *C′* responses are given when black and white colors imply "gloom," "coldness," or somber moods. The *K* type responses, on the other hand, are more often said to represent anxiety. These (as depth or vista responses) may show insecurity within the self, a three-dimensional "how do I stand in relation to?" sort of feeling.

Another category, *apperception,* demonstrates the patient's approach to a new situation or shows how he organizes new knowledge in relation to old.

Study of the subject's associations (*content* analysis) can discover areas of preoccupation, reveal hostility, etc.

Score for *originality* indicates superior performance (+) or bizarre fantasy (−); *popular* responses indicate ability to think as other persons do.

The circular diagrams in Figure 3 are arranged in general so that the symbols situated peripherally tend to indicate abnormality whereas those toward the center of the circle represent a more normal trend. This diagrammatic portrayal of Rorschach symbols and their approximate meanings enables one to see at a glance the main personality facets explored in this test procedure and to gain some immediate idea of their interrelationships.*

The picture of the subject revealed by the test is said to

*From Ulett, G. A.: Rorschach introductory manual, St. Louis, 1960, Bardgett Printing & Publishing Co.

show those basic elements of personality structure which, for the most part, remain fixed. It is possible to corroborate or suspect the diagnosis of psychiatric disease entities by the patterns of response to this test.

The validity of the Rorschach Test as a scientific method is still questioned and Rorschach experts admittedly lean heavily upon clinical experience. However, the test has gained wide acceptance and is often worth while to administer if only because of its ability to lower defenses, put the patient "off guard," and hence bring to light material that might otherwise have been seen only after weeks of clinical interviewing.

Sentence Completion Test. Various tests have been devised which require that the patient complete sentences beginning in some such way as "I become very angry when . . ." or "Other people think I . . ." Although this type of test is more transparent than most projective tests and generally does not utilize uniform scoring instructions, it is a useful supplementary source of data on how the patient wishes to present his attitudes about himself and toward others. Both mood and content are noted in relation to such areas as home, work, sickness, immediate family, etc.

The Draw-A-Person Test. This test, originated by Goodenough and further explored by Machover, is believed to provide data about the patient's feelings and perceptions of bodily image. The subject is asked to "draw a person" and later to draw the opposite sex. Intuitive analysis is carried out concerning structural factors (placement of figure on the page, etc.) and content factors (parts of body used, emphasized or de-emphasized, etc.).

Word Association Test. The word association test popularized by Jung consists of a series of 50 or more words which are presented to the subject one at a time. Mixed in the list are words assumed to be related to conflicts of this patient or words which generally produce emotional reaction. The type of association given to these words, together with signs of emotional disturbance such as delayed responses, suggests that the key word is related to a hidden complex.

Picture-Frustration Study (P-F). This test, developed by Rosenzweig, consists of 24 cartoonlike pictures, each representing two persons who are involved in a mildly frustrating situation of common occurrence. One figure in each picture is shown saying certain words which either frustrate the other individual or help to describe what is frustrating him. After examining the picture the subject writes in the blank space the first reply that enters his mind. The answers are scored in terms of the direction and type of aggression (i.e., *extrapunitive* if directed out upon the environment, *intrapunitive* if directed upon himself, or *impunitive* if the aggression is turned off). Similarly the responses are scored in terms of whether the patient is concerned more with the nature of the frustrating situation *(obstacle-dominant)*, with protecting himself *(ego-defensive)*, or with which solution of the problem is most important *(need-persistive)*. Interpretation is in relation to group norms and is suggested as giving some indication of the patient's usual behavior when under frustration.

INVENTORIES

In addition to tests of intellectual functions and projective tests, various self-administered inventories may be helpful. Not only are such paper-and-pencil tests economical in time but, because of their structure, they are also more reliable sources of personality data with many patients than are projective tests.

General personality scales

Two examples will be cited here of the large number of general personality inventories available to the psychologist.

Minnesota Multiphasic Personality Inventory (MMPI). The patient is asked to consider 566 statements about himself and to answer, if possible, whether each statement seems "true" or "false." ("Cannot say" is also available.) In the analysis a variety of scales are applied to the items. These include four validity scales: the L (lie), the F (failure of normal response), the K (test-taking attitude), and the ? (evasiveness) scale. The clinical scales include the Hs (hypochondriacal), D (depression), Hy (hysteria), Pd (psychopath), Ma (mania), Mf (masculinity-femininity), Pa (paranoid), Pt (psychasthenic), and Sc (schizophrenic). An Si (social introversion) scale is also available. The patient's score on all of these composes the MMPI profile. The experienced psychologist makes his diagnoses by scanning the profile and giving weight to the various scoring combinations that occur. Overall, the Minnesota Multiphasic Personality Inventory is a useful adjunct to other diagnostic techniques in defining self-attitudes, certain aspects of ego functioning, and types of symptomatology.

Guilford-Martin Temperament Profile. This is a more recent inventory, not dissimilar to the MMPI and aimed at predicting various types of job and social performances as well as uncovering tendencies toward self-preoccupation, shyness, depression, emotional lability, leadership potential, inferiority feelings, etc.

Symptom check lists

If the psychiatrist is faced with the need to screen rapidly a large number of reasonably cooperative patients, for the presence or absence of psychiatric disorder, a symptom check list may be useful. The following two instruments are but illustrations from a large group which have been designed for use under a variety of special circumstances.

Saslow Screening Test. This test differentiates with reasonable reliability between the psychoneurotic-psychophysiological group of patients and normal persons.

Cornell Index. This is a similar but longer test that has been used with large numbers of persons.

Behavior rating scales

Another method of measuring the patient's psychological and social performance is the behavior rating scale. Hospital personnel often find this is a convenient way of following simple changes in the patient through time. On occasion it may be used by psychiatrists or psychologists as a concrete way of describing major disturbed behaviors and of following surface manifestations of improvement or relapse.

Currently used scales for rating the behavior of hospitalized patients include (1) the *Social Ineffectiveness Scale* by Parloff, Kelman, and Frank, (2) *L-M Fergus Falls Behavior Rating Scale* by Lucero and Meyer, (3) Cutler and Kurland's *Clinical Quantification of Depressive Reactions*, (4) *Ward Behavior Rating Scale* by Burdock et al., (5) Ellsworth's *MACC Be-*

Table 2. Psychological test characteristics of psychiatric patients[*]

	Depression	*Schizophrenia*	*Manic-excitement*
Wechsler Intelligence scales	Performance scales lower than Verbal scales; difficulty in maintaining concentrated effort; Comprehension and Similarity tests generally low; low Digit Span; verbal productions frequently short; distorted and morbid Picture Arrangement stories	Vocabulary and Information subtests generally hold up well; other subtests fall below; Comprehension and Arithmetic both impaired; Performance scales with greatest impairment are Picture Arrangement, Picture Completion, and Object Assembly; qualitatively, responses to any subtest may be peculiar, revealing distortion of thought and perceptual processes; interest scatter is wide	It may not be possible to obtain test results due to the patient's easy distractibility, flight of ideas, and disruption of productive effort because of stimulation of the test; qualitative signs are most predominant, with patient associating to various test stimuli; tests calling for prolonged and concentrated effort pose greatest difficulty
Rorschach	Few responses; prolonged reaction time; low or absent M responses; low or absent color responses; high F+%; emphasis on D and Dd; few W responses; A% high; uncertainty, self-correction, self-depreciation, and qualification of responses	Abnormal responses (contamination, position responses, confabulation, perseveration, queer verbalization, personal references, descriptions, edging); many W responses, poor quality; bizarre and unusual details (Dd); M below normal; C and CF high; color naming (Cn); few popular responses; blocking; increased original (O+ and O−); stereotypy; increased A%	Poor quality (F−); poor W responses (confabulatory DW); increase in M and color responses; decrease in D responses; A% high with FM

[*]This table was prepared by Richard B. Cravens, Ph.D. Like any other tests or laboratory fin indicators. Particularly, the individual signs may not be meaningful in themselves but onl may give valuable and helpful clues in the diagnosis and management of patients with a ment

Paranoid	Psychoneurosis	Character disorders	Organic psychoses
atterning is similar protocol produced schizophrenic atient; Information d Vocabulary hold well; Comprehen- on also fairly well aintained; Digit pan suffers, as does cture Arrangement d Object Assembly; ay be close atten- on paid to irrelevant rts of test stimuli d meaning ascribed purpose of the test	Different neurotic conditions produce different patternings; in obsessive-compulsive conditions Information, Similarities, and Vocabulary tend to remain high, with Comprehension falling less than Information; Verbal Scale elevated over Performance Scale; hysterics generally show Comprehension elevated over Information; lower Vocabulary; Performance Scale score higher than Verbal Scale; depressive reactions show long reaction time; Verbal Scale elevated over Performance Scale; lowered Arithmetic Digit Span	Test-taking attitude important as diagnostic indicator; attitude may be breezy, all knowing, but without depth, cavalier; impression created that patient could tell more about a subject (answer to a test question) if time permitted; Performance Scale significantly elevated over Verbal Scale; Information tends to be low along with Arithmetic and Similarities, although all Verbal scales may be low; Picture Arrangement and Object Assembly elevated	Tests most sensitive to organic conditions are Digit Span, Similarities, Arithmetic, Digit Symbol and Block Design (all low); Vocabulary may remain high along with Information; Verbal Scale higher than Performance Scale; may be statements of perplexity and impotence; evidence of confusion and perseveration; fatigue frequently in the picture
ntroversive Erlebnistypus with high ; high F% and +%; high circumtantial elaboration f relationship of ards (similarities and ifferences); abstract ersonal references	Rejection; no FC; shading shock; not over 1 M; color shock; high F%; over 50% animal or anatomical; not over 25 responses; FM greater than M; (in anxiety: shading, preoccupation, K, k, c); increase in m; overawareness of symmetry; increase in details, Hd, and Ad	Low number of responses; Erlebnistypus constrictive; high F%; poor form level (low F+%); FM greater than M; CF greater than FC; C/F and CF and C; may have difficulty with cards VIII, IX, and X; few original responses; easy W and popular Anatomical, with crude sexual preoccupation; S responses; rejection of cards; suspicious inquiry; antisocial trends (few H); sadomasochistic coloring; egocentricity	Impotence (gives inadequate responses, unable to correct); perplexity (indecisive, seeks reassurance); automatic phrases, repetition, color naming (Cn); F+% low; total responses low; prolonged reaction time; M low

ngs used in clinical medicine, these patterns and signs are suggestive but not absolute diagnostic vhen seen in patterns or in conjunction with other findings and observations. As such, they lisorder.

Continued.

Table 2. Psychological test characteristics of psychiatric patients–

	Depression	*Schizophrenia*	*Manic-excitement*
TAT	Themes of despair, lack of success, failure, loss of love, and death are frequent; stories usually short and pessimistic in attitude; outcomes bleak; picture may cause patient to cry	Themes range from peculiar to bizarre, with private, cryptic meanings, sudden shifts in story, and lack of consistency or guiding story in the plot; sexual references common; length of story tends to be average but rarely may consist of several pages	Possibility of obtaining protocol may be doubtful; stories may ramble on and on as both the picture and the patient's own story serve as a stimulus; stories thus disjointed and contain references to sexual prowess, business success, conquests and other ego-inflating experiences, many of which are drawn from patient's life, real or imagined
MMPI	High D scale; high Pt scales; high F scale; low Ma scale; difficulty in completing tests	Neutral to positive slope; bimodal curve; high F; low K; elevated neurotic triad (Hs, D, Hy) with Pt, Sc, and Pa higher than the neurotic triad	Doubtful that such a patient could focus energy and attention long enough to complete the test; high F; all other scales may be irregularly elevated with a solitary peak of 80 or more on Ma

havioral Adjustment Scale (Form II), (6) *Normative Social Adjustment Scale* by Barrabee, Barrabee, and Finesinger, (7) Malamud and Sands' *Psychiatric Rating Scale*, (8) Wittenborn's *Psychiatric Rating Scales*, (9) *Phenomena of Depressions* by Grinker et al., (10) *Brief Psychiatric Rating Scale* by Overall and Gorham, (11) Hamilton's *Rating Scale for Depression*, (12) Lorr's *Inpatient Multidimensional Psychiatric Scale*, (13) *Symptom and Adjustment Index* by Gross et al., (14) *Katz Adjustment Scales*, (15) *Clyde Mood Scale*, (16) Lorr's *Psychotic Reaction Profile*, (17) the *MMHC Depression Rating Scale* by Greenblatt, Grosser, and Wechsler, (18) *Psy-*

ont'd

Paranoid	Psychoneurosis	Character disorders	Organic psychoses
...ories short; fre-...uent questioning as ... purpose of test; ...me pictures reacted ... in highly personal ...ay; patient ques-...ons source of picture ... in some way re-...tes picture to an ...pect of his life; ...ories guarded, full ...f suspicion and dis-...rust of motives of ...thers; reference to ...eople not viewed in ...icture; things may ...e happening to per-...on that are beyond ...is control	Stories range in length from below average for hysteric to usually above average for obsessive-compulsive; stories free of bizarre elements and tend to be complete, having plot and ending; may be precise and detailed description of picture per se as in case of obsessive-compulsive; gloomy, sad themes as in depressive reaction, or unsophisticated naïve plots as created by hysteric	Stories short, uncompli-cated, and without depth; breezy quality; reference to alcohol, drugs, or criminal activities of major or minor nature, with hero escaping punishment; stories may consist of few lines (description); refusal to tell story and questioning purpose of the test	Themes short, fre-quently limited to pic-ture description with no story or plot; un-certainty expressed as to outcome; confusion, fatigue, and persevera-tion from one picture to next; illness com-mon theme; reference to loss of ability or functioning
Neutral or positive ...ope, bimodal curve, ...igh F; low K; Pa ...5; Sc and Pt 58; ...levation on Ma	Validity scales within limits; negative slope; elevated neurotic triad peaking at D (Hs, D, Hy); inverted neurotic triad (high Hs, low D, high Hy) suggests psy-chosomatic symptoms	Typical profile is double spike curve peaking first at Pd and then Ma; neurotic triad (Hs, D, Hy) low	This profile similar to neurotic profile but may contain secon-dary peak at Sc; Mf, Pa, and Ma are low; profile may also be sawtooth in appear-ance, with peaks at F, D, Pd, Pa, and Sc

chiatric Judgment Depression Scale by Overall et al., and (19) the *Hospital Adjustment Scale* by Ferguson, McReynolds, and Ballachey.

Measures of social performance

Particularly in dealing with more seriously disturbed pa-tients, when one is planning treatment, it is helpful to de-cide the degree to which the patient's illness has interfered with economic self-sufficiency and with effectiveness on the job, in the immediate family, with spouse, and with friends. At the present time no scales for measuring social performance have found wide employment. Perhaps the clinically most useful hypotheses in defining the social performance expected at various levels of maturity have been developed by Erikson.

Vineland Social Maturity Scale, Revised. This scale, devised by E. A. Doll, consists of a graduated series of item clusters, each of which expresses a slightly higher level of social maturity. These are rated from data derived from a structured interview situation held with someone close to the patient. The scale was constructed primarily for assessing severity of mental deficiency but may be used to express gross social performance in any child or adolescent.

BRIEF TESTS

If time does not permit the psychiatrist recourse to psychological consultation, he may himself employ selected items from tests to obtain a "thumbnail impression" of certain personality functions. For example, in searching for evidences of the schizophrenic's tendency toward loose associations, over-generalized patterning of concepts, and defects in abstract thinking, questions borrowed from the *Comprehension* and *Similarities* subtests of the WAIS are clinically useful. If the patient is asked how a bicycle is like a wagon, a good reply would be in terms of function (i.e., they are both means of transportation). An answer which may indicate a tendency toward concrete thinking would be in terms of structure (i.e., they both have wheels). A poor answer would be either a failure to see any similarity or the use of bizarre or overinclusive type of similarity (i.e., they are both used outside the home).

Proverbs. In addition to the above, proverbs are commonly employed by clinicians to test for evidences both of schizophrenic distortions and of concretization or sterility of associations found in the patient with organic brain damage. If, upon being asked to explain the proverbs "A rolling stone gathers no moss," "All that glitters is not gold," and "A bird in the hand is worth two in the bush," a patient with normal I.Q. replies only in terms of stones, gold, and birds and he cannot comprehend the application of these proverbs to human affairs, abstract thinking may be assumed to be impaired.

Subtracting Serial Sevens. A brief method of measuring

attention and concentration abilities is to ask the patient to subtract 7's serially, starting from 100. Most persons can complete the task with no more than two errors in sixty seconds.

General Information. Questions testing general information (e.g., "How far is it from San Francisco to New York?" "Who is governor of your state?") are useful indicators of both cultural and intellectual factors.

Memory for Digits. Having the patient repeat after the examiner a series of unrelated digits is a brief test of attention and memory. Most individuals should be able to do this forward up to six or seven digits and backward up to four or five digits.

Kent E-G-Y Test. A number of brief tests of personality function have been devised. An example of a brief adult intelligence scale giving a simple, rough indication of both mental age and quality of thinking is the Kent E-G-Y Test.

Kent E-G-Y questions

		Points*
1.	What are houses made of? (Any material you can think of.)	1-4
2.	What is sand used for?	1, 2, or 4
3.	If the flag blows to the south, where is the wind coming from?	3

*Points assigned in scoring:

Total points	"Mental age" rating	Total points	"Mental age" rating
10-13	8	21-23	12
14-16	9	24-27	13
17-18	10	28-31	14
19-20	11	32-36	14+

1. One point for each item up to four.
2. One point for "play" or "scrubbing." Two points for any construction use. Four points for "glass."
3. Three points for "north"; no partial credits.
4. One point each, up to four.
5. Three points for "noon."
6. One point each, up to four. "New York is counted as a city unless another state has been mentioned.
7. Two points for "moon is lower down." Three points for "nearer" or "closer." Four points for generalized statement that nearer objects look larger than distant objects.
8. Two points for "steel." Four points for "iron."
9. Four points for "southwest"; no partial credits.
10. Two points for "13." Anyone who responds "50" should have his attention called to his mistake and should be permitted to try again. If he responds "7," it should be made clear that both red and white stripes are included.

4. Tell me the names of some fishes.   1-4
5. At what time of day is your shadow shortest?   3
6. Give the names of some large cities.   1-4
7. Why does the moon look larger than the stars?   2, 3, or 4
8. What metal does a magnet pick up?   2 or 4
9. If your shadow points to the northeast, which way is the sun?   4
10. How many stripes in the American flag?   2

SUGGESTED READINGS

Ames, L. B., Metraux, R. W., and Walker, R. N.: Adolescent Rorschach responses; developmental trends from 10 to 16 years, New York, 1959, Paul B. Hoeber, Inc., Medical Book Department of Harper & Bros.

Anastasi, A.: Psychological testing, ed. 3, New York, 1966, The Macmillan Co.

Anderson, H. H., and Anderson, G. L., editors: An introduction to projective techniques, Englewood Cliffs, N. J., 1951, Prentice-Hall, Inc.

Beck, S. J.: Rorschach's test, ed. 3, New York, 1961, Grune & Stratton, Inc., vols. 1 to 3.

Clyde, D. J.: Clyde Mood Scale manual, Coral Gables, Fla., 1963, University of Miami Biometric Laboratory.

Cronbach, L.: Essentials of psychological testing, ed. 3, New York, 1960, Harper & Row, Publishers.

Gilbert, J.: Clinical psychological tests in psychiatric and medical practice, Springfield, Ill., 1969, Charles C Thomas, Publisher.

Hathaway, S., and Meehl, P.: An atlas for clinical use of the MMPI, Minneapolis, 1951, University of Minnesota Press.

Klopfer, B., and Davidson, H.: The Rorschach technique: an introductory manual, New York, 1962, Harcourt, Brace & World, Inc.

Lanyon, R.: A handbook of MMPI group profiles, Minneapolis, 1968, University of Minnesota Press.

Lorr, M., and others: Inpatient multidimensional psychiatric scale, Palo Alto, Calif., 1963, Consulting Psychologist Press.

Lyerly, S. B., and Abbott, P. S.: Handbook of psychiatric rating scales (1950-1964). Bethesda, Md., NIMH, National Institutes of Health, PHS Publication no. 1495.

Mensh, I. N., and Hunt, W. A.: Abbreviated psychological measures, psychiatric unit operational procedures, rev. ed., Washington, D. C., 1954, Neuropsychiatry Branch, Professional Division, Bureau of Medical Surgery, Navy Department.

Pascal, G., and Suttell, B.: The Bender-Gestalt test, New York, 1951, Grune & Stratton, Inc.

Rapaport, D., Gill, M. M., and Schafer, R.: Diagnostic psychological testing, New York, 1968, International Universities Press, Inc.

Saslow, G., Counts, R. M., and DuBois, P. H.: Evaluation of a new psychiatric screening test, Psychosom. Med. 13:242, 1951.

Schafer, R.: Projective testing and psychoanalysis, New York, 1968, International Universities Press, Inc.

Smith, W. L., and Philippus, M. J.: Neuropsychological testing in organic brain dysfunction, Springfield, Ill., 1969, Charles C Thomas, Publisher.

Terman, L., and Merrill, M.: Measuring intelligence, New York, 1937, Houghton Mifflin Co.

Thelen, M. H., Varble, D. L., and Johnson, J.: Attitudes of academic clinical psychologists toward projective techniques, Amer. Psychol. **23:**517, 1968.

Ulett, G. A.: Rorschach introductory manual, St. Louis, 1960, Bardgett Printing & Publishing Co.

Wechsler, D.: The measurement and appraisal of adult intelligence, ed. 4, Baltimore, 1958, The Williams & Wilkins Co.

Wittenborn, J. R., Holzberg, J. D., and Simon, B.: Symptom correlates for descriptive diagnosis, Genet. Psychol. Monogr. **47:**237, 1953.

Wolff, H. G.: Non-projective personality tests; Cornell Indices and Cornell Word Form Application, Ann. N. Y. Acad. Sci. **46:**589, 1946.

Zubin, J., Eron, L. D., and Schumer, F.: An experimental approach to projective techniques, New York, 1965, John Wiley & Sons, Inc.

8
Psychodynamic concepts of personality development

The term *psychodynamic* ("dynamic") refers to the study of the causative factors and motivations of human interpersonal behavior. It stresses the importance of past and current interhuman relationships as opposed to organic (anatomical and physiological) factors as most important in determining the variables of personality in mental illness. Originally almost synonymous with "psychoanalytic," the term is currently more broadly conceived. In this section will be mentioned briefly a few common psychodynamic concepts which psychiatrists find useful in relating patients' childhood experiences to their adult emotional illnesses. Often it seems clear not only that constitutional factors and immediate life stresses have operated as possible causes but also that the groundwork for later illness was laid in chronically maladaptive attitudes and behaviors unwittingly fostered by the human environment of childhood.

By means of a series of systematic changes, personality develops stepwise from the neonatal period through the stages of adult life. Each period of adaptation contains fairly uniform biological and social conditions that challenge the individual to learn new behaviors and roles and to give up former expressions and identifications appropriate to an earlier life stage. The infant-mother tie in the first week involves different issues from those of the infant-mother tie in the third month of life, just as the adolescent-parent relationship involves different problems at 14 years of age than those at age 19. The study of personality development consists in defining these stage-specific challenges and in trying to understand how the genes, the brain, the previous experience of the person, and the environment have influenced adaptation by setting limits to change and by providing alternative possibilities for new behaviors and experiences.

At present there is no coherent theory of personality. A variety of incomplete theoretical positions exist, each of which clarifies limited problems. Neurophysiology, theories of conditioning and reinforcement, psychoanalysis, concepts of social role, ideas about ecological and cultural influences, and concerns with each person's uniqueness and essential moral potentials all attend to different aspects of personality. In our ignorance we are like the proverbial six blind men, each examining a different part of an elephant—no one has had the imagination or the facts to construct a balanced picture of the whole.

The psychoanalytic philosophy of human functioning puts the patient's wishes in the center of theoretical focus. Within Freud's study of dreams as well as within his psychotherapeutic technique, the patient's frustrated yearnings and hopes were the starting point for understanding the illness. Whether intentionality is conceived in terms of biologically structured *instincts,* conditioned secondary *drives,* psychic *needs,* socialized *role functions,* or moral *requirements,* using any view of personality, the psychiatrist understands the patient's symptoms as by-products of maladaptive, inappropriate patterns of goal-directed behavior. Therefore, a person's health or illness is linked to (1) the nature of his goals (realistic or unrealistic, infantile or stage-appropriate), (2) his repertoire of interpersonal behaviors for pursuing these goals (coping or defense mechanisms), and (3) his available modes of experiencing relationships and situations. Following are two pathological illustrations of this connection: (1) Depressive illnesses are said to occur in depressive personalities who, since childhood, have tended to set unreliable perfectionistic goals followed by withdrawn behavior and with hopelessness, envy, and repressed rage; (2) schizophrenic illnesses are reported to occur in disorganized personalities who, since childhood, have lacked clarity and conviction about inner needs and realistic goals, who too quickly have experienced confusion in the face of the unexpected, and who have used unworkable behaviors to meet daily situations. In a number of experimental studies developmental psychologists have shown that children function best when environmental stimuli conform to the child's expectations and when the child is encouraged to have aspirations that are, in fact, capable of being fulfilled. In several studies parents of disturbed offspring have been found to have disorders of thinking, perception, and attention which may make it difficult for them to present meaningful and consistent views of experience to their children.

PERSONALITY DEVELOPMENT

The outer limits of personal capabilities and sensitivities as well as certain general temperamental tendencies (energy

Table 3. Stages of personality development

Age	Stage	Developmental issues*
0-3 mo.	Neonatal	Psychophysiological patterning and maternal management of infant's tension; basis for autonomic stability or instability
3-6 mo.	Preattachment	Visual and auditory recognition; familiarity responses and strangeness anxiety begin; sociability and smiling; basis for trust or distrust
6-12 mo.	Attachment	Interpersonal vocalization; selective demand for mother; separation anxiety begins; basis for hope or hopelessness
1-2½ yr.	Early individuation (anal)	Walking, toilet training, exploration, verbalization, self-assertiveness, anxiety over self-control; basis for autonomy or doubt
2½-4 yr.	Late individuation (phallic)	Mastery of own body, communication, imaginative production; basis for socialized conscience or punitive and defective superego formation

*The terms listed are intended to indicate only in a general way a few salient intrapsychic, behavioral, and psychosocial changes characteristic of but not limited to each stage.

level, degree of passivity or activity in relationships, intellectual power, sensitivity to emotional arousal, and so on) are assumed to be settled by the arrangement of genes at the moment of conception. Predisposition to inherited disorders is also settled or influenced at this time. During fetal life it is known that certain maternal physiological influences can have an impact on later personality. Pavlovian conditioning can take place in the fetus. Disorders such as maternal rubella, placenta previa, and toxemia of pregnancy are associated with an increased incidence of cerebral palsy, epilepsy, mental retardation, and childhood behavior disorders. Prematurity or perinatal cyanosis, anoxia, or high neonatal serum bilirubin levels from any cause are also associated with these conditions.

Personality development can best be thought of as a series of life's stages (Table 3), in each of which specific adaptive

Table 3. Stages of personality development—cont'd

Age	Stage	Developmental issues
4-7 yr.	Oedipal	Learning to read; family role definition; basis of comfortable sex identification or castration anxiety and penis envy
7-9 yr.	Latency	Industry and work habits, attainment of concrete logical thinking, role in school and neighborhood, friendships; basis for self-esteem or sense of inferiority
9-12 yr.	Preadolescence	Discipline of memory, attainment of abstract logic, gang and clique formation, homoerotic exploration
12-16 yr.	Early adolescence	Puberty, disillusionment with family myths, intellectual autonomy, and availability of complex or intuitive judgment
16-20 yr.	Late adolescence	Identity formation, career choice, esthetic and religious preference, heterosexual relationships
20-30 yr.	Early adulthood	Intimacy, commitment to parenthood, worldly competition
30-65 yr.	Maturity	Social responsibility, generativity, leadership
Over 65 yr.	Old age	Integrity or despair

changes usually occur. During the initial 3 to 6 weeks of life infants vary considerably in arousal level and sleepiness, in intensity of hunger, in social responsiveness, in their sensitivity to contact, taste, smell, postural change, sights, and sounds. The principal developmental change here is the *stabilization of vital functions* of eating, sleeping, and tension management through rocking, stroking, bathing, and comforting sounds. If a reasonably stable relationship occurs between a comfortable, intelligent, and observant mother and an infant who has no unusual sensitivities or tendencies to tension buildup and overreactivity, a sound basis for later development is provided. In a similar fashion each later developmental stage has primary change processes. An infant or child may begin early to show his characteristic mode of dealing with new situations, a mode that may become a lifelong style of personality. Kagan and Moss, for example, show that passive, inhibited infants predict dependent unassertive young adults. Studies now have demonstrated that immediately after birth males and females have a different repertoire of response styles. With the maturation of new abilities, however, or with the occurrence of serious conflict at a later developmental stage, the style of personality may be altered considerably.

Careful observation of newborn infants has identified the presence of expressive behavior patterns, including smiling, although the social smile is first seen in most infants between 3 and 7 weeks of age. By 3 to 4 months considerable perceptual competence has developed and sensorimotor coordination of the fingers, hands, eyes, mouth, and head is seen. About this time the infant can begin to notice the difference between the familiar and the unfamiliar. A strange object appearing before him may lead to an anxious sobering. By 5 or 8 months of age "stranger anxiety proper" develops in some infants, presumably indicating that the infant now can perceive clearly the difference between his family and strange persons. It is assumed that during the second 6 months of life the infant clarifies the difference between the inside and outside of his body and between himself and other persons. This comes about as the infant attaches himself more and more specifically to his mother. He may begin in the third 6 months of life to experience increasing separation anxiety when she is away from his presence.

Between 9 and 14 months of age the child stands and shortly thereafter begins to walk. In the subsequent developmental period of 12 to 15 months the child for the first time is prevented from carrying out his goals (stopped from knocking over things) and begins to hear "No." This development facilitates his capacity not only to differentiate perceptually between himself and others (a capacity presumed to have appeared at about 2 to 3 months of age) but also to deal with himself as a separate person and to treat his own impulses with some beginning objectivity. From 18 to 36 months, cognitive capacities and early interpersonal patterns emerge, particularly focused about control of bowel and locomotor functions and about the pleasure in manipulating and sensing the diversity of the physical world. Language capacity matures and the use of fantasy play becomes a major mode for self-expression and for internalization of new learnings about family life. From 4 to 7 years of age the child experiences with intense affect the forces of love and anger and the habitual family defenses against anxiety, and he may attempt to exert his or her own powers to intervene in sibling or parental transactions. A phase of overestimation of his own power to seduce or to overwhelm other family members gives way to a more realistic self-appraisal, except in the instance of an emotionally disturbed youngster. This facilitates movement of the child into the community, via school, and the gradual attenuation through the next few years of the intense family bonds set up in the earliest period of life.

In recent years developmental psychologists have noted that the child develops in a healthy manner when the home and social environment do not contain too many contradictions and when the environment supports the development of new capacities in the child that are appropriate to his age. Certain environmental requirements may be stated for each developmental stage. For example, 3- to 4-year-old children are generally more responsive to and rewarded by women than by men; 6- or 7-year-old children tend to be rewarded more by the opposite sex parent, and, at least for a larger group of children, as they grow older, the same sex parent tends to function as the model and as the person who shapes behavior. Social class and subcultural differences are important here. In middle class families in industrial countries the child's aggression tends to be disciplined by the same sex parent, whereas in families in which the father is unskilled the mother expects him to be the disciplinarian for all the children and expects herself to be the nurturant support.

In *Three Contributions to the Theory of Sex,* Freud schematized these complex developments by the concepts of *oral, anal,* and *phallic* phases of *pregenital development.* The classical Freudian position has been that during each phase a primary instinctual impulse strives for discharge. Each impulse has a specific *aim* (the act, such as sucking, which would provide a mode of discharge and pleasurable reduction of tension), a specific *object* (the breast), and a specific *source* (the erogenous zone—in the oral phase, the mouth of the infant). On the basis of Freudian theory, you would assume that character traits referable to trust, self-confidence, narcissism, and auto-eroticism have been dealt with in the oral phase (age 0 to 18 months); that traits of ambivalence, orderliness or sloppiness, punctuality, defiance, submission and impulse control have been dealt with in the anal phase (age 18 months to 3 years); and that in the phallic phase (age 3 to 5 years), in which the child is preoccupied with the significance of having or not having a penis (the *castration complex*), traits of sexual identity or fears, self-esteem, sex role definition, and social facility would begin to be salient. On the basis of the form these early pregenital experiences take and, in particular, upon the manner in which the child resolves them for himself during the *oedipal period* (age 4 to 7 years), the superego is said to be formed. This intrapsychic agency, contained within the ego, represents those aspects of the parental images which the child takes as his own lifelong automatic guideposts to moral and social values.

During *preadolescence* the individual becomes more effective as a worker and strives for the first time to achieve some individuality and intimacy outside the family with his peers. It is usual at this period for the child to find a confidant of the same sex with whom he explores and tests many questions about life. Homosexual experiences are normal here.

With the advent of *adolescence*, an internal upheaval is brought about by the biological pressure of sexual maturation and the social pressure to become emancipated from the family. The ensuing struggle to find a new psychological equilibrium tests the strength of earlier ego development and normally produces, to some degree, symptoms which in the adult would be judged neurotic.

The young family man or woman faces genuine testing of abilities to take economic and emotional responsibilities for others. Here a degree of self-centeredness or self-love *(narcissism),* which may have been consistent with outward mental health in earlier years, can lead to trouble. Or, if chronic tendencies to misperceive reality or to mistrust oneself or others remain, the increasingly intimate and complex relationships at home and at work will be stressful and lead to symptoms.

Finally, as the mature individual grows older, sufficient self-respect and autonomy must have developed to permit the natural social and biological changes of approaching senescence to be accepted with calm (as in serene old age) rather than alarm (as in involutional melancholia).

At any stage of life, disorganizing symptoms may appear for the first time. But the clinician, upon sensitive and careful inquiry into the patient's past, will note lifelong trends in reacting to certain types of events as though they were threatening; he will see that the patient—instead of solving certain types of problems—finds it necessary to bring into play some pathological defense mechanisms. Thus, though symptoms may have been absent, the overuse of certain defense mechanisms has heralded potential mental illness for years.

Prominent characteristics in the developmental pattern are summarized in Table 3.

MECHANISMS OF DEFENSE

A well-adjusted individual frequently reaches conclusions and resolves conflictual situations through a rational consideration and weighing of the facts before making his decision. The person who is emotionally disabled and finds conflicts very anxiety-provoking seeks to escape from the dilemma through one or a variety of behavioral gambits that have been termed "mechanisms of defense." While such mechanisms are clearly seen in psychoneurotics and psychotics, they also exist to some degree in everyone. Such patterns of action, if commonly used, may "character-ize" the individual who comes to rely upon them more or less automatically for handling his anxieties and in resolving interpersonal problems. For such reasons it is useful to have knowledge of these psychological mechanisms that are called upon for the self-defense of the person in times of conflict.

MECHANISMS OF DEFENSE

compensation Mechanism in which an approved or admirable character trait is developed to conceal either the absence of some other or the presence of an opposite one. The latter may exist only in the unconscious. A person who has no capacity as an athlete may compensate in scholarship.

complex formation Interassociation of a number of related or even unrelated ideas in the unconscious, in such a way that any threat to one brings out the emotional tone and defense of the whole.

condensation Expression of a whole group of ideas with a single word, phrase, or thought.

conversion Attempt to keep a disturbing wish from realization, through inhibition of motor and/or sensory activities—either partial (blindness, paralysis) or complete (generalized paralysis or refusal to move).

denial Bland disregard of a disturbing reality situation or intense inner affect. Mutually incompatible thoughts can exist side by side in *logic-tight compartments* or be completely *isolated* as in circumscribed amnesia.

displacement Substitution of a different object upon whom affect is then centered or released. The emotional investment (cathexis) is transferred from the unacceptable ideas to other, associated ideas that can appear in consciousness without causing anxiety.

dissociation Separation in which one idea or several groups of ideas become split off from the main body of thought. Dissociated ideas are not accessible to consciousness.

dreaming Repressed material appears and conflicts are "worked through" or solved in one's dreams.

fantasy identification One adapts or patterns behavior after that of an image or ego ideal whose behavior one admires.

inhibition In aim inhibition the aim or goal of an instinctual drive is modified but the original drive is satisfied to some extent. Thus a desire in the child for sexual relations with a parent may change to an attitude of love or respect in which there is no overt sexuality.

introjection The object is, as it were, ingested by the mind so that the psychic energies of the ego appear to be organized as if they were under the control of the introject. The experience of a feared or a desired person being inside the self.

introversion Introversion occurs when a person withdraws from environmental context and indulges in excessive fantasy. This is usually followed by marked regression.

isolation The impulse to action, the thought, or the act is isolated from the associated affect and the wider associations connected with it. The thought, for example, is conscious but minus the distressing associations or affect. This defense is found in obsessional neurosis.

projection. Displacement of one's wishes, fears, or desires upon another person.

reaction formation Transformation of one drive into seemingly the exact opposite, as in expressing extreme consideration toward one for whom hostile feelings are held.

regression Abandonment of mature behavior patterns for increasingly immature or infantile ones. Extreme retreat into fantasy life *(autism)* can lead to escape from upsetting realities through *delusion formation.*

repression Total exclusion of the idea from consciousness.

somatization Conflict is repressed and becomes represented by physical symptoms involving parts of the body innervated by the autonomic nervous system.

sublimation Substitution of a more socially acceptable activity for one that is unacceptable.

symbolization An object or an act represents a complex group of objects or acts.

undoing The disturbing thought or action is allowed to occur and is then followed by the opposite throught or act, which cancels the effect of the first thought or act in a magical way. This mechanism is especially seen in obsessions and compulsions.

ROLE OF DEFENSES IN SYMPTOM FORMATION

Defense mechanisms are utilized to some extent by all persons in their day-to-day living but are seen in extreme form in mental disorder, where frequently one type of mechanism, used predominantly, fosters a symptom picture characteristic for that disorder.

In many adult patients it appears that the current life situation has evoked long-forgotten, unresolved anxieties from an earlier period, which in turn foster inappropriate defenses and symptom formation. Thus, for example, the complex emotional attachment to the first object of one's affection, mother, with its attendant fluctuating, mixed (ambivalent) feelings toward father, who threatens or at least partly usurps that mother love, is often never fully understood or solved by the child. If this occurs, the unacceptable (to society and the superego) feelings of love and hostility (Oedipus complex) are repressed instead of accepted. At a later time, under the pressure of similar affectionate feelings toward an adult lover or similar competitive feelings toward a business rival, anxiety may be experienced; in psychoanalytic theory this is considered to stem from the fact that in the early family situation these similar feelings, instead of being accepted and mastered, were repressed.

When such anxiety related to repressed complexes occurs, symptoms or behaviors appear which are determined in part by the defense employed. For example, with *reaction formation* the individual may feel a need to be excessively considerate of and polite to his rival; or the offending feelings might be *displaced* and experienced openly in relation to political figures or chance or distant acquaintances rather than in relation to their real human object. If the anxiety were to be dealt with still more pathologically, perhaps compulsive acts, obsessive thoughts, or delusions might become related in the patient's mind to the rival or lover.

SUGGESTED READINGS

Benedek, T.: Parenthood as a developmental phase, J. Amer. Psychoanal. Ass. 7:389, 1959.

Blos, P.: On adolescence, New York, 1962, The Free Press of Glencoe, Inc.

Bowlby, J.: Nature of the child's tie to his mother, Int. J. Psychoanal. 39:350, 1958.

Erikson, E. H.: Identity and the life cycle, Psychol. Issues 1:169, 1959.

Erikson, E. H.: Childhood and society, ed. 2, New York, 1963, W. W. Norton & Co., Inc.

Freud, A.: Concept of developmental lines, psychoanalytic study of the child, New York, 1963, International Universities Press, Inc.

Freud, S.: Outline of psychoanalysis, New York, 1949, W. W. Norton & Co., Inc.

Hartmann, H.: Ego psychology and the problem of adaptation, New York, 1958, International Universities Press, Inc.

Hess, R. D., and Handel, G.: Family worlds, Chicago, 1959, University of Chicago Press.

Jessner, L., and Pavenstedt, E.: Dynamic psychopathology in childhood, New York, 1959, Grune & Stratton, Inc., chaps. 2, 3, 4, and 6.

Kagan, J., and Moss, H.: Birth to maturity, New York, 1962, John Wiley & Sons, Inc.

Kessen, W., and Kuhlman, C.: Thought in the young child, Monogr. Soc. Res. Child Develop. 27(2):3, 1962.

Pasamanick, B., Rogers, M. E., and Lilienfeld, A. M.: Pregnancy experience and behavior disorder, Amer. J. Psychiat. 112:613, 1956.

Piaget, J.: Play, dreams and imitation in childhood, New York, 1962, W. W. Norton & Co., Inc.

Rapaport, D.: Structure of psychoanalytic theory, Psychol. Issues 2:1, 1960.

Reich, W.: Character analysis, ed. 3, New York, 1949, Orgone Institute Press.

Scott, J. P.: Process of primary socialization in canine and human infants, Monogr. Soc. Res. Child Develop. 28(1):2, 1963.

Solnit, A. J., and Provence, S. A.: Modern perspectives in child development, New York, 1963, International Universities Press, Inc.

Sullivan, H. S.: The interpersonal theory of psychiatry, New York, 1953, W. W. Norton & Co., Inc.

9
Symptoms of psychiatric disorders

Behavior, both normal and pathological, derives from sources which include instinctual and hereditary drives, as well as environmentally and socially determined forces. *Instincts* have been defined as inherited neuronal (probably diencephalic) patterns of behavior, which are present at birth and which alter with growth, cerebral myelinization, hormonal development, and the modifying impact of intellect and acquired social patterns. *Emotion* accompanies and colors behavior as a result of the facilitation and impeding of instinctual drives. *Conation* is the inherent urge to all activity, mental as well as physical; its level varies widely from sluggish to hypomanic but is characteristic for any individual throughout his life.

Consciousness can be defined as the organism's capacity to react to stimuli and is displayed in degrees of awareness or *attention* to the surrounding environment. The five senses serve as means for *perception* of all sensory stimuli, which are *recognized* or identified in terms of previous experiences. Such recognized sensations are organized into *concepts* which, subject to intelligence, judgment, and wisdom, are put into function through *motor action*. *Will* is the crystallization of cognition and thought that leads to behavior. *Personality* is the resultant picture of all the habitual patterns displayed by the individual, from a fusion of his genetic endowment and the sum of experiential modifications. A wide variety of normal variations and the combination of behavioral symptoms make up identifiable character types and form the basis for clinical syndromes.

Many different terms have been used to describe the infinite variety of symptoms that are the *psychopathology* of mental disorders. Some of these are but adaptational adjustments that may occur to a lesser degree in the coping behavior of normal persons. Others are the florid manifestations of a malfunctioning brain. Although usually described as disturbances of "separate functions of the mind," it is well to remember that because the organism functions as a whole this designation is merely a convenient fiction.

DISORDERS OF PERCEPTION

The avenues of perception include sight, hearing, touch, taste, and smell—of which the disorders are classically *illusions* and *hallucinations*. An *illusion* is a false interpretation or misinterpretation of a real sight, sound, or other sensation. It may express a hoped for or feared event or be simply the result of a delirious, toxic, or febrile state. A *hallucination* is a false perception for which there exists no actual sensory basis. So-called *pseudo hallucinations, hypnagogic* and *hypnopompic hallucinations,* occur while persons are falling asleep and awakening, respectively. These lack the vividness and clarity of *true hallucinations*. Most common are hallucinations of hearing. The auditory type may be *elementary hallucinations,* consisting of noise and music, or more complex *hallucinatory voices (phonemes)*. Special cases include *"Gedankenlautwerden,"* in which the patient hears his own thoughts spoken aloud, and *functional hallucinations,* with the phonemes occurring only if there is some external source of noise (e.g., running water). *Hallucinations of vision* may be elementary, consisting only of flashes of light, or be more organized (persons and things) in flashback memories, and even *mass hallucinations* of groups of persons in active scenes. In *heautoscopy ("Doppelgänger")* the subject sees and recognizes himself. *Extracampine hallucinations* are ones identfied as outside the visual field (e.g., "behind me"). Other visual hallucinatory experiences include *macropsia,* seeing things enlarged, and *micropsia (lilliputian hallucinations)* in which things seem smaller. *Hallucinations of smell* are usually of disagreeable and noxious odors, while *hallucinations of taste* often refer to poisons "and dope in the food." *Hallucinations of touch* are often interpreted as insects crawling over the skin (e.g., cocaine bug) but may involve *sexual hallucinations* of erection, orgasm, et cetera. *Hallucinations of deep sensation* and of *vestibular sensation* include feelings such as twisting or flying. A special case of hallucinations is that of *"phantom limb"* arising from sensations of an amputated stump. So-called *negative hallucinations* in which something present is perceived as being absent occur in hysteria and as a phenomenon readily demonstrated under hypnosis.

DISORDERS OF CONSCIOUSNESS, ORIENTATION, AND ATTENTION

These disorders are closely related to those of perception. *Apperception,* for instance, is the comprehension of what is perceived, or perception supplemented by *recognition* and *interpretation.* The ability to perceive and apperceive depends upon the *state of attention* or focusing ability, which may be hyperactive *(startle) distractible,* easily diverted, or tenaciously adherent to some single stimulus. *Confusion* is a state of impairment of the sensorium which can vary all the way from a slight *clouding of consciousness* to a deep *stupor.* The term *coma* refers to a profound degree of unconsciousness from which the patient cannot be aroused and which usually results from some general organic or cerebral condition. *Disturbances of orientation* (time, place, and person) are those in which the patient does not know where he is, what time it is, or how to identify himself and those around him. This most often occurs with states of toxic delirium but can be seen in *dream states* of psychogenic or unknown origin. Sometimes listed under alteration of consciousness are states of *heightened suggestibility* and *negativism;* in the former the subject is influenced with uncritical acceptance, as in hypnosis and some types of "folie à deux," but in the latter any suggestion produces just the opposite reaction.

DISORDERS OF MEMORY

Disorders of memory involve the mechanisms for the reception and registration of ideas, for their retention, and for later recall and reproduction. These mechanisms show three major types of disorders: *hypermnesia, amnesia,* and *paramnesia.* Hypermnesia is an abnormal mnemonic capacity seen in mild manic and paranoid conditions. The term *amnesia* refers to a loss of memory. In *organic amnesia,* as for example in the aging brain, *recent memory* may be lost while memory for remote past events is retained. In *psychogenic amnesia* recall is inhibited for psychological reasons. There may be a *generalized* or a *selective* type of amnesia in which inconvenient events or topics are forgotten. *Anterograde amnesia* is one that continues progressively, parallel with ongoing activity in which the subject appears to act normally but later has no recollection of his behavior. In *retrograde amnesia* the loss of memory extends backward, as for a period preceding trauma to the head. *Paramnesia* refers to a falsification of memory, commonly observed in Korsakov's syndrome as *confabulation* in which the patient simply fills in the gaps of his memory by fabrications which have no basis in fact. *Retrospective falsification* occurs when the patient unconsciously distorts or "embroiders" his memories of past life experiences in response to some emotional needs. The illusion of memory known as "déjà vu" refers to a false feeling of familiarity for some new scene; "jamais vu" is the term for a false feeling of unfamiliarity.

DISORDERS OF THINKING

The production of *rational thinking* is complicated business and depends upon the smooth coordinated functioning of very complicated brain mechanisms. Even at best, "normal humans" show frequent lapses from logic *(parapraxis);* and as Freud pointed out in his *Psychopathology of Everyday Life,* emotion is commonly betrayed *(lapsus linguae)* and can interfere with intellectual functioning. When thinking is obviously guided by processes beyond awareness and finds its origin in complexes, wishes, and other motivations not under conscious recognition, it is called *autistic* or *dereistic thought.* Disturbances in *progression* of thought *(stream of thought)* include *flight of ideas,* in which one thought follows another in quick succession but with little progress toward a single goal idea. This may be associated with an inner-push *distractibility* and often involves words having a similar sound *(clang associations).* In the opposite vein, speech and thinking may be *retarded* or manifest *blocking* with sudden obstructions, which may be removed as suddenly as they appeared. In schizophrenics there may be *fragmentation* or *scattering* of speech to the point of incoherence; thoughts may be so *tangential* as to be barely related to each other, or entirely new and unusual words *(neologisms, word salad)* may be produced. *Perseveration* occurs when an idea is abnormally repeated and continued, particularly in the retarded, epileptic, or senile. *Circumstantiality* occurs when a person's sequence of spoken words unnecessarily elaborates trivial details. In persons less disabled one finds evidence of extreme *volubility (logorrhea)* and in some a tendency to brood over abstract matters or take refuge in scientific terms *(intellectualization)*. Belief that specific thoughts can lead to the fulfillment of wishes or can ward off evil *(magical* or *superstitious thinking)* is found commonly in children and in less sophisticated cultures. Disturbances in the content of thought include preoccupation *(trends)* and overdetermined ideas resulting more from affective factors than from logical reasoning. Ideas that persistently thrust themselves into consciousness are termed *obsessions*. Allied to these are *phobias, fears, doubts,* and *indecisions. Fantasy* occurs in the form of ideas that are hoped for but recognized as unreal. *Pseudologia fantastica* is different from normal *daydreams* in that the patient *(impostor* and *pathological liar)* believes his ideas sufficiently to act upon them. A *delusio*n is a false belief not founded upon logical inference and one which cannot be corrected by adequate proof of its falsity. Most common are *delusions of persecution* in which the patient believes that various persons or forces are attempting to harm or manipulate him with hostile intent. Such beliefs may be vague and poorly organized *(unsystematized delusions)* or may be in the form of an elaborate fixed or systematized delusion. Closely related to these are *ideas of reference,* in which the patient falsely interprets remarks and actions of people around him as ridiculing or depreciatory of him. *Litigious behavior* may occur, with the involvement of lawyers and courts. A commonly related everyday phenomenon is *pathological jealousy.* Patients who feel they have great powers, religious significance, or special identity demonstrate *delusions of grandeur.* Patients heavily burdened with feelings of unworthiness develop delusions of *self-accusation,* ideas of guilt, sin, poverty, and the like. *Delusions of disease* arise from extreme hypo-chondriasis.

DISORDERS OF AFFECT

Disorders of *affect* constitute a large segment of mental illness with changes in emotion or *feeling tone*. (The term *mood* is used for sustained affect). *Depression* is a state of melancholy in which the patient views the world around him with sadness and pessimism. Depression as a symptom occurs in all degrees and with many types of psychiatric illness. *Anaclitic depression* refers to depression in infants who have been deprived of a suitable mother figure. The exact opposite of depression are states of *pleasurable affect, elation, euphoria, hypomania,* and *mania. Exaltation* merges into *ecstasy* as the peak of rapture and is seen in acute schizophrenia with states of religious mysticism. *Ambivalence* refers to the simultaneous coexistence of antithetical emotions, ideas, or wishes toward, and at the same time away from, a given object or situation. Particularly in schizophrenia, affect may appear to be *flat* (absence of feeling tone) or it may be *inappropriate* to the situation (e.g., giggles without reason). *Depersonalization* occurs when the patient has a feeling that things around him seem "unreal" or that the world has undergone a profound change. *Anxiety* is a feeling of apprehension and uneasiness. If it cannot be attributed to any particular idea or object it is labeled *"free-floating anxiety." Tension* is prolonged anxiety. *Panic* is severe overwhelming anxiety which can lead to terror and utter disorganization.

DISORDERS OF THE MOTOR ASPECT OF BEHAVIOR

Behavior disorders may show themselves as disturbances of *conation* or *volition* and *will, attitudes,* and *disposition* toward carrying out some behavior; as *ambivalence* in making decisions; and in aggressive displays of hostility from frustration and "pent-up" emotions. *Motor behavior* may be increased *(drivenness)* or decreased *(psychomotor retardation, painful effort).* Repetitious activities include *stereotypy* (persistent repetition) and *automatic obedience (echopraxia*—imitation of the movement of others—or *echolalia*—repetition of the phrases of others). *Cerea flexibilitas* describes a high degree of susceptibility in which the subject's limbs may be molded like wax into any position. *Grimaces, tics, peculiarities of gait,* and *other types of mannerisms* occur. *Compulsions* are morbid and often irresistible urges to perform certain acts. *Negativism* refers to a refusal to do what is asked or even a performance of the exact opposite. The term *aversion* refers not simply to passive unwillingness but rather to self-assertive negative reaction characterized by sullen uncooperativeness.

In addition to all the above there may be seen disturbances in appearance, decoration, dress, demeanor, and, indeed, the total life pattern, including the patient's relationship to family, work, and society and his attitudes toward many aspects of the community in which he lives. From these symptoms are derived patterns of behavior, the syndromes of specific diagnosable mental illnesses.

SUGGESTED READINGS

Barbizet, J.: Human memory and its pathology, San Francisco, 1970, W. H. Freeman & Co.

Chapman, A. H.: Textbook of clinical psychiatry, Philadelphia, 1967, J. B. Lippincott Co.

Eaton, M. T.: Psychiatry, Flushing, N. Y., 1969, Medical Examination Publishing Co.

Fish, F. J.: An outline of psychiatry for students and practitioners, ed. 2, Baltimore, 1968, The Williams & Wilkins Co.

2

CLINICAL SYNDROMES

10
Problem of classification

The classification of mental disorders is based upon a description of behavioral symptoms and varies over the years with changes in psychological theory. In the following pages we have sought, where practical, to indicate not only the latest official psychiatric nomenclature but also some of the names popularly used as roughly equivalent terms.

A. P. A. Standard nomenclature	*Common equivalents*
Mental retardation	{ Exceptional children Feebleminded
Organic brain syndromes a. Psychoses associated with organic brain syndromes (disorders caused by or associated with disturbance of brain tissue function)	Organic psychoses
b. Nonpsychotic organic brain syndromes	{ Organic behavioral disorders
Psychoses not attributed to (known) physical conditions	Functional psychoses
Neuroses	Psychoneuroses
Behavioral disorders of children and adolescents	{ Emotional disorders of children
Psychophysiological disorders	{ Psychosomatic disorders Organ neuroses
Personality disorders and certain other nonpsychotic disorders Transient situational disorders	{ Personality and character disorders, traits and maladjustments

The terms "psychosis" and "neurosis" have been used to dichotomize serious and "major" from less serious or "minor" psychiatric disorders respectively. Such dichotomy is misleading, as many chronic neurotic disorders are more crippling than some transient psychotic states. The concept of psychosis, traditionally similar to the legal term "insanity," usually implies an emotional (mental) illness whose seriousness is measured by behavior so unacceptable as to necessitate the withdrawal of social privileges. The concept, however, applies not only to the popularly conceived, chronic hallucinatory, delusional, and withdrawn states but also to fleeting states of mental incompetence such as the deliria which accompany various infectious, metabolic, and toxic ills.

A group of behavioral disturbances which interfere to no catastrophic extent with social functions are called *psychoneuroses*. In these disorders the symptoms may include anxiety, depression, obsessions, or fears, as well as a host of autonomic disturbances. Where the symptomatology is primarily visceral in nature, the terms "organ neurosis" and "psychophysiological disorder" have been applied.

The category *psychopath* was once used as the wastebasket of psychiatry. Cases of dubious diagnosis not clearly psychotic or psychoneurotic were often classified under this heading. More frequently, now, the term "psychopath" is used to refer only to asocial or antisocial behavior disorders classed under the term "sociopathic" personality disorder. The concept *personality disorder* is now used for a category within which the classic psychopath is but one type.

Each patient's mental disorder is a highly individual affair. Often exact categorization of an individual case is so fraught with difficulty as to appear impossible. If followed over a period of time, the patient may seem to pass from one diagnostic category into another. With some reservations, however, categorization of mental disorder proves useful in estimating the type of risk and problems likely to be encountered in planning therapy and in judging prognosis.

It should be borne in mind that a single dramatic symptom taken by itself can lead to erroneous diagnosis. Depression and anxiety can occur to some extent in many mental disorders, and the occurrence of paranoid symptomatology does not always mean schizophrenia, as paranoid delusions may occur also in general paresis, involutional or senile psychosis, acute alcoholic hallucinosis, and other conditions.

In understanding the production of behavioral abnormalities, the roles of genetic predisposition, organ dysfunctions, and the exogenous and endogenous toxins must be emphasized, as well as social tensions, defects in family social structure or environmental attitudes, and traumatic childhood experiences. The complex interplay of these factors must be grasped by the psychiatrist who, therefore, finds it impossible to settle upon a single etiological factor to explain any behavior disorder.

The following chapter on diagnostic terms is reproduced for your convenience from the *Diagnostic and Statistical Manual* prepared by the American Psychiatric Association. For full definition of each term, reference should be made to that *Manual*. In the chapters which follow, we have not devoted space to all of the syndromes but have tried to include those conditions which are commonly encountered in general psychiatric practice or which represent unusual diagnostic problems.

SUGGESTED READINGS

Cooper, J. E., Kendell, R. E., Gurland, B. J., Sartorius, N., and Farkas, T.: Cross-national study of diagnosis of mental disorders: some results in the first comparative investigation, Amer. J. Psychiat. **125**:21, 1969.

Diagnostic and statistical manual of mental disorders, ed. 2, Washington, D. C., 1968, American Psychiatric Association.

Ewalt, J. R., and Farnsworth, D. L.: Textbook of psychiatry, New York, 1963, McGraw-Hill Book Co.

Fenichel, O.: The psychoanalytic theory of neurosis, New York, 1945, W. W. Norton & Co., Inc.

Henderson, D. K., and Batchelor, I.: Textbook of psychiatry for students and practitioners, ed. 10, London, 1969, Oxford University Press.

Katz, M. M., Cole, J. O., and Lowery, H. A.: Studies of the diagnostic process: the influence of symptom perception, past experience, and ethnic background on diagnostic decisions, Amer. J. Psychiat. **125**:937, 1969.

Lusted, L. B.: The introduction to medical decision making, Springfield, Ill., 1968, Charles C Thomas Publisher.

Mayer-Gross, W., Slater, E., and Roth, M.: Clinical psychiatry, ed. 3, Baltimore, 1969, The Williams & Wilkins Co.

Menninger, K.: A guide to psychiatric books with a suggested basic reading list, ed. 2, New York, 1956, Grune & Stratton, Inc.

Menninger, K., Mayman, M., and Pruyser, P.: The vital balance, New York, 1963, The Viking Press, Inc.

Muncie, W.: Psychobiology and psychiatry, ed. 2, St. Louis, 1948, The C. V. Mosby Co.

Noyes, A. P., and Kolb, L. C.: Modern clinical psychiatry, ed. 7, Philadelphia, 1968, W. B. Saunders Co.

11
Standard nomenclature of mental disorders*

In this chapter is presented the standard nomenclature of mental disorders, as prepared by the Committee on Nomenclature and Statistics of the American Psychiatric Association.

I. ORGANIC BRAIN SYNDROMES (O.B.S.)
A. Psychoses
Senile and presenile dementia

290.0   Senile dementia
290.1   Presenile dementia

Alcoholic psychosis

291.0   Delirium tremens
291.1   Korsakov's psychosis
291.2   Other alcoholic hallucinosis
291.3   Alcoholic paranoid state
291.4   Acute alcoholic intoxication
291.5   Alcoholic deterioration
291.6   Pathological intoxication
291.9   Other alcoholic psychosis

Psychosis associated with intracranial infection

292.0   General paralysis
292.1   Syphilis of central nervous system
292.2   Epidemic encephalitis
292.3   Other and unspecified encephalitis
292.9   Other intracranial infection

Psychosis associated with other cerebral condition

293.0   Cerebral arteriosclerosis
293.1   Other cerebrovascular disturbance

---

*Adapted from Diagnostic and statistical manual of mental disorders, ed. 2, Washington, D. C., 1968, American Psychiatric Association.

Psychosis associated with other cerebral condition—cont'd

293.2	Epilepsy
293.3	Intracranial neoplasm
293.4	Degenerative disease of the C.N.S.
293.5	Brain trauma
293.9	Other cerebral condition

Psychosis associated with other physical condition

294.0	Endocrine disorder
294.1	Metabolic and nutritional disorder
294.2	Systemic infection
294.3	Drug or poison intoxication (other than alcohol)
294.4	Childbirth
294.8	Other and unspecified physical condition

B. Nonpsychotic O.B.S.

309.0	Intracranial infection
309.13	Alcohol (simple drunkenness)
309.14	Other drug, poison, or systemic intoxication
309.2	Brain trauma
309.3	Circulatory disturbance
309.4	Epilepsy
309.5	Disturbance of metabolism, growth, or nutrition
309.6	Senile or presenile brain disease
309.7	Intracranial neoplasm
309.8	Degenerative diseases of the C.N.S.
309.9	Other physical condition

II. PSYCHOSES NOT ATTRIBUTED TO PHYSICAL CONDITIONS LISTED PREVIOUSLY

Major affective disorders

296.0	Involutional melancholia
296.1	Manic-depressive illness, manic
296.2	Manic-depressive illness, depressed
296.3	Manic-depressive illness, circular
296.33	Manic-depressive, circular, manic
296.34	Manic-depressive, circular, depressed
296.8	Other major affective disorder

Schizophrenia

295.0	Simple
295.1	Hebephrenic
295.2	Catatonic
295.23	Catatonic type, excited
295.24	Catatonic type, withdrawn
295.3	Paranoid
295.4	Acute schizophrenic episode
295.5	Latent
295.6	Residual

Schizophrenia—cont'd

295.7	Schizoaffective
295.73	Schizoaffective, excited
295.74	Schizoaffective, depressed
295.8	Childhood
295.90	Chronic undifferentiated
295.99	Other schizophrenia

Paranoid states

297.0	Paranoia
297.1	Involutional paranoid state
297.9	Other paranoid state

Other psychoses

298.0	Psychotic depressive reaction

III. NEUROSES

300.0	Anxiety
300.1	Hysterical
300.13	Hysterical, conversion type
300.14	Hysterical, dissociative type
300.2	Phobic
300.3	Obsessive compulsive
300.4	Depressive
300.5	Neurasthenic
300.6	Depersonalization
300.7	Hypochondriacal
300.8	Other neurosis

IV. PERSONALITY DISORDERS AND CERTAIN OTHER NON-PSYCHOTIC MENTAL DISORDERS
Personality disorders

301.0	Paranoid
301.1	Cyclothymic
301.2	Schizoid
301.3	Explosive
301.4	Obsessive compulsive
301.5	Hysterical
301.6	Asthenic
301.7	Antisocial
301.81	Passive-aggressive
301.82	Inadequate
301.89	Other specified types

Sexual deviation

302.0	Homosexuality
302.1	Fetishism
302.2	Pedophilia
302.3	Transvestitism
302.4	Exhibitionism

Sexual deviation—cont'd

302.5	Voyeurism
302.6	Sadism
302.7	Masochism
302.8	Other sexual deviation

Alcoholism

303.0	Episodic excessive drinking
303.1	Habitual excessive drinking
303.2	Alcohol addiction
303.9	Other alcoholism

Drug dependence

304.0	Opium, opium alkaloids, and their derivatives
304.1	Synthetic analgesics with morphinelike effects
304.2	Barbiturates
304.3	Other hypnotics and sedatives or tranquilizers
304.4	Cocaine
304.5	Cannabis sativa (hashish, marihuana)
304.6	Other psychostimulants
304.7	Hallucinogens
304.8	Other drug dependence

V. PSYCHOPHYSIOLOGICAL DISORDERS

305.0	Skin
305.1	Musculoskeletal
305.2	Respiratory
305.3	Cardiovascular
305.4	Hemic and lymphatic
305.5	Gastrointestinal
305.6	Genitourinary
305.7	Endocrine
305.8	Organ of special sense
305.9	Other type

VI. SPECIAL SYMPTOMS

306.0	Speech disturbance
306.1	Specific learning disturbance
306.2	Tic
306.3	Other psychomotor disorder
306.4	Disorders of sleep
306.5	Feeding disturbance
306.6	Enuresis
306.7	Encopresis
306.8	Cephalalgia
306.9	Other special symptom

VII. TRANSIENT SITUATIONAL DISTURBANCES

307.0   Adjustment reaction of infancy
307.1   Adjustment reaction of childhood
307.2   Adjustment reaction of adolescence
307.3   Adjustment reaction of adult life
307.4   Adjustment reaction of late life

VIII. BEHAVIOR DISORDERS OF CHILDHOOD AND ADOLESCENCE

308.0   Hyperkinetic reaction
308.1   Withdrawing reaction
308.2   Overanxious reaction
308.3   Runaway reaction
308.4   Unsocialized aggressive reaction
308.5   Group delinquent reaction
308.9   Other reaction

IX. MENTAL RETARDATION

310   Borderline
311   Mild
312   Moderate
313   Severe
314   Profound
315   Unspecified
        With each: following or associated with
        .0   Infection or intoxication
        .1   Trauma or physical agent
        .2   Disorders of metabolism, growth or nutrition
        .3   Gross brain disease (postnatal)
        .4   Unknown prenatal influence
        .5   Chromosomal abnormality
        .6   Prematurity
        .7   Major psychiatric disorder
        .8   Psychosocial (environmental) deprivation
        .9   Other condition

X. CONDITIONS WITHOUT MANIFEST PSYCHIATRIC DISORDER AND NONSPECIFIC CONDITIONS
Social maladjustment without manifest psychiatric disorder

316.0   Marital maladjustment
316.1   Social maladjustment
316.2   Occupational maladjustment
316.3   Dyssocial behavior
316.9   Other social maladjustment

Nonspecific conditions

317   Nonspecific conditions

No mental disorder
318   No mental disorder

XI. NONDIAGNOSTIC TERMS FOR ADMINISTRATIVE USE
319.0   Diagnosis deferred
319.1   Boarder
319.2   Experiment only
319.3   Other

Fifth digit qualifying phrases

Section I   .x1   Acute
                 .x2   Chronic

Section II   .x6   Not psychotic now

Sections
III-VIII   .x6   Mild
                 .x7   Moderate
                 .x8   Severe

All disorders
                 .x5   In remission

12
Organic brain syndromes (O.B.S.)

This classification of mental disorders includes a broad group of illnesses of both known and unknown etiology. Some, as *general paralysis,* are the direct result of a known brain infection; others result from organic brain changes due to head trauma, growth of neoplasms, toxic agents, or (like *presenile dementia*) from some other as yet poorly defined or unknown cerebral condition. Under this heading too are disorders of the brain that result from general physical conditions such as systemic infection, metabolic change, or endocrine disorder. The number of such conditions is very large but examples of the more important will be given.

In this section we will discuss both acute and chronic brain disorders. We would here stress the similarities among the toxic and organic psychoses and point out that, although some rather characteristic differences can occur with a specific agent or anatomical predilection of lesion, yet perhaps more striking are the similarities which produce a basic syndrome consisting of (1) impairment of orientation; (2) impairment of intellectual functions, including comprehension, calculation, knowledge, learning, judgment, and recent memory (remote memory being at times preserved); and (3) lability and shallowness of affect.

Differences in the clinical picture may occur. Presumably differences in personality structure account for the appearance of such types as paranoid, depressed, manic, etc., listed under individually described psychoses due to widely different agents.

The term "acute brain disorder" has been used for organic

brain syndromes from which the patient recovers. They are the result of temporary, reversible, diffuse impairement of brain tissue function such as is present in acute alcoholic intoxication or acute delirium. The basic disturbance of the sensorium may release other disturbances, such as hallucinations, poorly organized transient delusions, and behavior disturbances of varying degree.

These disorders are subclassified according to the cause of the impairment of brain tissue function. Some of the more commonly seen acute brain disorders are discussed in this section. They may be associated with such conditions as intracranial infections, systemic infections, trauma, circulatory disturbances, metabolic disorders, etc. These typically reversible, toxic psychoses may also, on occasion, when the brain damage is severe, progress to an irreversible organic syndrome.

Organic brain disorders are considered *chronic* when they result from relatively permanent and usually diffuse impairment of function of cerebral tissue. While the underlying pathological process may subside or respond to specific treatment, as in syphilis, there remains always a certain irreducible minimum of brain tissue destruction which cannot be reversed, even though the loss of function may be almost imperceptible clinically. As time passes, the chronic brain syndrome may become milder, vary in degree, or progress; but some disturbance of memory, judgment, orientation, comprehension, and affect persists permanently.

These disorders are classified according to the cause of the impairment of brain function. Some of the diagnostic categories are identical with those of the acute brain syndromes; the differentiation is based on the permanent impairment of brain function in the chronic group.

Finally, there is a group of conditions with organic brain change and behavior disorder but in which the behavioral symptoms are not of a degree to warrant the term "psychosis." For such, the term "nonpsychotic organic brain syndrome" is used. Such a diagnosis may often be appropriately applied in the case of children where mild brain damage may result in hyperactivity, short attention span, easy distractibility, and impulsiveness. Other children with this diagnosis may be withdrawn, listless, apathetic, or unresponsive.

GENERAL MANAGEMENT OF
ORGANIC BRAIN DISTURBANCES

The management of organic brain disturbances is a problem often faced by both the psychiatrist and the general practitioner. The term "delirium" is commonly used for acute brain disorders which, although classed as psychoses, are more or less temporary conditions characterized by disorientation and accompanied by illusions and hallucinations and a predominant affect of fear. Disturbances in brain metabolism may be of infectious, toxic, vascular, nutritional, or traumatic origin and are usually reversible, so that complete recovery may occur.

The symptoms of delirium seem to *depend* on underlying personality and life experiences of the subject. For example, paranoid misinterpretations are not uncommon in persons known to have been of suspicious nature.

The *chief complaint* is usually indicated in a referral by private physician or by family, stating that the patient is becoming restless and uneasy and shows increasing tendency to emotional instability and sensitivity to light and sound. *History* may reveal evidence of some underlying infectious, metabolic, or nutritional illness, a head injury, or chronic drug ingestion. One suspects delirium in a patient over 40 years of age, when hospitalized for cardiac decompensation, kidney or liver disease, hypertension, or metabolic disorder, or following surgical procedures, particularly those involving the eyes or ears. The administration of barbiturate sedation may be the final insult in those patients whose sluggish circulation is laden with other medication.

From the *behavioral* standpoint there is outstanding disturbance in intellectual functions, with disorientation as to time, place, and person, poor recent and remote memory, defects in fund of general information, and defects in ability to calculate and in judgment. Illusions and hallucinations (predominantly visual, sometimes tactual) may be present. Unsystematized paranoid ideas are not infrequent. The mood is usually fearful although elation and depression can occur. A patient may jump out of the window to his death in a sudden attempt to escape envisioned attackers. Speech may be indistinct. The patient may be restless and irritable, with insomnia and a tendency to emotional instability if seen early, but later he may be semicomatose or in coma. On *physical* examination tremors, incoordination, urinary incontinence, dehydration, malnutrition, signs of vitamin deficiency, and elevated temperature are found. *Laboratory* reports indicate leukocytosis, albuminuria, glycosuria. The EEG often shows slowing of basic rhythms.

Prognosis. Prognosis is good with active treatment, but the ultimate course depends upon the underlying disease and the extent of arteriosclerotic and senile change.

Treatment. Precautions against suicide are essential.

Stop sedatives and all other nonvital drugs.

Promote rest and sleep. Do not disturb when asleep. Hydrotherapy, 95° to 96° F., may be useful.

Avoid wet packs if circulatory difficulties exist; use no mechanical restraints.

Give parenteral fluids if patient is dehydrated—and as long as urine output can increase (1000 ml. 10% glucose in H_2O, I. V.).

Get patient up as soon as medical condition permits. Provide constant companionship and a light in the room while the patient is awake.

Do not joke about hallucinations. Urge the patient to accept them as bad dreams (note content, as it may give clues for later psychotherapy).

Sedate with paraldehyde orally or by nasal or rectal tube. A good mixture consists of 40 ml. paraldehyde per 10 ml. compound spirits of orange. Give one tablespoon in iced tea and then repeat, one teaspoon per hour, until asleep.

This condition fluctuates. The patient may be clear in the morning but confused as the evening shadows fall. The harm that comes to the patient from yelling is little when compared to the possible toxic effects of medication that not only may fail to make him quiet but actually may also make him worse.

SUGGESTED READINGS

Cohen, M. E.: The management of disturbed cardiac patients, Mod. Conc. Cardiovasc. Dis. 22:182, 186, 1953.

Cohen, S.: The toxic psychoses and allied states, Amer. J. Med. 15:813, 1953.

Fantus, B., and Kraines, S. H.: The therapy of acute delirium, J.A.M.A. 115:929, 1940.

Levin, M.: Delirium: gap in psychiatric teaching, Amer. J. Psychiat. **107**:689, 1951.

Lipowski, Z. J.: Delirium, clouding of consciousness and confusion, J. Nerv. Ment. Dis. **145**:227, 1967.

Wolff, H. G., and Curran, D.: Nature of delirium and allied states, Arch Neurol. Psychiat. **33**:1175, 1935.

PSYCHOSES ASSOCIATED WITH ORGANIC BRAIN SYNDROMES

Senile and presenile dementia

Senile dementia (and psychoses with cerebral arteriosclerosis)

Although the processes of both arteriosclerosis and senile degeneration not infrequently affect the same brain, it is usual for one to predominate over the other. The two disorders are to some degree clinically distinguishable, they represent separate pathological entities, and each may exist without the other. Relative to the size of the population from which mental disturbances are drawn, the senile and arteriosclerotic psychoses are by far the most frequent of all psychoses. Senile psychosis is twice as common in women and psychosis with cerebral arteriosclerosis three times as common in men.

Anamnesis. The *chief complaint* is given by the family, who may state that the patient's behavior (confusion, delusions, weakness, incontinence, etc.) is no longer manageable. The *history* in both disorders reveals gradual onset over previous months or years—of forgetfulness, failure of efficiency, exaggeration of previous personality weaknesses, deterioration of judgment and personal habits, loss of emotional control, and physical weakness. Social changes may precipitate a worsening of symptoms. A history of headache, dizziness, explosive emotional outbursts, syncopal attacks, or cardiac disturbance strongly suggests arteriosclerotic psychosis, whereas predominance of personality disturbance favors a diagnosis of senile psychosis.

Examination. Examination reveals one of a great variety of clinical pictures appearing in the sixth to ninth decade which have in common progressive signs of organic mental deficit, an exaggeration of the aging process. In the *behavioral* patterns we find untidiness of dress, easy emotionality with fluctuations, restlessness and confusion at night, and defects in recent memory appearing early. During initial stages the failure of memory for recent events causes excessive reminiscence of past life, which may lead the family to think the patient has a keen mind. Fabrication, disorientation, and rambling incoherent speech develop later. Patients show poor judgment and tend to hoard objects of little worth. Prolonged depression, periods of confusion which remit, dizziness, aphasias, apraxias, fainting spells, and convulsive seizures are useful diagnostic signs, since they are rare in senile cases but not uncommon with cerebral arteriosclerosis. The picture of gradual, progressive deterioration of intellectual functions (rather than a sudden exacerbation of symptoms) usually indicates a senile psychosis. The illness may release traits that caricature the prepsychotic personality. Neurotic trends with hypochondriasis are common. Results from *physical* tests indicating hypertension and peripheral arteriosclerosis do *not* favor either diagnosis. In the end there results a completely bedridden organism, responding with primitive reflexes and suffering malnutrition, generalized weakness, incontinence, fractures, and decubitus ulcers. Early loss of abstract thinking and inability to organize and retain new observations are revealed by *psychological* tests.

Pathological examination frequently reveals no correlation between the degree of brain damage and symptomatology. Senile psychosis presents a diffuse atrophy of cortical convolutions and individual nerve cells with preservation of cortical architecture. Senile plaques which stain with silver are found in great number throughout the cortex. The Alzheimer type of neurofibril change is sometimes seen. Cerebral arteriosclerosis presents a great variety of focal lesions accompanied by atherosclerosis (large vessels are rarely spared), arteriolosclerosis, and capillary fibrosis. Anemic or hemorrhagic areas of softening occurring in any part of the brain are usual. There is no correlation between arteriosclerosis of the brain and of other body areas.

Prognosis. In senile cases the total course of illness may be from 1 to 10 years; death occurs from infection (pneumonia, bacteremia from decubitus ulcers, etc.). In arteriosclerotic cases the course is extremely variable and depends on the state of vessels in vital organs.

Treatment. In very early stages the family should prepare for the resulting failing judgment with tactful suggestions of retirement. Limit work routine within the tolerance of the patient.

Provision of a protected physical and social environment with proper diet, simple activities, and quiet companionship pays dividends. Regularity and hobbies should be encouraged.

Recently the role of a high-nitrogen diet (including powdered milk and egg) has been advocated to overcome the negative nitrogen balance that occurs in the aged. Hydergine (dehydrated ergot preparation) sublingual tablets have been given 6 to 8 per day with reported good results. Metrazol alone, 0.1 Gm. orally, 1 to 2 tablets t.i.d., and in combination with nicotinamide, 400 mg. daily, has been reported to aid in relieving the confusion seen in these patients.

Paraldehyde or barbiturates, sparingly employed, relieve restlessness and insomnia. Avoid daytime catnaps.

Immobilization in bed—even in case of fractures—is to be avoided, as it hastens confusion and physical deterioration.

Occupational therapy and group psychotherapy have been found useful even in fairly advanced states of deterioration. Often the earliest action to be taken is the removal of major occupational, financial, and family responsibilities. Frequently the failure of judgment requires the appointment of a guardian.

Beware of risking injuries through falling.

Avoid sexual stimulation which may lead to difficulties with children of opposite sex. These patients recognize a child's sex but ignore age.

The alert physician who detects the onset of senility may save the family shame and disgrace by advising for trust funds and competent legal guardianship before the onset of poor business and social judgment. Remember these conditions are characterized by fluctuation both in intellectual function and in mood. The diagnosis is best made in the evening hours, when the patient is fatigued and shadows fall.

SUGGESTED READINGS

Busse, E. W.: Findings from the Duke geriatrics research project on the effects of aging upon the nervous system. In Blumenthal, H. T., editor: Medical and clinical aspects of aging, New York, 1962, Columbia University Press.

Corsellis, J. A. N.: Mental illness and the ageing brain, Maudsley monograph no. 9, London, 1962, Oxford University Press.

Cowdry, E. V.: Care of the geriatric patient, ed. 4, St. Louis, 1971, The C. V. Mosby Co.

Gregory, I.: Nicotinic acid therapy in psychoses of senility, Amer. J. Psychiat. **108**:888, 1952.

Hoch, P. H., and Zubin, J., editors: Psychopathology of aging, New York, 1961, Grune & Stratton, Inc.

Hofstatter, L., et al.: Pharmaceutical treatment of patients with senile brain changes, Arch. Neurol. Psychiat. **75**:316, 1956.

Palmore, E.: Normal aging, Durham, N. C., 1970, Duke University Press.

Post, F.: The clinical psychiatry of late life, New York, 1965, Pergamon Press, Inc.

Presenile dementia

Abnormalities of behavior which occur in middle life as a result of permanent loss of brain substance include two generally recognized clinical entities: *Alzheimer's disease* and *Pick's disease*. Although there apparently are clinical differences, the differential diagnosis between the two can be made definitely only at autopsy, where the distinguishing characteristics are seen on microscopic examination of the brain. Some authorities believe these disturbances originate from a metabolic disorder. On the basis of pathological data, a close relationship between Alzheimer's disease and senile psychosis has been postulated.

Anamnesis. The *chief complaint* made by those around the patient is that he has been showing a poorly defined personality change over the previous 1 to 10 years. Forgetfulness, carelessness in dress or work habits, apathy, antisocial or unethical acts (usually of minor importance, such as increased use of profanity, pilfering, etc.), and a tendency to repeat ideas or statements have appeared gradually. Occasionally the initial *history* may, instead, present the picture of a sudden onset of confusion or apathy following severe emotional or physical trauma. But careful inquiry in these cases will reveal preceding changes of the type noted above. In a small percentage of cases *family history* reveals other cases of organic brain damage appearing before senescence. Onset occurs in the third to the sixth decade of life and both syndromes occur more frequently in females than in males.

During the first years of the illness, only careful history and observation will prevent mistaken diagnosis of psychogenic disturbance.

Examination. In the early stages, the patient's *behavioral* pattern tends to show affability, periods of mild euphoria and depression, defects in recent memory, with perseverative ideas and behavior. Frequently a complete denial of these symptoms may necessitate relying on careful observation for diagnosis. In later stages, confusion, inertia, protracted states of panic, or psychotic symptoms develop. Making a differential diagnosis on the basis of clinical observations is fraught with difficulty. There is a tendency in Alzheimer's disease to show a greater loss of memory and a greater confusion at the onset of the illness. After the syndrome is well developed, the presence of confabulation, motor restlessness, tremors, and epilepsy also favors the diagnosis of Alzheimer's disease. In the early stages, patients with Pick's disease may show only slight defects in recent memory with the predominating defects being loss of initiative, difficulty in attention, and stereotypy of behavior. In advanced stages, patients with Pick's disease tend toward marked inertia. Confabulation is rare, and even in advanced cases memory is likely to be less affected. No abnormalities appear on *physical* examination in early cases. Weight loss, aphasia, gait disturbances, changes in muscle tonus, and other focal neurological signs occur in advanced cases. Pneumoencephalograms as *diagnostic* tests are valuable principally to demonstrate cortical atrophy, not to differentiate the type. Localized atrophy over frontal or temporal lobes suggests Pick's rather than Alzheimer's disease. In Alzheimer's disease *pathological* findings are as follows: There is a generalized marked atrophy of the cortex with approximately one third of the cells showing fibrillary degeneration (of Alzheimer). Microscopically these cells and the characteristic miliary plaques accompanied by hyaline degeneration of small blood vessels present the diagnostic features of Alzheimer's disease. In Pick's disease the gross pathology shows visible atrophic areas circumscribed to a single convolution or a lobe, with the lesion often occurring symmetrically. Microscopically, all that is seen is cell degeneration, which may be localized over the frontal and temporal lobes and usually involves the first three layers of cortical ganglia.

Prognosis. Two to twenty years' total duration of illness.

Treatment. No specific treatment. Eventual hospitalization is inevitable. At that time helping the family to accept the situation aids in the patient's hospital adjustment.

SUGGESTED READINGS

Alpers, B. J., editor: The pre-senile dementias—symposium, Trans. Amer. Neurol. Ass. **89:**9, 1964.

Newton, R. D.: Identity of Alzheimer's disease and senile dementia and their relationship to senility, J. Ment. Sci. **94:**225, 1948.

Williams, G. R.: Genetics of the pre-senile dementias, Trans. Amer. Neurol. Ass. **89:**9, 1964.

Zawuski, G.: Die Erblichkeit der Alzheimerschen Krankheit, Arch. Psychiat. Nervenkr. **201:**123, 1960.

Ziegler, D.: Cerebral atrophy in psychiatric patients, Amer. J. Psychiat. **111:**454, 1954.

Alcoholic psychoses

The personality difficulties that lead to alcoholic addiction may include various types of emotional and behavioral disorders. Of these conditions, immoderate drinking is but a symptom. The present section will be concerned, however, not with addiction to alcohol but rather with the psychotic disturbances that result from states of alcoholic intoxication which have been prolonged or repeated and often associated with dietary deficiencies.

Delirium tremens. This is a type of delirium occurring in about 5% of chronic alcoholics, characteristically with sudden onset at night associated with a period of heavy drinking. Symptoms occur characteristically with the withdrawal of alcohol. Hallucinations and illusions are predominantly visual, typically moving, colored, and with large numbers of the same objects or small animals. Patients are usually disoriented, although they may sense the unreality of their illusions. There is a hypersensitivity of sensory perception and a predominant mood of fear. They are restless and hyperactive and have insomnia. There is a coarse arrhythmic tremor of the tongue, face, fingers, legs, eyes, and even trunk. These may early be felt more readily than seen. Convulsions occur in 9% of cases. Nausea, vomiting, and dehydration may occur. There is fever in 90% of cases and albuminuria at the height of the delirium. This condition can, in itself, be fatal and is often complicated by head injuries, unrecognized fractures, pneumonia, and cardiac decompensation.

Korsakov's psychosis (alcoholic). This amnestic polyneuritic syndrome can be caused by other toxins but occurs in about 1 per 100 chronic alcoholics, in women more frequently than in men, and with mean age of onset at 51 years. The condition begins insidiously, and it may be difficult to detect the intellectual impairment. Anterograde amnesia is typical, but remote memory and learning ability may also be impaired. There may be disorientation for time and place with attempt to cover defects by confabulation. Aphasia, agraphia, and stereotyped speech occur; mood is indifferent or may be euphoric. Polyneuritis occurs, usually symmetrical, involving both upper and lower extremities and with sensory and motor deficit. Mortality is high.

Other alcoholic hallucinosis. Only one fifth as common as delirium tremens, this occurs after a shorter period of drinking, typically in younger persons with family or personal history of psychopathology. There is a prodromal period of anxiety, headache, insomnia, and increased sensitivity to sounds. Patients are well oriented. There are occasional cutaneous sensations but more typical are auditory hallucinations in which voices talk about the patient in the third person. Such hallucinations may be delusionally rationalized by the patient. Fear is the predominant mood and suicidal attempts are common. Prognosis is good for the individual attack, but symptoms may last several months or the condition may become chronic.

Alcoholic paranoid state. This term is used to describe the occurrence of paranoid ideas but without other changes due to chronic drinking.

Acute alcoholic intoxication. Uncomplicated intoxication with or without delirium, mood change, or tremor is often seen as one of many acute episodes in the course of chronic alcoholism.

Alcoholic deterioration. The continued excessive use of alcohol over a period of time may result in deterioration, with brutality, ethical dulling, labile affect, impaired memory, diminished will power, dilated facial vessels, tremor, and "rum fits." *Alcoholic encephalopathy,* or *Wernicke's syndrome,* shows clouding of consciousness, opthalmoplegia, and ataxia. Pathologically lesions are in the periventricular nuclei. Beginning with delirium, the condition may end fatally or with a residual Korsakov's syndrome.

Pathological intoxication. This is seen in 1% of alcoholic hospital admissions as a reaction of blind rage and confusion or paranoid feelings with acts of violence or occasionally an ecstatic state of a few minutes' to a few hours' duration with later amnesia for the attack. Symptoms of intoxication may be transitory or absent and the condition is independent of the amount taken. It occurs most frequently in persons with psychopathic character traits.

Other alcoholic psychosis. Marchiafava's disease is a rare, progressive mental decadence which may end in confusion, dementia, and epileptiform seizures. It occurs in middle or later years, typically in persons of Italian extraction and following the consumption of large quantities of red wine. There is degeneration of the corpus callosum.

SUGGESTED READING

McNichol, R. W.: The treatment of delirium tremens and related states, Springfield, Ill., 1970, Charles C Thomas, Publisher.

Psychosis associated with intracranial infection
General paresis

General paresis is a chronic spirochetal meningoencephalitis which severely disturbs the function of the cerebral cortex, thereby producing clinical neurological signs, including marked changes in personality and mental abilities, often a psychosis characterized by depression, expansiveness, or agitation, and terminally a dissolution of mental and physical capacities.

Types. The following distribution has been observed: (1) simple deteriorating (40%), (2) depressed (25%), (3) expansive (15% to 20%), (4) manic (10% to 15%), and (5) paranoid (less than 10%).

Anamnesis. Occasionally the onset may be sudden with a person apparently in the best of health developing a classic paretic syndrome or with sudden onset of a cerebral accident, aphasia, hemiplegia, convulsion, or psychotic episode which may be of but a few hours' or days' duration and precede the classic psychiatric mental picture by months or years. More often the onset is insidious, with the development of forgetfulness, discourtesy, carelessness of personal appearance, unsound judgment, periods of depression, undue optimism, and overactivity. The consequences of these symptoms for the individual have led this period of onset to be termed the "medicolegal period."

In fully developed paresis the psychotic symptoms occur, and although the syndromes produced are multiform in variety, the types listed above have been classically delimited on the basis of the most conspicuous symptoms. The age of onset is usually between 30 and 50 years, and a period of 5 to 15 years often elapses between the initial syphilitic infection and the development of paresis.

Examination. The essence of paretic neurosyphilis, *behaviorally,* is mental deterioration with confusion, memory defect, impaired judgment, and lability of mood occurring in all forms; but these may be masked by more dramatic symptoms. The classic expansive paretic syndrome (less common than popularly believed) is characterized by delusions of grandeur in which the patient brags of great riches or power, with an accompanying euphoria. The patient is often hypersuggestible and can be persuaded to do almost anything that is asked of him. Depressed and manic forms may both show agitation and are often like similar states of other etiology. A paranoid type is occasionally seen, with systematized delusions and with good retention of most intellectual faculties.

On *physical* examination, neurological abnormalities are not essential for the diagnosis of early paretic neurosyphilis. Pupillary disorders are common. Advancing infirmity of the body is manifested by slouching carriage, hypotonia, and flattening and smoothing out of the facial lines (paretic facies). Tremors of the facial muscles, extended tongue, and outstretched fingers occur early. Highly typical of paresis is the speech disorder characterized by faulty enunciation, slurring of consonants with rapid speech, poor articulation with elision, and mispronunciation. Handwriting typically shows defects, with evidence of tremor, poor spacing and spelling, and transposition and omission of letters. The tendon reflexes may be normal, increased, decreased, or absent at any stage of the disease.

By *laboratory* tests, blood serology is usually positive. Cerebrospinal fluid is clear under normal or slightly increased pressure and shows pleocytosis (25 to 75 cells/c.mm.); globulin test is positive, and protein is increased 50 to 100 mg./100 ml.; the colloidal gold reaction is markedly abnormal with a first-zone curve (i.e., 5555443211); there is usually a strongly positive Wassermann reaction (over 95% of cases positive if two or more tests used). EEG's show high-voltage slow waves in cases with severe mental impairment, the EEG pattern usually improving with treatment. *Psychometric* examination may demonstrate an organic picture and decrease in I.Q. which usually fails to improve with treatment.

In macroscopic studies of *pathology* are seen thickened and opaque meninges, cerebral atrophy shown by widening of sulci and dilatation of ventricles, and granular ependymitis. Microscopically, there are meningeal and perivascular infiltrates (lymphocytes and plasma cells), loss of and degenerative changes in nerve cells, reaction of microglia (rod cells) and astrocytes, and presence of the organism *Treponema pallidum*.

Prognosis. Without treatment the disease is progressive. The grandiosity, mania, depression, agitation, and paranoid ideas recede into the background. The patient is less active and dementia becomes the outstanding characteristic. This period of decline may take a few weeks or 2 or 3 years, and the patient terminally becomes bedridden and paralyzed, with development of emaciation and decubital ulcers, with death from intercurrent infection, or with convulsive seizures. With adequate treatment complete recovery is possible, the best results occurring with early institution of therapy.

Differential diagnosis. The mental disturbance of meningovascular syphilis may be indistinguishable from that of the meningoencephalitic form. A differential diagnosis may be possible in those cases in which the history, signs, and symptoms, including serology, suggest a primary and predominating involvement of the meninges and blood vessels rather than of the parenchyma of the nervous system. Suggestive of this type of syphilis, rather than of general paresis, are comparatively early onset after infection, sudden onset of mental disturbance, focal signs, particularly cranial nerve palsy, apoplectiform seizures, very high spinal fluid cell count, positive blood and spinal fluid serology, and prompt response to general systemic and antisyphilitic treatment.

Treatment. Penicillin (10 million to 25 million units I.M.) is administered over a 14-day period. The minimum effective penicillin concentration is 0.03 unit/ml. serum for 2 weeks. When the patient is sensitive to penicillin, other antibiotics are used. Relapses may occur 4 to 9 months after a course of therapy, and all patients should have an examination of cerebrospinal fluid within at least 2 years.

Fever therapy was frequently used until recent years: (1) malaria, *plasmodium vivax*, 10 to 12 paroxysms (total of 150 hours above 100° F.) or (2) fever cabinet, 10 treatments (total of 5 hours at 106° F.).

SUGGESTED READINGS

Harrison, T. R., et. al.: Principles of internal medicine, ed. 5, New York, 1966, McGraw-Hill Book Co.

Merritt, H., Adams, R., and Solomon, H.: Neurosyphilis, New York, 1946, Oxford University Press, Inc.

Timberlake, W. H.: Neurosyphilis, Amer. J. Psychiat. 111:524, 1955.

Psychosis associated with other cerebral conditions
Cerebral arteriosclerosis

See under "Senile dementia (and psychoses with cerebral arteriosclerosis)," p. 98.

Epilepsy

Psychotic states that are neither seizures nor postictal phenomena may occur in epileptics. They are thought to result from chronic alteration of the brain as a result of severe and repeated seizures. Such conditions occur after several years of seizures and usually after a bout of several convulsions. Overactivity, speech abnormalities, wide variations in mood, visual and auditory hallucinations, delusions, and lack of insight characterize the condition.

Of considerable importance not only in connection with epilepsy but also regarding the pathogenesis of schizophrenia are the schizophrenic-like psychoses of epilepsy. These occur in persons with otherwise normal personalities, save for epileptic personality changes in cases where the seizure disorder was of long duration. The genetic background is of epilepsy rather than schizophrenia. The average age of onset is 30 years. The psychosis is usually of insidious onset after many years (average 14) of epilepsy. Onset in some cases can be acute and the symptoms may improve or become chronic; and although the seizure disorder may tend to improve, the psychiatric illness runs toward an end state of general impairment of an organic type. Paranoid features are common, and typical schizophrenic type delusional formation and hallucinary experiences with clear consciousness occur frequently. Flatness of affect, catatonic features, and schizophrenic thought disorders are regularly seen.

SUGGESTED READING

Slater, E., Beard, A. W., and Glithero, E.: The schizophrenia-like psychoses of epilepsy, I to V, Brit. J. Psychiat. **109**:95, 1963.

Intracranial neoplasm

Too frequently overlooked in admissions to chronic hospitals and unrecognized until autopsy are those cases whose mental symptoms may occur at any stage of growth of a cerebral neoplasm. Slight behavior alteration, irritability, forgetfulness, and lack of interest are primary symptoms. Disturbance of sensorium may occur with consequent delirium. Affect is labile, with euphoria and facetiousness (*Witzelsucht*), seen particularly in frontal lobe lesions. Depression and anxiety may occur. Intellectual functioning declines. Simple auditory hallucinations of whistles, bells, etc. or visual hallucinations of flashing or colored lights may be a clue to focal pathology. Uncinate gyrus tumors may give olfactory or déjà vu symptoms.

SUGGESTED READINGS

Bilckiewicz, A., and Gromska, J.: Diagnostic value of mental disorders in temporal lobe tumors, Neurol. Neurochir. Psychiat. Pol. **13**:397, 1963.

Guvener, A., Bagchi, B. K., Kooi, K. A., and Calhoun, H. D.: Mental and seizure manifestations in relation to brain tumors—a statistical study, Epilepsia (Amst.) **5**:166, 1964.

Remington, F. B., and Rubert, S. L.: Why patients with brain tumors come to a psychiatric hospital: a thirty year survey, Amer. J. Psychiat. **119**:256, 1962.

Selecki, B. R.: Intracranial space occupying lesions of all patients admitted to a mental hospital, Med. J. Aust. **1**:383, 1965.

Huntington's chorea

A heredofamilial degenerative disease of the nervous system, Huntington's chorea occurs in adult life (35 to 40 years) and is distinguished by persistent and progressive choreiform movements and mental deterioration. The earliest mental symptoms are of emotional lability with irritability and temper, sexual assault, or destructive violence. Psychotic episodes may occur, resembling manic-depressive psychoses or hebephrenic type of schizophrenia. Feelings of unworthiness and self-accusation may lead to suicidal attempts. Memory becomes poor and there is inattention. Suspicion, jealousy, and paranoid trends and later agnosias, apraxia, and disorientation are apparent. The pathological picture includes leptomeningitis, brain atrophy, and dilatation of ventricles.

SUGGESTED READINGS

Goldman, D.: New treatment for hereditary (Huntington) chorea, Amer. J. Med. Sci. **224:**573, 1952.

Stone, C. S.: Huntington's chorea, a sociological and genealogical study of a new family, Ment. Hyg. **15:**350, 1931.

Wilson's disease

Wilson's disease is a familial disease usually with onset in adolescence and fatal in 2 to 7 years, with cirrhosis of the liver and glial proliferation of the globus pallidus (hepatolenticular degeneration). Intention tremor, athetosis, dysarthria, dysphagia, contractures, muscle weakness, progressive dementia, and emaciation are observed. Beginning with facile laughter, the patients may become silly and noisy. Instability of mood, irritability, excitement, hallucinations, and even a picture resembling schizophrenia have been described.

This disease has recently been considered the result of an inborn error of mineral metabolism. The blood and liver of the patients show high copper content. It has been reported that treatment with dimercaprol (BAL) resulted in an increased elimination of copper with a decrease in symptoms and improvement in the EEG.

Jakob Creutzfeldt disease

Jakob Creutzfeldt disease (cortical-striatal-spinal degeneration) is a rapidly developing dementia associated with extrapyramidal disorders and sometimes with lower motor neuron disorders. Ataxia, dysarthrias, spasticity, choreoathetoid movements, tremor, cogwheel rigidity, and muscular wasting occur. Death occurs within 6 months to 2 years of the onset.

SUGGESTED READING

Wilson, S. A. K.: Neurology, ed. 2, Baltimore, 1955, The Williams & Wilkins Co.

Multiple sclerosis

Multiple sclerosis, like any brain disease with scattered degenerative foci, may produce a variety of psychiatric pictures. Paranoid, depressive, hypomanic, and schizophrenic-like states have been described and seem to be related both to the site of the lesion and to the previous personality patterns. In early cases a differentiation from hysteria is sometimes a problem, due to the apparent indifference of the patient to his disease. Thus eutonia sclerotica, or false sense of physical well-being, has been attributed (along with the frequent lability of mood) to the typical subependymal periventricular lesions in the region of the thalamus. Schilder points out, however, that such eutonia is but one manifestation of the attitude not infrequently found in many who are gravely ill.

SUGGESTED READINGS

Baldwin, M.: A clinico-experimental investigation into the psychologic aspects of multiple sclerosis, J. Nerv. Ment. Dis. **115:**299, 1952.

Braceland, F., and Giffin, M.: The mental changes associated with multiple sclerosis, Proc. Ass. Res. Nerv. Ment. Dis. **28:**450, 1950.

Harrower, M.: The results of psychometric and personality tests in multiple sclerosis, Proc. Ass. Res. Nerv. Ment. Dis. **28:**461, 1950.

Hartstein, J., and Ulett, G.: Galactose treatment of multiple sclerosis (a preliminary report), Dis. Nerv. Syst. **18:**1, 1957.

Langworthy, O., and LeGrand, D.: Personality structure and psychotherapy in multiple sclerosis, Amer. J. Med. **12:**586, 1952.

Pratt, R. T. C.: An investigation of the psychiatric aspects of disseminated sclerosis, J. Neurol. Neurosurg. Psychiat. **14:**326, 1951.

Ulett, G.: Geographic distribution of multiple sclerosis, Dis. Nerv. Syst. **9:**342, 1948.

Brain trauma

We are concerned here with the psychic sequelae of a head injury. In describing the acute injury itself the term "concussion" is properly used only when some amount of amnesia is present. States of impaired consciousness following head injury are described as confusion (mild, moderate, or severe), subcoma, or coma. Following head injuries of varying degrees of severity, there may occur deliria, amnesic states, the "posttraumatic constitution" of Meyer (i.e., easy reaction to alcohol, influenza, etc.), lasting vasomotor neurosis (with headaches, irascibility, and hysterical or even epileptic episodes), traumatic defect conditions such as the aphasias, and even marked progressive cerebral degeneration.

It has been pointed out that in most cases posttraumatic symptoms are substantially receding by 3 months following the injury. In one series approximately 15% of patients had symptoms persisting 1 year or longer. It is felt that patients with pretraumatic psychoneurotic personalities are more likely to develop posttraumatic psychiatric symptoms, but patients with normal pretraumatic personalities are not uncommon. A high correlation has been found between the existence of persistent complicating psychosocial factors—such as continuing compensation, pending litigation, occupational stresses, persistent associated bodily injuries, etc.—and the severity and persistence of psychiatric sequelae.

SUGGESTED READINGS

Brock, S., editor: Injuries of the brain and the spinal cord and their coverings, ed. 4, New York, 1960, Springer Publishing Co., Inc.

Garrett, J. F., and Levine, E. F.: Psychological practices with the physically disabled, New York, 1962, Columbia University Press.

Kamman, G.: Traumatic neurosis, compensation neurosis or attitudinal pathosis? Arch. Neurol. Psychiat. 65:593, 1951.

Rowbotham, G. F.: Acute injuries of the head, ed. 4, Edinburgh, 1964, E. & S. Livingstone, Ltd.

Psychosis associated with other physical conditions
Pernicious anemia

Minor mental symptoms are extremely common in patients with pernicious anemia. Psychotic reactions have been reported in up to 15% of patients from some clinics. Delirium, delusions, hallucinations, depression, agitation, and signs of organic deterioration may all occur. The role of associated vitamin deficiencies may be a factor. The psychiatric symptoms tend to disappear with treatment of the anemia.

SUGGESTED READINGS

Betts, W. C.: The use of electroshock therapy in psychosis associated with pernicious anemia, N. Carolina Med. J. **13**.321, 1952.

Lewin, K. K.: Role of depression in the production of the illness in pernicious anemia, Psychosom. Med. **23**:23, 1959.

Samson, D., Swisher, S., Christian, R., and Engel, G.: Cerebral metabolic disturbance and delirium in pernicious anemia, Arch. Intern. Med. (Chicago) **90**:4, 1952.

Paralysis agitans

Paralysis agitans is characterized by degenerative lesions in the globus pallidus and substantia nigra, due to either senile or vascular parenchymatous changes. Similarly the syndrome may occur with virus encephalitis, carbon monoxide poisoning, or following trauma. Progressive muscular rigidity, immobile facies, flexion of neck, trunk, and extremities, a propulsive gait, and slow rhythmic tremor characterize the syndrome. In many patients there are no mental symptoms. Most patients are good natured but some react to their disability with irritability, peevishness, and dissatisfaction. In others senile or vascular changes may produce psychotic symptoms.

SUGGESTED READING

Prichard, J., Schwab, R., and Tillmann, W.: The effects of stress and the results of medication in different personalities with Parkinson's disease, Psychosom. Med. **13**:106, 1951.

Pellagra

Pellagra occurs with a polyavitaminosis of the B complex. It tends to appear in communities where dietary standards are low, and it may develop in institutionalized persons who are already psychotic. Neuronal and capillary changes are found throughout the neuraxis, usually most marked in the cerebrum. Stomatitis, glossitis, achlorhydria, and diarrhea are common. In early cases erythema of the skin, especially on the extensor surfaces of the extremities and the inner thighs, is followed by scaling and red-brown pigmentation. The early mental symptoms include irritability, headache, restlessness, lassitude, insomnia, emotional instability, difficulty in concentration, apprehension, and forgetfulness. Later, memory defects, confusion, disorientation, delirium, and finally dementia may occur. Late in the disease severe neurological complications develop with stupor, incontinence, varied sensory disturbances, irregular involuntary movements, convulsions, rigidity, and paralyses. Niacin is the specific therapeutic agent given, 100 mg. t.i.d. in mild cases and in severe cases 1200 to 1500 mg. per day. Brewer's yeast, 40 to 200 Gm., is added to a liberal diet.

SUGGESTED READINGS

Sebrell, W. H., Jr., and Harris, R. S., editors: The vitamins: chemistry, physiology, pathology, New York, 1954, Academic Press, Inc., vol. 1.

Spillane, J. D.: Nutritional disorders of the nervous system, Baltimore, 1947, The Williams & Wilkins Co., especially chaps. 2, 5, 6, and 13.

Porphyria

Acute porphyria is said to occur in families in which psychiatric disorders run rife. Occurring most frequently in women and in the third or fourth decades of life, the attack may be precipitated by sulfonal or barbiturates. Beginning with colicky abdominal pains and the appearance of a urine which darkens to a port-wine color on standing, the condition advances rapidly to the production of convulsions, paralyses, and sensory disturbances whose bizarre character (e.g., transient amaurosis) may be confused with symptoms of conversion hysteria. Transient confusional psychoses are common.

SUGGESTED READINGS

Markowitz, M.: Acute intermittent porphyria. A report of five cases and a review of the literature, Ann. Intern. Med. 41:1170, 1954.

Roth, N.: The neuropsychiatric aspects of porphyria, Psychosom. Med. 7:291, 1945.

Sikes, Z. S.: Electroencephalographic abnormalities and psychiatric manifestations in intermittent porphyria, Dis. Nerv. Syst. 21:226, 1960.

Tschudy, D. P.: In Conn, H. F., editor: Porphyrias—current therapy, Philadelphia, 1965, W. B. Saunders Co.

Drug or poison intoxication
Bromide intoxication

A very common cause of delirium in psychiatric practice is the ingestion of bromide medication, usually as a sedative. With an excessive amount, unsteadiness, confusion, memory loss, and hallucinations occur and in some cases an acneform eruption.

Anamnesis. Among early symptoms, *chief complaints* are fatigue and sleepiness with generalized ataxia which the patient himself may bring to the physician's attention. Later, symptoms of brain dysfunction develop. The *history* is commonly one of underlying personality disorder, with increasing nervousness and ingestion of Bromo Seltzer, B. C., Neurosine, or some "salty liquid preparation." Too often the patient will deny any history of medication. The elderly, arteriosclerotic, chronic alcoholic or patient with cardiorenal disease has a lower tolerance for bromides. In such individuals 2 Gm. per day may produce intoxication in a few weeks. Weight loss, constipation, and insomnia occur.

Examination. In the *behavioral* picture, confusion, memory loss, delusions, and hallucinations occur frequently; the latter are predominantly visual and often of colors, lights, and large animals. There may be excitement, fear, or depression. As *physical* symptoms, ataxia, weakness, and slurred speech may occur. In some cases (10%) acneform eruption is present. This seems dependent more upon a dermatological predisposition than upon amount of drug ingested. Weight loss, cachexia, and even stupor can result. Based on *laboratory* tests, a serum bromide level of 150 mg./100 ml. is cited as the average at which symptoms begin, although as little as 75 mg./100 ml. or as much as 200 to 300 mg./100 ml. may be required. The tolerance is directly dependent upon the ingestion of salt in the diet, 10 to 15 Gm. chloride being necessary for elimination of each gram of bromide ingested. A simple test for the presence of bromide is to add 1 Gm. of animal charcoal to 20 to 25 ml. urine and filter for a few minutes. To 5 ml. of the filtrate, add 1 ml. trichloracetic acid and 1 ml. 0.5% gold chloride. Brown color indicates the presence of bromides.

Prognosis. Good. In any patient with elevated blood bromide it is wise to withhold the final diagnosis of other psychosis until the blood bromide has returned to normal. Excretion is much slower than uptake. Mental symptoms may persist after the removal of bromide from the blood by as much as 2 weeks or more. With good chloride intake bromide level may fall 50% in 7 days. Excretion is principally via kidneys.

In general, the higher the blood bromide, the more intense are the symptoms. A routine blood bromide test can be of as great diagnostic value as a routine serological examination in patients admitted to a psychiatric service.

Treatment. Force fluids.

Give oral NH_3Cl, enteric-coated, up to 8 Gm. per day (in divided doses); 1000 to 2000 ml. physiological saline solution, I.V.

Sedate with chloral hydrate or paraldehyde if necessary. Chlorpromazine, 50 mg. I.M. q. 4 h., may be used cautiously.

SUGGESTED READINGS

Cornbleet, T.: Bromide intoxication treated with ammonium chloride, J.A.M.A. **146**:1116, 1951.

Hodges, H. H., and Gilmour, M. T.: The continuing hazard of bromide intoxication, Amer. J. Med. **10**:459, 1951.

Levin, M.: Toxic psychoses. In Arieti, S., editor: American handbook of psychiatry, New York, 1959, Basic Books, Inc., Publishers, vol. 2.

Perkins, H. A.: Bromide intoxication. Analysis of cases from a general hospital, Arch. Intern. Med. (Chicago) **85**:783, 1950.

Barbiturate intoxication

In recent years the barbiturate compounds have been favorite chemical agents for suicide. *Acute barbiturate intoxication* occurs in 1 out of every 1900 patients admitted to a general hospital and requires careful attention to medical as well as psychiatric factors, as death occurs in 7% to 15% of such cases.

Examination. The patient is brought to the emergency room in a coma with respiratory depression, followed by shock, a state clinically indistinguishable from uremia or opium poisoning. Hypothermia develops unless secondary pneumonitis has produced a rise in temperature. All neurological signs are sluggish, including pupillary reaction. Cyanosis and airway obstruction often supervene, followed by death due to central respiratory inhibition.

Diagnosis. Diagnosis is usually made on the basis of history of ingestion of barbiturates plus finding barbiturates by chemical analysis of the urine. This method is preferable to testing the blood or stomach contents.

Treatment. If patient is seen within the first hour, remove any drug from the stomach by aspiration. Do not use emetics. Blood pressure, pulse, and respiration must be closely watched and frequently recorded. Suction apparatus and oxygen resuscitator should be at the bedside when symptoms indicate their usefulness. Good nursing care is essential with the emphasis on the prevention of complications. The patient should be kept warm, position frequently changed, and prophylactic antibiotics administered.

For stimulation of depressed respiratory center, use amphetamines; Benzedrine given intravenously at the rate of 1 mg./min. seems to be the drug of choice. Maintain an open airway and give oxygen as necessary to support respiratory exchange. Tracheotomy set should be quickly available. Maintain adequate cardiovascular circulation. Hypotension may be relieved by subcutaneous Neo-Synephrine, 1 to 5 mg., given when blood pressure falls below 90 mm. Hg systolic or 50 diastolic. Recent experience from Denmark seems to indicate that the treatment of choice relies upon maintenance of a stable cardiovascular state by the use of oxygen, blood, or plasma expanders and by forced diuresis in seriously ill patients. Osmotic diuretics (urea, mannitol) may be used intravenously. Hemodialysis may be accomplished by means of the artificial kidney or by the simpler procedure of intermittent peritoneal lavage with the addition of albumin to the peritoneal fluid to expedite the removal of barbiturate bound to the plasma protein.

SUGGESTED READINGS

Blachly, P., and Brookhart, J.: Studies on the analeptic action of electrical stimulation in barbiturate poisoning, Anesthesiology 16:151, 1955.

Clemmeson, C., and Nilsson, E.: Therapeutic trends in the treatment of barbiturate poisoning, Clin. Pharmacol. Ther. 2:220, 1961.

Cohn, R.: Barbiturate intoxication, a clinical EEG study, Ann. Intern. Med. 32:1049, 1950.

Fraser, H. F., Wikler, A., Essig, C. F., and Isbell, H.: Degree of physical dependence induced by secobarbital or pentobarbital, J.A.M.A. 166:126, 1958.

Fraser, H. F., and others: Chronic barbiturate intoxication, Arch. Intern. Med. (Chicago) 94:34, 1954.

Matthew, H.: Acute barbiturate poisoning, Amsterdam, 1971, Excerpta Medica Foundation.

Robie, T. R.: Treatment of acute barbiturate poisoning by nonconvulsive electrostimulation, Postgrad. Med. 9:253, 1951.

Childbirth

Psychosis with childbirth is classed among the psychoses associated with other physical conditions such as those of endocrine, toxic, infectious, or metabolic origin. However, pregnancy brings not only the internal stress of dramatic physiological changes but also the external stresses of new social responsibilities and emotional readjustments within the family. It is a natural breaking point for women with vulnerabilities of personality and is the situation in which up to 8% of psychoses in women occur. This category includes schizophrenic, manic-depressive, and toxic reactions which descriptively and from a therapeutic and prognostic point of view do not differ greatly from these disorders occurring in other life situations.

Clinical types. Distribution is approximately as follows: schizophrenic (30% of cases), schizoaffective (20% to 25%), manic state (20%), depressive state (15%), and toxic psychoses (10%).

Anamnesis. The *chief complaint* is usually the observation by others that the patient has undergone a change in behavior 1 to 6 weeks following delivery, although in about one fifth of the cases the onset is before parturition. *History* reveals the onset of irritability, crying spells, insomnia, somatic complaints, and seclusiveness beginning in the first trimester. Except in toxic psychoses, no correlation exists with prolonged labor, toxemia of pregnancy, anemia, infection, or anesthetic complications, but in a sizeable percentage the child is basically unwanted or even illegitimate. Most studies do not indicate any correlation with the sex of the infant. Repeated pregnancies not uncommonly bring a repetition of symptoms. *Past* history may reveal a young woman who is not emotionally free from her mother, who was emotionally upset at the menarche, and who is sexually frigid with her husband. *Family* history reveals 14% with psychoses among parents or siblings.

Overall *behavior* does not differ from that in classic schizophrenic, manic, depressive, or toxic disorders except in content of thought. Fears of one's own and the baby's death, delusions of the baby's being deformed, dead, or not yet born—or even a complete denial of pregnancy and marriage—are not unusual. *Physical* examination frequently reveals signs of dehydration and malnutrition. As shown on *laboratory* tests, anemia, hypoproteinemia, and elevated nonprotein nitrogen may occur.

Treatment. Symptoms of mild or moderate emotional disturbance early in pregnancy should be treated immediately with psychotherapy as a preventive measure. Psychotic symptoms are treated with all the techniques of modern psychiatry, including phenothiazines, when the clinical picture includes agitation or schizophrenic symptomatology. Both during and after psychosis, psychotherapy is essential. It is a good rule to avoid leaving the mother alone with the new baby if the patient is delusional, as infanticide is not rare. Frequently social service work is of value at the time the patient leaves the hospital, in making plans for the new infant, or in case work with the family. Some authorities have recommended sterilization as a preventive measure after a careful evaluation of personality assets to determine the likelihood of repeated psychosis with further pregnancies.

SUGGESTED READINGS

Arensten, K.: Postpartum psychoses, with particular reference to prognosis, Danish Med. Bull. **15**:97, April, 1968.

Brew, M. F., and Seidenberg, R.: Psychotic reactions associated with pregnancy and childbirth, J. Nerv. Ment. Dis. **111**:408, 1950.

Ekblad, M.: Induced abortion on psychiatric grounds; a follow-up study of 479 women, Acta Psychiat. Neurol. Scand. **99** (supp.):1, 1955.

Markham, S. A.: A comparative evaluation of psychotic and non-psychotic reactions to childbirth, Amer. J. Orthopsychiat. **31**:565, 1961.

Melges, F. T.: Postpartum psychiatric syndromes, Psychosom. Med. **30**:95, Feb., 1968.

Passenbarger, R., Steinmetz, C. H., Poolar, B. G., and Hyde, R. T.: The picture puzzle of the post-partum psychoses, J. Chronic Dis. **13**:161, 1961.

Wainwright, W.: Fatherhood as a precipitant of mental illness, Amer. J. Psychiat. **123**:40, 1966.

NONPSYCHOTIC ORGANIC BRAIN SYNDROMES
The epilepsies

Introduction. These *seizure* disorders are of importance to the neuropsychiatrist not only because they are common afflictions (0.5% of the population) but also because they present a wide variety of deviations from normal behavior whose pathophysiology aids our understanding of the functioning of the central nervous system. The term "convulsive disorders" (introduced to avoid the odious label of "epilepsy") is misleading, because many seizures occur without motor (convulsive) manifestations. In the older terminology "grand mal" referred to seizures in which a major convulsion occurred, and the term "petit mal" was reserved for all lesser seizures. Observation of the seizure states by means of the electroencephalograph has disclosed that abnormal electrical disturbances of the brain (paroxysmal cerebral dysrhythmias) occur during all types of seizures and often in the resting record between seizures. The spread of such brain disturbance to the motor cortex can produce motor symptoms and generalized convulsions. Sensory, visceral, and other varieties of submaximal seizures occur when the brain disturbance remains focal in other than motor areas of the brain.

It is clinically useful to regard the seizure as a symptom, thus directing one's attention both to the possible etiological mechanisms and to the part of the brain involved. Thus seizures limited to one side of the body or, for example, characterized only by motor symptoms of one limb give definite evidence of focal brain involvement. The cause of a seizure, however, can be injury, neoplasm, infection, or other agent which so alters the cells as to induce a focus of abnormal electrophysiological discharge. The spread of such an electrical seizure to, or its origin in, diencephalic centers seems responsible for obliteration of conscious awareness. Seizure discharges which originate from the temporal lobes can produce a variety of behavioral changes, often difficult to distinguish from symptoms occurring in some of the major psychotic reactions.

Studies made from electrodes inserted into brain tissue, at various depths below the cortex, have produced evidence that paroxysmal electrical storms can occur in the brain without being evident from conventional scalp or even from cortical recording electrodes. Reports have appeared relating such deep focal disturbance to the occurrence of hallucinations. *Psychic phenomena* in the form of lapses of consciousness are common to almost all seizures. Strange variations lasting a few seconds, minutes, or hours, such as dream states, a feeling of having experienced it all before (déjà vu), confusion, fugues, ecstasies, etc., are not uncommon. With focal, temporal lobe seizures the aura of the attack may consist of an illusion or hallucination which is related to the life experience of a patient (a remembered scene or dream experience), thus reaffirming that the acquired neuronal patterns of the temporal lobe have to do with the engrams of memories, thoughts, and feelings.

Postictal clouded states. After a seizure the patient may be confused and resistant, motor behavior returns but conscious control of it lags behind, and—if he is restrained—the patient may fight and injure those around him. With return of consciousness this behavior comes to an end.

Seizures in hysteria. Seizures may occur in hysterical patients without the usual widespread abnormal discharge in the EEG. The attacks usually begin in the presence of other persons and in a situation of emotional significance. The patient sinks to the ground without injury or tongue biting. Urinary incontinence is rare. The pupils usually react to light, consciousness is not entirely lost, and the patient responds to sensory stimulation. The duration of the attack may be prolonged, and its overall character is bizarre. One must not overlook the fact that hysterics are not immune to epilepsy and that both types of attack can occur in the same individual.

Personality and intellectual changes with convulsive disorders. Although repeated severe seizures may be associated with mental changes, this is by no means always the case. Of the 90% of epileptics who are outside institutions, the majority show no gross evidence of peculiar personality or unusual behavior. Of clinic and private patients only about 1 in 10 shows recognizable intellectual deterioration.

Where mental symptoms do exist, common brain pathology may produce both the seizure and the mental defect. Abnormalities of thinking may be the result of drug treatment, as may personality alterations, particularly discouragement and loss of initiative.

Etiology. The immediate cause of the clinical seizure is the underlying cerebral dysrhythmia. Precipitating causes include trauma, brain tumors, infections (encephalitis, abscess, meningitis), toxins, anoxia, and metabolic diseases.

The role of heredity, though often overemphasized, is an

important factor. Ten percent of epileptics have a family history positive for seizure disorder. In the case of children with febrile convulsions the family history is double this figure. The terms "idiopathic" and "cryptogenic" epilepsy refer to seizures of unknown cause and often to an inherited cerebral dysrhythmia.

Types. The most commonly seen seizures may be classified as (1) infantile spasms, (2) febrile convulsions, (3) petit mal, (4) petit mal variant, (5) grand mal, (6) focal motor and Jacksonian seizures, (7) myoclonic seizures, (8) focal sensory seizures, (9) thalamic and hypothalamic seizures, and (10) psychomotor seizures.

Infantile spasms. These are frequent, brief, jerking or quivering spells seen during the first year of life and lasting up to the fourth year. There may be eye rolling and an upward flinging of the arms. The accompanying brain wave disturbance of almost continuous high-voltage slow waves and spikes with shifting multiple foci has been termed hypsarrhythmia. The condition is seen in boys more frequently than in girls. Eleven percent die before the third year, and 87% of those who live are feebleminded. The usually ascribed causes are encephalitis, anoxia, and birth trauma.

Febrile convulsions. These are convulsions occurring during fevers associated with a variety of illnesses. This term is reserved for those cases in which repeated episodes occur. Seen in the third to tenth year, the condition carries a relatively good prognosis. The interseizure EEG is usually normal.

Petit mal. These seizures typically are brief (up to 15 seconds) laspses of consciousness, accompanied by rhythmic blinking of the eyes, nodding of the head, jerking of the arms, sudden loss of posture, or staring. Such attacks are accompanied by the classic 3/sec. spike and wave pattern in the EEG. Attacks occur frequently, from 5 or 6 to over 100 per day (pyknolepsy). Appearing before puberty, they tend to decrease and disappear with increasing age and rarely are carried into adult life. In those cases in which grand mal convulsions also occur or where the EEG shows a strong grand mal (spike) component the prognosis is more guarded, as the latter type of seizure may persist into adult life. Hereditary factors are the same as for other types of seizure. Encephalitis is believed to be a common cause.

Petit mal variant. This diagnosis is made from an EEG pattern in which the spike and wave complex is atypical and occurs at a frequency other than 3/sec. There occur tonic or tonic-clonic convulsions, brief attacks of impaired consciousness, or sudden losses of posture. It differs from petit mal by an earlier age of onset and is frequently associated with evidence of organic brain damage and the occurrence of intellectual impairment.

Grand mal. This term is applied to the generalized convulsive seizure. In usual sequence, with or without some premonition or transient sensory experience (aura), the patient loses consciousness, muscles become rigid (tonic), respiration is suspended, and he falls. Jerking (clonic) movements then occur, respiration returns, and consciousness is gradually recovered. Loss of sphincter control and minor injury such as tongue biting are common. During the seizure the EEG shows high-voltage spiking activity that is often indistinguishable from the electrical component of the muscle discharge; later the record becomes almost flat. Voltage returns with slow activity which increases in frequency as consciousness is gained. The interseizure records may show spiking activity, but more usually show high-voltage slow waves, often occurring paroxysmally. Forty percent of persons with grand mal seizures have relatively normal EEG tracings during the interseizure period. The etiology of this condition is varied and such seizures occur following trauma, oxygen lack, vascular disease, encephalitis, toxins, neoplasms, or metabolic disease, or they result from an inherited cerebral dysrhythmia.

Focal motor and Jacksonian seizures. These are sometimes called partial seizures and may occur with involvement of one extremity with or without loss of consciousness. A convulsion beginning locally and spreading on one side of the body is termed "Jacksonian." From such focal beginnings a spread to the opposite side of the body may occur, with production of a generalized seizure. The EEG may show localized spike discharges. Surgical intervention with removal of a focal lesion or focus of abnormally discharging brain tissue should be considered in these patients.

Myoclonic seizures. Sudden single jerking of the head, limbs, or trunk may occur, associated with multiple high-voltage spikes in the EEG, with or without mixed slow waves. Consciousness is not noticeably impaired. This phenomenon is commonly associated with major seizures (64%). Symptoms are often accentuated upon awakening or on going to sleep.

Focal sensory seizures. These seizures may occur either as aurae (premonitory symptoms of a generalized seizure) or as an independent attack. Visual, auditory, or olfactory seizures may occur with focal involvement of the corresponding cortical area.

Thalamic and hypothalamic seizures. Paroxysmal brain disorder in these regions should be considered with the occurrence of attacks of vertigo, dizziness, cardiac palpitation, pain, or paresthesia, associated with loss of consciousness or convulsive phenomena. Sweating, vomiting, respiratory distress, and urge to micturate, as well as attacks of uncontrollable rage, have been described. Positive spike patterns of 14/sec. and 6/sec. may occur in the EEG associated with this clinical picture. These electroencephalographic patterns are seen most often in adolescents, are accentuated in light stages of sleep, and often have a temporal or occipital focalization. In patients with these symptoms, the paroxysmal nature of the complaint may be overlooked and the case be misdiagnosed as one of neurosis, gastric migraine, neurotic headache, behavior disorder, and the like. Trauma and encephalitis are among the commonest etiological factors.

Psychomotor seizures. The term "psychomotor" (psychic or epileptic equivalent) has been used to describe attacks of epilepsy in which the subject becomes confused but does not, as a rule, completely lose consciousness. There may be accompanying emotional displays of rage or fear and such behavior as negativism, staring, groping, chewing, swallowing, smacking of the lips, laughing, crying, rubbing, plucking, undressing, showing confusion in his speech, or exhibiting other complex behavior for which he is later amnesic.

Neurophysiologically this type of epilepsy has been linked to the limbic system. The EEG may disclose a temporal spike focus which is sometimes seen only during the sleeping record. If the abnormal discharge remains localized in the anterior part of the temporal lobe, no clinical symptoms occur. When, however, it spreads, high-voltage 6/sec. and flat-topped 4/sec. waves are seen in distant cortical areas and the typical clinical manifestations occur.

This type of epilepsy occurs most commonly in adults but is found, rarely, in young children. It is often seen in combination with other types of convulsive disorder. It has been estimated that approximately half of the patients with anterior temporal foci have more or less continuous psychiatric symptoms, either as personality disorder or as psychosis. The etiology of the irritated temporal lobe focus may be traumatic, with birth trauma a common offender. Other types of focal lesions are less commonly found. Surgical intervention in selected cases may be of value.

Diagnosis. The EEG is a definite aid to diagnosis in about 50% of cases. In an additional group, recording during sleep may elicit focal patterns, particularly anterior temporal spikes and 14/sec. and 6/sec. positive spiking. The precipitation of spike and wave activity, with or without a seizure, and less commonly the elicitation of other diagnostic patterns or convulsive phenomena by strong hyperventilation can be of distinct diagnostic aid. Other activation procedures (Metrazol, photo-Metrazol, and photic stimulation) are of questionable diagnostic significance. A search for the cause in every case of seizure should include complete neurological examination, x-ray films of the skull, spinal fluid examination, and—where indicated—arteriography and/or pneumoencephalography.

Treatment. In general it can be stated that no two cases of seizure disorder are alike; therefore, treatment must be individualized. Total management requires cooperation on the part of the patient and his family, patience on the part of the doctor, and a mulifaceted treatment approach.

Anticonvuslant therapy. The safest drug with fewest side effects should be tried first and the dose rapidly increased to tolerance. If one is ineffective, another drug should be substituted; if partially effective, a second drug added and likewise systematically evaluated. Complete seizure control may require continued high dosage. Only when seizures are controlled is it wise to reduce the dosage of those drugs with annoying side effects.

Table 4. Anticonvulsant drugs*

Seizure pattern	Drug	How supplied	Gm./day maximum		Dosage limited by‡	Idiosyncrasy§
			Child	Adult		
Generalized, convulsive, focal Jacksonian, or autonomic	Phenobarbital	Tab. 15, 30, and 100 mg. Elix. 15 mg./tsp.	0.1 Gm.	0.3 Gm.	—	Irritability
	Mebaral	Tab. 30, 100, and 200 mg.	0.2 Gm.	0.5 Gm.	—	Irritability
	Bromides	Tab. and sol.		3.0 Gm.	—	Bromide intoxication
	Mysoline	Tab. 250 mg.	0.1 Gm.	2.0 Gm.	Unsteadiness	Nausea, giddiness
	Mesantoin	Tab. 100 mg.	0.1 Gm.	0.8 Gm.	Unsteadiness	Bone marrow depression, lymphadenopathy
	Dilantin	Cap. 30 mg., 100 mg. Enteric-coated 0.1 Gm. cap. Loz. 50 mg. Susp. 100 mg./tsp.	0.1 Gm.	0.6 Gm.	Vomiting, unsteadiness	Gum swelling, hirsutism
Psychomotor attacks	Peganone	Tab. 250 mg., 500 mg.	1.0 Gm.	4.0 Gm.	Anorexia, insomnia	Hepatitis, psychosis
	Phenurone	Tab. 500 mg.	1.0 Gm.	4.0 Gm.		
	Celontin	Cap. 300 mg.	0.3 Gm.	2.5 Gm.	Headache, anorexia	
	Milontin	Cap. 500 mg. Susp. 300 mg./tsp.	1.0 Gm.	3.0 Gm.		
Petit mal triad (absence, akinesia, myoclonus)	Tridione	Cap. 300 mg. Dulcet (loz.) 150 mg. Sol. 150 mg./tsp.	0.9 Gm.	3.0 Gm.	Hiccups	Photophobia, bone marrow depression
	Paradione	Cap. 150 mg., 300 mg. Sol. 300 mg./ml.	0.9 Gm.	3.0 Gm.	Hiccups	Photophobia, bone marrow depression
	Diamox	Tab. 250 mg.	0.2 Gm.	1.0 Gm.	Anorexia, thirst	
	Zarontin	Cap. 250 mg.	0.5 Gm.	1.5 Gm.	Nausea	Psychiatric symptoms, bone marrow depression

*Modified from table used by the Seizure Unit of the Children's Medical Center, Boston, Mass.

Mebaral (mephobarbital), Mysoline (primidone), Mesantoin (methylphenylethylhydantoin), Dilantin (diphenylhydantoin), Peganone (ethotoin), Phenurone (phenacemide), Celontin (methsuximide), Milontin (methylphenylsuccimide), Tridione (trimethyloxazolidinedione), Diamox (acetazolamide), Zarontin (ethosuximide).

Dosages: Usually 25% to 50% of the maximum is prescribed initially and is given in two to three doses every day with meals. At 2- to 4-week intervals the dosage is increased by small steps as needed and tolerated until either seizures are eliminated or toxic symptoms appear.

Combinations: When drugs used singly fail to control seizures, combinations may succeed; e.g., Dilantin 3 parts, phenobarbital 1 part, or Dilantin 1 part, Tridione 3 parts. Amphetamines may be added as needed to combat mild sedation. Some believe that amphetamine has a beneficial effect on petit mal seizures. Occasionally Dilantin will aggravate petit mal seizures and Tridione or Atabrine, convulsive seizures. To simplify evaluation of therapy, *only one drug should be changed during a 2-week period.* Librium (chlordiazepoxide) and Valium (diazepam) have some anticonvulsant properties and are useful when given in combination with other anticonvulsants. They are preferred over phenothiazines, which lower convulsive threshold.

Essential observations:

†Monthly wbc count and differential smear are obligatory because of possible bone marrow depression.
‡Sedation or grogginess is usually the factor which limits dosage in all except Dilantin.
§Rash. All drugs have produced rash in sensitive patients, usually after 8 to 12 days of treatment.

Complications: Bone marrow depression, erythematous rash, liver toxicity, or *psychosis* requires immediate withdrawal of the offending drug, and a maximal dose of phenobarbital is given daily for 2 weeks to prevent precipitation of status epilepticus.

Tranquilizers may be helpful to reduce hypermobility and agitation, especially in children and in patients with psychomotor seizures. In combination with anticonvulsants, tranquilizers may add to the somnifacient effects of phenobarbital, Mesantoin, Tridione, etc., such that dosages of the latter may be reduced. Beware the occasional convulsant properties of some tranquilizers. For a summary of important drugs see Table 4.

Antibiotics. Antibiotics should be given a trial in all cases with a history or question of encephalitis, and especially in those cases with a progressive worsening or multiple EEG foci. A course of 4 or 5 weeks of Achromycin, Terramycin, or Chloromycetin may be tried.

Surgical treatment. Surgical treatment consists of removal of epileptogenic focus localized by EEG.

Psychotherapy. Decisions regarding the type of psychotherapy used should be governed entirely by the needs of the patient. A type of supportive therapy is probably given by every doctor who treats epileptics and recognizes their need to accept the illness and to adjust to chronic medication and the limitation of certain activities. The adjustment to life in which the possibility of a convulsion is always potentially present may lead to a neurotic, chronic invalidism more restrictive than epilepsy. Some attempt should be made to discuss the emotional relationship of the patient to the physician and to encourage emotional expression as well as reeducation in life goals and patterns. Group therapy for epileptics has been found to be worthwhile, and a reorientation of attitudes of the patient's relatives and employers.

The condition of *status epilepticus,* which occurs in about 8% of epileptics, requires vigilant nursing care, intravenous glucose and saline, and catheterization as necessary. Diphenylhydantoin (Dilantin sodium, Steri-Vial or ampule) is useful. Inject intravenously at a rate not to exceed 50 mg./min. Most episodes are controlled by 250 mg. This dose may be repeated or 250 mg. be given intramuscularly at 4- to 6-hour intervals for 2 to 3 days. Continue orally when patient is conscious. Paraldehyde, 5 ml. (mixed with 10 ml. of vegetable oil), per 15 pounds of body weight, can be given by rectum. Barbiturates which may be used are sodium Amytal, 0.5 Gm. I.V., or

Luminal sodium, 0.3 Gm. I.V. *Repeat only with great caution, as oversedation can be more dangerous than status.* Alternatively, magnesium sulfate, 10 ml. of 25% solution I.V., or Avertin with amylene hydrate in an anesthetic dose per rectum, 60 to 80 mg./kg. of body weight, may be given.

SUGGESTED READINGS

Barker, W., and Barker, S.: Experimental production of human convulsive brain potentials by stress-induced effects upon neural integrative function: dynamics of the convulsive reaction to stress, Proc. Ass. Res. Nerv. Ment. Dis. 29:92, 1950.

Cobb, S.: Borderlands of psychiatry, Cambridge, Mass., 1943, Harvard University Press.

Falconer, M. A.: Serafitinides, A., and Corsellis, J. A. N.: Etiology and pathogenesis of temporal lobe epilepsy, Arch. Neurol. (Chicago) 10:233, 1964.

Flor-Henry, P.: Schizophrenic-like reactions and affective psychoses associated with temporal lobe epilepsy etiological factors, Amer. J. Psychiat. 126:400, 1969.

Gastaut, H., Jasper, H., Bancaud, J., and Waltregny, A.: The physiopathogenesis of the epilepsies, Springfield, Ill., 1969, Charles C Thomas, Publisher.

Gibbs, F., and Gibbs, E. L.: Atlas of electroencephalography, Reading, Mass., 1952, Addison-Wesley Publishing Co., Inc., vol. 2.

Gibbs, F. A., and Gibbs, E. L.: Borderlands of epilepsy, J. Neuropsychiat. 4:287, 1963.

Lennox, W. G., and Lennox, M. A.: Epilepsy and related disorders, Boston, 1960, Little, Brown & Co., vols. 1 and 2.

Penfield, W., and Jasper, H.: Epilepsy and the functional anatomy of the human brain, Boston, 1954, Little, Brown & Co.

Rodin, E. A.: The prognosis of patients with epilepsy, Springfield, Ill., 1968, Charles C Thomas, Publisher.

Slater, E., Beard, A. W., and Glithor E.: The schizophrenia-like psychoses of epilepsy, Brit. J. Psychiat. 109:95, 1963.

Stevens, J. R.: Psychiatric implications of psychomotor epilepsy, Arch. Gen. Psychiat. 14:461, 1966.

Tresser, T. D. A.: The psychiatric patient with an EEG temporal lobe focus, Amer. J. Psychiat. 120:765, 1964.

13

Psychoses not attributed to known physical condition

Definition. Among those mental disorders classified as "of psychogenic origin or without clearly defined physical cause," the ones labeled as psychoses cause the most catastrophic interference with normal patterns of behavior. They are characterized by a varying degree of personality disintegration and failure correctly to evaluate external reality. Individuals with such disorders show defect in their ability to relate themselves effectively to other people or to their own work. Although outbursts of antisocial, dangerous, or self-destructive behavior may be important symptoms, the special features of much psychotic behavior are its bizarre, withdrawn, or asocial qualities.

Onset may occur at any time from infancy to old age, is common during adolescence, and frequently appears in persons who have, since childhood, been "different." Duration of the psychosis may vary from a few hours to several decades or even most of a lifetime.

Although a great deal of research has been carried out on these patients, psychotic disorders remain a huge enigmatic public health problem the world over. Available evidence suggests that some psychoses are probably constitutional in origin and dependent in some way upon as yet undiscovered physiological and biochemical dysfunctions. Other psychoses appear to be of psychosocial origin and related to severe chronic emotional stress originating within the infant and childhood family milieu. Probably the best assumption is that most psychoses result from a complex interaction of both of these types of etiological factors.

Classification. These psychotic disorders are divided into two principal groups, depending upon whether *affective* (affective psychoses) or *thinking* (schizophrenic and paranoid psychoses) disturbances are more prominent. On close examination, however, all such patients suffer from meaningfully related disturbances of both affect and cognition.

Major affective disorders

This presentation will follow the classification of the A.P.A. Standard Nomenclature, which divides affective disorders into *involutional, manic-depressive,* and *other types.* However, it should be emphasized that categorization of this group of illnesses is not yet definitive. Depression as an isolated mood symptom is universal and becomes a sign of illness only by degree. As an initial step, affective disorders can be classified as *primary,* depression or mania occurring in a person never before psychotically ill, or as *secondary,* disturbance that occurs in the course of and is considered in connection with some other illness (such as psychoneurosis, alcoholism, or organic brain disease).

Primary affective disorders may be divided into the *endogenous-reactive continuum* or be seen as a *bipolar-unipolar* dichotomy. The term *endogenous* refers to depressions usually "serious" or "psychotic" based upon hereditary or constitutional factors and including symptoms of guilt, psychomotor retardation, melancholia, feeling of hopelessness, nihilism, suicidal behavior, sleep, appetite, and sexual disturbances, together with ideas of reference and hallucinations. *Reactive depression* (often used synonymously for "neurotic depression") refers to disorders believed to be provoked by some physiological or social stress. A common example of this is a syndrome seen for two to three months after bereavement, with some or all of the following symptoms: depressed mood, sleep disturbance, crying, difficulty in concentration, loss of interest in daily events, anorexia, and weight loss.

Recently clinical and genetic data have been martialed (Winokur, Perris, Angst, et cetera) to support a dichotomy seen in hospitalized patients with primary affective disorders into *bipolar* (manic-depressive) and *unipolar* (depressive) disease. In the bipolar class the patient must have experienced an episode of mania, while in the unipolar type only depression need have occurred. In the majority of patients the episodes are without precipitating psychological or physical incident. Depressive episodes generally last longer than manic, and unipolar depression is reported of longer duration than bipolar. Over half of the patients with bipolar disorders become ill prior to 30 years of age; unipolar onsets reach their peak a decade later. Electroconvulsive therapy, with and without antidepressant drugs, significantly improves the prognosis of depression, particularly in older age. Modern treatments have decreased earlier mortality rates for mania (reported to be over 20%), but suicide still accounts for 13% to 17% of patient deaths. Recovery rate for mania (95%) is higher than for depression (80%). About half of patients with first admission for mania or depression do not have a second attack; patients with bipolar disturbances have more episodes than those with a unipolar type.

Involutional melancholia

Mental disorders associated with the climacteric include those psychotic and neurotic conditions that may also occur at earlier ages, and some authors feel that these reactions are really a variant of the manic-depressive reaction. At this period there occur marked changes in family and job roles, general decline in mental and physical strength and endurance, loss of orgastic potency in the male, and vasomotor changes. All these factors, together with a loss of the capacity to have babies in the female, produce a specific psychological coloring of the melancholias occurring in this age group so that they are often considered as a distinct entity. The term "agitated depression" describes the intensely fearful overactive condition which is a characteristic behavioral trait in many of these *involutional melancholias* and which helps differentiate them from the more usually retarded, manic-depressive illness (depressed type) reactions. Those who believe that these are but a part of an overall single category, "affective psychoses," point to the fact that, like the manic-depressive reactions, involutional melancholia occurs more often in women and in those of Hebrew origin, has an inherited tendency, and shows at least equally good response to electroconvulsive therapy.

The illness is seen typically in women between the ages of 40 and 55 years and somewhat later in men. The incidence is 5 to 10 times as frequent in women as in men. Accompanying the common physiological symptoms of the climacteric (vasomotor instability, insomnia, emotional lability), depressive symptoms occur. In some patients, in addition to the depression, delusions of a paranoid nature are seen. When these are the main feature of the illness, the term "involutional paraphrenia" is properly used.

Anamnesis. The symptoms often begin with a *chief complaint* of early morning awakening and difficulty in falling asleep. Slow onset is usual, with gradually increasing agitation, melancholia, feelings of unreality, somatic delusions, dramatic self-accusations, and the feeling of having committed the world's worst sins. These lead the relatives to seek medical aid for the patient. *History* typically reveals a woman who has been rigid and unadapting, subnormally assertive, overmeticulous, or worrisome yet whose personality has been sufficiently stable not to have disrupted earlier in life with manic-depressive or schizophrenic symptomatology. Marriage of a child, death of a loved one, or financial reverses are frequent precipitating factors. *Family history* reveals other major psychoses and emotional instability.

Examination. In the *behavioral* status, orientation and intellectual functioning are usually intact, although judgment may become defective and insight is usually lacking. In severe cases there may be a superimposed delirium with auditory and visual hallucinations. The mood is melancholic but this is usually complicated by overt anxiety manifestations such as hand wringing. Feelings of unreality extend to body parts which seem strange and changed. Almost constant hypochondriacal and nihilistic delusions may be often repeated (rut-formation) and include such typical statements as "My body is rotten, my bowels are filled with concrete, I am going down to Hell," etc. Paranoid delusions lack the grandiose quality seen in schizophrenia, and involutional patients do not usually fear or resist their delusional persecutors but rather look upon them as meting out rightful punishment for their sins. Other schizophrenic signs such as thought blocking are absent. Impotence and loss of libido are frequent. *Physical* examination frequently reveals loss of weight, dehydration, and tachycardia. Constipation and cessation of menses do occur.

Treatment. Electroshock (8 to 15 treatments) shortens the course of the illness to less than 90 days and, most important of all, minimizes the danger of suicide. Effort in this age group should be made to achieve gradual onset of the convulsions (glissando) and to soften the convulsions through the use of sodium Amytal, succinylcholine chloride, and other relaxants. Chlorpromazine and reserpine may relieve agitation and diminish the intensity of paranoid preoccupation. Such drugs, however, must be used with caution as they can intensify depressive symptoms, especially in patients showing primarily serious symptoms of depression. The antidepressant drugs, especially imipramine, amitriptyline, desipramine, and nortriptyline, offer an alternative to a course of convulsive treatments, which is often not without complications in this older group of patients. Reeducative and supportive psychotherapy, with encouragement to accept the pleasures of the later years, is important. The paranoid type often requires up to 20 electroshock treatments and has a poorer prognosis.

Prognosis. Hospitalized patients will remit within 9 months (80% to 85%) without electroshock therapy. With ECT, hospitalization is reduced to but a few weeks. Best results occur in younger patients with a rapid onset of illness, with accompanying anxiety and agitation, with severe depression, and with the prospect of return to a favorable environment.

Involutional melancholics are said to manifest the most intense of all psychic pain. Suicide is a real danger (25% to 50% in untreated cases), and, because of this, once the diagnosis is made, the patient should not be left alone and the institution of treatment should be as immediate as with any other medical or surgical emergency.

SUGGESTED READINGS

Bellak, L.: Manic-depressive psychosis and allied conditions, New York, 1952, Grune & Stratton, Inc.
Campbell, J.: Manic-depressive disease, clinical and psychiatric significance, Philadelphia, 1953, J. B. Lippincott Co.

Greenblatt, M., Grosser, G. H., and Wechsler, H.: Differential response of hospitalized depressed patients to somatic therapy, Amer. J. Psychiat. **120**:935, 1964.

Henderson, D. K., and Batchelor, I.: Textbook of psychiatry for students and practitioners, ed. 9, London, 1962, Oxford University Press.

Hollister, L. E., Overall, J. R., Shelton, J., Pennington, V., Kimbell, I., and Johnson, M.: Drug therapy of depression, Arch. Gen. Psychiat. **17**: 486, 1967.

Huston, P. E., and Locher, L. M.: Involutional psychoses, Arch. Neurol. Psychiat. **59**:385, 1948.

Perris, C.: A study of bipolar (manic depressive) and unipolar recurrent depressive psychoses, Acta Psychiat. Scand. **42**:1, 1966.

Rado, S.: Psychodynamics of depression from the etiologic point of view, Psychosom. Med. **13**:51, 1951.

Rosenthal, S. H.: The involutional depressive syndrome, Amer. J. Psychiat. **124**(supp.):21, 1968.

Rusch, K.: Involutional melancholia, Hawaii Med. J. **11**:152, 1952.

Simon, R. K.: Involutional psychoses in Negroes, Arch. Gen. Psychiat. **13**:148, 1965.

Ulett, G., and Parsons, E. H.: Psychiatric aspects of carcinoma of the pancreas, J. Missouri Med. Ass. **45**:490, 1948.

Wittenborn, J. R., Plante, M., Burgess, F., and Maurer, H.: A comparison of imipramine, electroconvulsive therapy and placebo in the treatment of depressions, J. Nerv. Ment. Dis. **135**:131, 1962.

Manic-depressive illness

In some nosological formulations all disorders in which depression or mood change is the primary symptom are considered as part of a single disease entity—affective psychosis. Other authors tend to categorize several separate affective illnesses. Within any such grouping, however, the manic-depressive psychoses form a large and well-defined entity.

Types. The very name *manic-depressive* is misleading, as it implies a cyclothymic swing between two extremes of mood. Within a single patient, followed through the years, isolated attacks of both mania and depression may occur but this is by no means always the case, as patients frequently have attacks of only one type. Attempts to classify have led to a welter of terms which are often more useful in briefly characterizing an attack rather than a patient.

Terms used include *manic-depressive illness, manic type,* ranging from hypomania to delirious mania; *manic-depressive illness, depressed type,* ranging from simple retardation to stuporous melancholia; and *manic-depressive illness, cir-*

cular type, having manic and depressive phases follow or alternate in some regular or irregular manner.

The terms *manic-depressive, manic,* and *manic-depressive, depressed,* may be used to signify the phase of attack of an individual with circular type disorder. At times symptoms of manic and depressive phases appear to mix, and in the literature one finds such terms as "agitated depression," "maniacal stupor," etc. Such mixing occurs particularly when a depression or a mania changes into the opposite mood.

Anamnesis. At the *onset* in the *manic type,* early rising, impatience with delay, good humor, and press of social and business duties characterize the hypomanic as a "live wire." As the manic tendency progresses, his family may notice his tendency to monopolize the conversation, increasing irritability, and intolerance of restraint. Poor judgment coupled with plans and schemes and increased sexual drive may lead to excesses that bring the family to seek a physician's aid. In the *depressed type,* insomnia and early awakening, failure to eat, and weight loss may precede the onset of extended mood disturbance, with self-accusation, slow thinking, motor retardation, and melancholia. There are feelings of guilt, self-accusation, and inability to accept responsibility and perform daily tasks. Libido is lost; there are suicidal ruminations and body- and self-preoccupation.

Similar attacks, either of mania or of depression or of both, may be revealed in the *history* and indeed a definite diagnosis may be possible only after previous attacks. Of great importance is the recognition of cases of mild manic-depressive illness in which symptoms of headache, blurry vision, dyspnea, palpitation, anorexia, weight loss, nausea, abdominal pain, weakness and/or other generalized symptoms may bring the patient to his family physician. In such cases the history is not psychologically spectacular and the symptoms may remit without the true nature of the illness being recognized. Since such cases are commonly seen in the medical clinic and general hospital and labeled as neurotic, the physician must be constantly alert for the minimal signs that clearly delineate the illness as an attack of manic-depressive disorder. Such symptoms include insomnia, difficulty in concentration, obsessions and phobias (including the fear of insanity), suicidal ideas, and psychomotor retardation.

Family history is important, for it has long been accepted that heredity plays a role in this illness (single autosomal dominant gene with incomplete penetrance). Available figures indicate an occurrence in the general population of 0.4% (1 in 250 persons) with about 25% occurrence in parents and full siblings of the patient. According to one authority, if one parent is afflicted, the illness occurs in 25% of the children, whereas with both parents manic-depressive two thirds of the children have definite manic-depressive illness and one third show mild affective psychopathy. Kallmann's studies of monozygotic twins revealed a 95% co-twin involvement.

There is some acceptance that the illness occurs with greater frequency in those of pyknic build. It occurs about twice as frequently in women. The illness is said to occur more commonly in Irish and Jewish persons and those of higher socioeconomic strata. The disease is seen at ages from 15 to over 70 years but with a peak onset between 35 and 39. Attacks may occur coincidentally with the frequent disturbances of mood seen at puberty, pregnancy, menstruation, and menopause.

The family history may be of suicide rather than of manic or depressive attacks. The premorbid personality may be given to mood swings but otherwise seemingly well adjusted. Typically there is no precipitating event although the common symptoms of guilt and desire for punishment may fixate upon any of a great variety of stressful episodes seemingly related to the incipiency of the attack. The illness follows a usual course of 6 to 18 months with manic cycles typically the shorter, depressive the longer. The course of the cycle varies with response to electroconvulsive or drug therapy.

Biochemical aspects of these disorders have received increasing attention in recent years. Particular attention has been given to changes in the metabolism of adrenal steroids, which has been reported to fluctuate with changes in mood. The effective antidepressant iproniazid is a monoamine oxidase inhibitor. This class of agents effectively increases brain levels of norepinephrine and serotonin, thus supporting the theory that depression is caused or accompanied by a decrease in brain catecholamines. Imipramine (a tricyclic compound and not a monoamine oxidase inhibitor) decreases cell permeability to norepinephrine, thus preventing its inactivation through binding of the cells. Thus both of the agents effectively increase the available concentration of norepinephrine. They both also reverse the sedation brought about by reserpine, which is believed to act through depletion of brain serotonin and norepinephrine. Such findings may well represent important steps to unraveling the etiology of the affective disorders.

Examination. In the *manic type* the three cardinal symptoms *behaviorally* are (1) flight of ideas, (2) increase of psychomotor activity, and (3) emotional excitement. Distractibility, rhyming, punning, and clang associations are seen. Bizarre dress, shameless hypersexuality, hallucinations, grandiose delusions, pressure of activity, and even delirium may occur. *Physically,* exhaustion, fever, and mild bodily injuries may be present. *Psychological* examination in the early stages shows increased M and C on the Rorschach with lowered form-level and increased original productions.

In the *depressed type* the cardinal symptoms *behaviorally* are (1) difficulty in thinking, (2) psychomotor retardation, and (3) emotional depression. These patients move slowly, speak slowly, and in a low tone. They prefer to answer in monosyllables. Consciousness is not clouded and they are well oriented. Self-accusation, hypochondriacal and nihilistic delusions, and hallucinations may occur, being more marked in cases of longer duration. (Depressives accept the delusion as rightful punishment for their sins, whereas the paranoid resents his persecutors). The condition can progress to stupor. *Physically,* one sees a depressed countenance and downcast eyes or weeping. Constipation (danger of impaction) and urinary retention occur; appetite, sleep, and circulation are poor; and there is a decline in potency and libido. Menstrual disorders are common. On the Rorschach *psychological* examination responses are few, reaction time is prolonged, and high F+% is seen, with Dd emphasis and low M and C. Test behavior is characterized by improverishment of thought and action, with painful uncertainty, rejection, pedantic self-correction, self-deprecation, and qualification of responses. One fears suicide when the Rorschach protocol shows superior intelligence, color shock, deep conflict, and signs of depression. Macabre content on card IV may also be significant.

With modern treatments, prognosis is good. The course of the untreated attack can vary from a few weeks to many years. The average duration of the first attack is 6 to 8 months. Most authors state that manic episodes are of shorter duration than depressive. As the patient grows older the attacks usually become longer. Either depression or mania may occur, or there may be an alternation or a mixture of types. In 85% of cases the second attack will be of the same type (manic or depressed) as the first. In some patients the attacks occur with predictable, clocklike regularity. In one series 92% of manics and 80% of depressives recovered after their first attack. In another series 79% had a second attack, 63% a third, and 45% a fourth. Patients with the first attack at 30 years of age are in great danger of a recurrence in 10 to 15 years. Prognosis is poor in patients over the age of 40 years. In patients with strong exogenous factors the illness tends to be shorter. *Suicide* risk is grave in depressions and during recovery from manic or depressive states. Whenever danger of suicide exists, the patient should be put under strict observation and possible suicidal instruments and medications be removed from reach. Windows should be guarded and the patient not left alone. Complaints of hopelessness and worthlessness of living signify serious danger. Guilt feelings and need for punishment (sometimes expressed in delusional form) may motivate suicide. Family history of suicide may be an attraction to similar attempts. Electroshock decreases the risk of suicide, increases the chance for recovery, and shortens the hospital stay by 6 to 12 months. Drug treatment with the psychic eneergizers may, in selected cases, produce similarly good results.

Treatment. Depending upon the severity of the illness and the stage of recovery, electroshock, drug therapy, and psychotherapy will all be found useful here.

Electroshock. Eight to twelve convulsive treatments may be given, at the rate of three times a week for depression and daily or twice a day in manic excitement.

Drug therapy. Symptomatic treatment includes use of hypnotics for insomnia. Long-acting barbiturates are given for

early morning awakening, short-acting barbiturates for difficulty in falling asleep. To avoid habituation, a shift to chloral hydrate may be helpful.

In mild cases specific mood stimulation with the amphetamines (Dexedrine in 5 mg. doses) is a useful morning medication. Recently a number of so-called psychic energizers have
been recommended for even severe depressions. The iminodibenzyl derivatives imipramine (Tofranil), amitriptyline (Ela-
vil), desipramine (Pertofrane, Norpramine), and nortriptyline (Aventyl) have been used with excellent results. Treatment is usually started with a dose of 25 mg. t.i.d. and may be
increased to 200 mg. (amitriptyline) or 300 mg. (imipramine) daily. The monoamine oxidase inhibitors, nialamide
(Niamid), phenelzine (Nardil), and isocarboxazid (Marplan),
are also used in the treatment of less severe depressions. Most
of these "energizers" require 1 or more weeks before achieving successful amelioration of symptoms. Therefore, electroconvulsive therapy (four to six treatments) is often given
during the initial phase of such drug therapy. Initial reports
seem to indicate that medication should be continued for at
least 3 months after discharge from the hospital.

Chlorpromazine and other tranquilizers may be useful in
manic states. Large doses may be necessary. Such drugs can
produce depressive symptoms and therefore must be used with
care in agitated depression. Tranquilizers have been successfully combined with electroconvulsive therapy in treating
both manic reactions and agitated depressions. Here, however, care must be observed, as these drugs can lower blood
pressure and thus increase the hazard of convulsive therapy.

Chlorpromazine is not indicated in cases of uncomplicated
depression where it may intensify the symptoms. It can, however, be used in combination with electroshock therapy in
doses from 50 to 600 mg. t.i.d for mania and for agitated depressions, where it seems both to control the agitation and
reduce the number of shock treatments needed. In mania it
may also be used without electroshock treatment.

Lithium salts have been administered with success in the
treatment of patients with manic psychosis. The suggested
dose range is 0.75 to 1.5 Gm. of lithium carbonate per day,
but if blood levels are not controlled (plasma level kept below

2 mEq./L.) toxic symptoms may occur; hence the the medication procedure must be closely monitored.

Nursing care should include spoon feeding or tube feeding (only if necessary), high caloric diet with vitamins, together with care of constipation and urinary retention in depressions. Occupational therapy and ward management should permit a pace designed to calm manic patients and to urge depressive ones to activity but with consideration of their diurnal mood rhythm (i.e., slowed in A.M. and more spontaneous in P.M.). Warm tubs (97° F., 1 to 2 hours once or twice daily) may be a useful adjunct to the treatment regimen.

In excited manic patients one must guard against sudden exhaustive death. This develops with fall in blood pressure, rapid pulse, weight loss, profuse perspiration, and hyperthermia.

Psychotherapy. Psychotherapy is extremely difficult in severe cases, and even in milder cases experienced therapists usually have achieved disappointing results. In this as in other recurrent psychotic disorders, however, it is to be emphasized that the rapid symptomatic relief afforded by the physical therapies is only part of a treatment plan, which should work toward an improved psychological condition. Such psychotherapeutic efforts may begin during abatement of the illness cycle and with the patient safely guarded in a watchful therapeutic institutional milieu. The value of such psychotherapy is as a prophylactic strengthening of defenses against future emotional stresses.

Studies by a few psychoanalysts have suggested that one difficulty in maintaining these patients in psychotherapy is the nature of the transference-countertransference situation which they tend to establish. These patients frequently have been quite willing to sacrifice latent mature capabilities in the service of gaining approval and dependent gratifications. Furthermore, if an attempt is made to relinquish the attitude of hopeless helplessness, the patient comes face to face with intense feelings of envy and competitiveness.

Psychotic depressive reaction

Patients suffering from a psychotic depressive reaction are severely depressed and manifest evidence of gross misinterpretation of reality, including—at times—delusions and hallu-cinations. This reaction differs from the manic-depressive reaction, depressed type, principally in (1) absence of history of repeated depression or of marked cyclothymic premorbid personality with excessive moodiness or mood swings and (2) presence of environmental precipitating factors. In this latter regard it has been reported that even in manic-depressive re-actions, depressed type, the incidence of precipitating events may be as high as 85%, and one might go even further and find in 100% of cases some "last straw that breaks the camel's back." It would, therefore, appear that the older, widely used term "reactive depression" is really without diagnostic sig-nificance, as the final evaluation of any possible precipitating event depends on the value systems of both patient and psy-chiatrist. The term was most commonly applied to psychoneu-rotic depressions where the time sequence of emotional reac-tion to stress was obvious. The term "psychotic depressive reaction" as described here best applies to those depressions of psychotic proportion occurring in the patient for the first time, and in direct relation to some obvious environmental disturbance such as death of a loved one or loss of love, prop-erty, or status, together with predisposing physical factors such as a viral infection, drugs, malnutrition, or mutilating surgery. Impact of reality testing and marked functional inadequacy distinguish these conditions from depressive neuroses.

The prognosis is good in these cases due to the lack of major psychopathology in the premorbid personality. Where psy-chotherapy alone is unable to produce an adequate working through of the traumatic situation in a short time and the patient remains severely handicapped by symptoms, antide-pressant medication or a course of electroshock treatments is indicated.

SUGGESTED READINGS

Angst, J., Weis, P., Grof, P., Baastrup, P., and Schou, M.: Lithium pro-phylaxis in recurrent affective disorders, Brit. J. Psychiat. 116:604, 1970.

Ayd, F. J.: Recognizing the depressed patient, New York, 1961, Grune & Stratton, Inc.

Azima, H., and Glueck, B. C., Jr.: I, Psychotherapy of schizophrenia and manic depressive states; II, Contributions of basic sciences to psychiatry, Psychiat. Res. Rep. Amer. Psychiat. Ass. 17:1, 1963.

Bellak, L.: Manic-depressive psychosis and allied conditions, New York, 1952, Grune & Stratton, Inc.

Bratfos, O., and Haug, J. O.: The course of manic-depressive psychosis, Acta Psychiat. Scand. 44:89, 1968.

Bunney, W. D., Jr., Mason, J. W., Roatch, J. F., and Hamburg, D. A.: A psychoendocrine study of severe psychotic depressive crises, Amer. J. Psychiat. 122:72, 1965.

Davies, E. B., editor: Depression, Cambridge, England, 1964, Cambridge University Press.

Dovenmuehle, H., and Verwoerdt, A.: Physical illness and depressive symptomatology; II, Factors of length and severity of illness and frequency of hospitalization, J. Geront. 18:260, 1963.

Grinker, R. R., Sr., Miller, J., Sabshin, M., and Nunnally, J. C.: The phenomena of depressions, New York, 1961, Hoeber Medical Division, Harper & Row, Publishers.

Kraepelin, E.: Manic depressive insanity and paranoia, edited by G. M. Robertson, Edinburgh, 1921, E. & S. Livingstone, Ltd.

Lindemann, E.: Symptomatology and management of acute grief, Amer. J. Psychiat. 101:141, 1944.

Maddison, D., and Duncan, G. M., editors: Aspects of depressive illness, Edinburgh, 1965, E. & S. Livingstone, Ltd.

Mendelson, M.: Psychoanalytic concepts of depression, Springfield, Ill., 1960, Charles C Thomas, Publisher.

Parkes, C. M.: Recent bereavement as a cause of mental illness, Brit. J. Psychiat. 110:198, 1964.

Pitts, F. N., Meyer, J., Brooks, M., and Winokur, G.: Adult psychiatric illness assessed for childhood parental loss, and psychiatric illness in family members—a study of 748 patients and 250 controls, Amer. J. Psychiat. 121 (supp.): i, 1965.

Prien, R. F.: Lithium carbonate in psychiatry, Washington, D. C., 1970, American Psychiatric Association.

Schildkraut, J. J.: The catecholamine hypothesis of affective disorder: a review of supporting evidence, Amer. J. Psychiat. 122:509, 1965.

Stewart, M. A., Drake, F., and Winokur, G.: Depression among medically ill patients, Dis. Nerv. Sys. 26:479, 1965.

Winokur, G.: The natural history of affective disorders (manias and depressions), Seminars Psychiat. 2:451, 1970.

Winokur, G., Clayton, P., and Reich, T.: Manic depressive illness, St. Louis, 1969, The C. V. Mosby Co.

Schizophrenia

Kraepelin (1896) isolated a number of psychiatric symptoms present in maladies characterized by poor prognosis and grouped them under the heading *dementia praecox*. Bleuler felt this an awkward term for a condition in which patients are not necessarily "demented" and in which they do not all become ill early in life. The term *schizophrenia* was chosen because a "splitting of different psychic functions" seemed an important characteristic. The term "group of schizophrenias" is better, for it is apparent that the group includes several diseases.

Schizophrenia constitutes the largest group of severe behavior disorders in our culture. Its victims occupy about 25% of all the hospital beds in the United States. One person in 100 will some time be hospitalized for schizophrenia, and, due to an increase in marriage and reproduction among schizophrenics, this number is increasing. Usually experiencing the onset of personality disorganization in adolescence or in early adult life, the schizophrenic patient has a lifelong struggle to gain internal security and to maintain relationships with other persons. Although often unrecognized, severe emotional problems, including a tendency to react to stress by withdrawal into a world of fantasy, arise early in life and often are associated with a failure to establish security with parental figures.

Although seen throughout the world and among persons of all cultures, schizophrenia occurs most frequently in individuals from lower socioeconomic groups. As demonstrated by Faris and Dunham, it occurs in areas of high mobility and social disorganization. Although occurring in persons of all ages, it is seen primarily in persons between 20 and 40 years of age, with a peak in the 25- to 34-year-old group.

The etiology of schizophrenic conditions is today unknown. Many theories abound, including genetic, biochemical, psychological, and social formulations.

Major genetic evidence has come from twin studies of Kallman and others which show identical twins both affected in 60% to 85% of instances, whereas with fraternal twins, both are affected in only 14% of cases, or about the same as sibling expectancy. In the general population, the incidence approaches 1%. Currently, geneticists propose "a specific inherited disease due to a single mutant inherited gene, either recessive, dominant, or intermediate." *Incomplete penetrance* and *constitutional resistance* are mentioned.

Some propose that the genetic factor is manifested through an "inborn error of metabolism," and Heath and co-workers speak of "taraxein" as a substance which ". . . impairs enzymatic activity in a pathway related to the metabolism of amines." Injected into the body, it produces abnormal electrical potentials from the limbic area or other brain areas.

Osmond and others predicted an abnormal pathway of epinephrine metabolism, with the production of psychotomimetic substances, adrenochrome, and adrenolutin. Another unproven report related schizophrenia to serum copper in the form of the metalloprotein ceruloplasmin, a test for which was developed by Akerfeldt. Wooley and Gaddum proposed, and later abandoned, a theory of central serotonin deficiency in schizophrenia.

A number of workers have demonstrated the adverse effects of schizophrenic serum and urine upon rope climbing and other task-learning and retention abilities of rats, upon web spinning of spiders, and upon behavior of tropical fish, tadpole larvae, and cells in tissue culture. Considerable work has been done in an attempt to identify such substances in blood and other body fluids (Heath, Gottleib, Martin, Bercel). An odorous substance has been found in the sweat of schizophrenic patients by Kathleen Smith, while Kety and others, working on an intoxication theory, have studied possible disturbances in transmethylation as related to exacerbation of schizophrenic symptoms.

Psychodynamic formulations since Freud's suggestion of a narcissistic psychosis have focused on ego disturbance, on an inability to achieve self vs. object differentiation, and on the disruptive effect on ego development resulting from unusual sensitivity to sensory input. Mednick and Schulsinger have studied children with schizophrenic mothers and have suggested that, in addition to heredity, factors that are predisposing to a "high risk for schizophrenia" include a history of severe paranatal distress and a poorly controlled hyperresponsive autonomic nervous system. A further hypothesis is that the latter comes about from damage to the hippocampus from anoxia at birth. Shakow pointed out perceptual problems with the inability to long maintain a major set. Mahler demonstrated in children a "symbiotic schizophrenic-like psychosis" in which the child was unable to differentiate from the mother, while others speak of the schizophrenogenic mother as a rejecting or an overprotecting person or as one unable to understand her child. Social psychiatrists impugn the total family as manifesting disturbed communication and interaction, marital schism, and placing the child in the double bind so that he "can't win."

Lacking today is a single coherent, well-formulated, and

testable hypothesis; hence it is widely accepted that schizophrenic conditions result from some genotypically determined traits that are either suppressed or elicited by other genotypic or environmental factors to produce the symptoms of schizophrenia.

The term "schizophrenia" is commonly used therefore to include a group of psychoses with a course which is at times chronic and at times marked by intermittent attacks and which can stop or retrogress at any stage but does not permit full *restitutio ad integram*.

The disease is characterized by a specific type of alteration of thinking, feeling, and relation to the external world. The term "splitting of psychic functions" includes the lack of integration of different strivings and complexes. Rather, one set of complexes or ideas dominates the personality for a time, while other groups of ideas or drives are split off and seem partly or completely impotent. Often ideas are only partly worked out, fragments of ideas are connected in an illogical way to constitute a new idea, and concepts lose their completeness. The process of association often works with mere fragments of ideas and concepts. This results in associations which appear incoherent, bizarre, and utterly unpredictable. Often thinking stops in the middle of a thought (blocking), at least as far as it is a conscious process. Instead of a continuing thought, new ideas crop out which neither the patient nor the observer can bring into connection with the previous stream of thought (so-called tangential thinking). Genuine interference with perception, concentration, or memory is not demonstrable, although these functions suffer qualitative distortions. In the most severe cases emotional and affective expression seems to be completely lacking; in other cases the feelings expressed are inappropriate or of less than ordinary intensity (flattening). Ambivalence of emotion with the simultaneous occurrence of good and evil thoughts is common.

In addition to the above *primary features,* many accessory or *secondary symptoms* are present: hallucinations, delusions, confusion, stupor, manic or melancholic fluctuations, and catatonic symptoms. It is to be remembered that in schizophrenic patients outside hospitals these secondary symptoms are less apparent and may be absent altogether.

Psychoanalytic theory considers the logic of schizophrenic associations to be closely related to the associative patterns in dreams, fantasies, and the imaginative productions of young children. This type of thinking, which is believed to be present at the preverbal stage of personality development before the child has socialized concepts of interpreting the world, has been called *primary process thinking*. In it, important wishes, self-attitudes, and communication of even very mundane needs may be in highly symbolic form; this form tends to be consistent for each individual, so that intuitive, observant hospital personnel may gradually learn that a certain bizarre gesture or word actually is a distorted but specific request.

Types. The question is not one of defining and delimiting different disease entities but of grouping symptoms. Type classification is not static, for a case which begins as hebephrenic may be classified as paranoid several years later.

Schizophrenia—simple type

In simple schizophrenia the accessory symptoms are absent. The patients simply become affectively and intellectually weaker; will power and the capacity for work and caring for themselves diminish. They appear stupid and finally show the picture of severe dementia. The condition progresses slowly over the years and may never be seen as a medical problem. Eventual adjustment is more commonly that of a vagabond, transient laborer, or alcoholic than of a hospital inmate.

Schizophrenia—hebephrenic type

The term "hebephrenic" is used to designate those acute psychoses with subsequent deterioration and without catatonic or paranoid characteristics. Onset is usually between ages 12 and 25 years. The picture is sometimes characterized by pronounced feelings of mental and physical incapacity, various pathological sensations, and areas of hypochondriacal concern which gradually induce the patients to renounce all activities. There may be sexual preoccupation, emotional dulling, and clowning or grotesque silliness; there is concern with abstruse philosophical problems but without formation of clear-cut delusional symptoms.

Schizophrenia—catatonic type

Catatonic schizophrenia is distinguished by symptoms of stupor, mutism, negativism, impulsivity, and peculiar motility. In hyperkinetic phases (catatonic type, excited) patients are given to random impulsive activity, cursing, self-disregard, sleeplessness, and much repetitious overactivity. In akinetic phases (catatonic type, withdrawn) they may manifest cerea flexibilitas, failure to swallow, and command automaticity. Onset is usually acute and may alternate between mania and melancholia. There is marked improvement in over half of the cases followed eventually by new thrusts, with more deterioration each time.

Schizophrenia—paranoid type

In the beginning, patients state that things seem different. They do not feel as they used to; they become suspicious and overuse projection to the point that completely indifferent events are referred to themselves; they believe there is a conspiracy against them; voices talk about them and finally to them. This may lead to violent action, as in turning upon or fleeing from supposed tormentors. As the disorder tends toward chronicity patients may experience diminishing affective disturbances, ideas of omnipotence, and delusions of grandeur.

Acute schizophrenic episode

The term "acute schizophrenic episode" is used for patients who show an acute onset of schizophrenic symptoms, often associated with confusion, perplexity, ideas of reference, emotional turmoil, dreamlike dissociation, and excitement, depression, or fear. These attacks frequently subside in a few weeks. Usually such remissions are followed by recurrences, or the illness may take on the characteristics of catatonic, hebephrenic, or paranoid schizophrenia, and then the diagnosis should be accordingly changed.

Meduna and McCulloch delimited from the group of acute schizophrenics those patients who showed confusion and disorientation, raised body temperature, and a pseudodiabetic glucose tolerance curve. The prognosis of this condition (labeled oneirophrenia) is good, but the finding of a defect in sugar metabolism has not been replicated by some workers.

Mayer-Gross described an oneiroid dreamlike state of clouded consciousness occurring in acute schizophrenic breakdown.

Previously these conditions were included under the term "acute undifferentiated schizophrenia."

Schizophrenia—latent type

The latent category is used for those patients who have clear symptoms of schizophrenia but no history of a previous psychotic schizophrenic episode. Terms sometimes used for this group of patients include "prepsychotic," "pseudopsychopathic," or "borderline" schizophrenia.

Schizophrenia—residual type

The residual category is for patients who show signs of schizophrenia but who, following a psychotic episode, are no longer psychotic.

Schizoaffective type

The schizoaffective category is intended for those cases showing significant admixtures of schizophrenic and affective reactions. The mental content may be predominantly schizophrenic, with pronounced elation (schizoaffective, excited) or depression (schizoaffective, depressed). Patients may show predominantly affective changes with schizophrenic-like thinking or bizarre behavior. The prepsychotic personality may be at variance with expectations based on the presenting psychotic symptomatology. On prolonged observation, such patients usually prove to be basically schizophrenic in nature.

Schizophrenia—childhood type

The diagnosis of schizophrenia in children is being made with increasing frequency. The prognosis of this condition diagnosed before puberty is poor. This illness presents as atypical and withdrawn behavior (autistic child), alteration of motor behavior, failure to develop identification separate from the mother (symbiotic psychosis of Mahler), and as general unevenness, gross immaturity, and inadequacy in development. Communication is poor. There is difficulty in establishing good relationship with persons around them, and behavior is often repetitive and stereotyped. This may result in a picture of general mental retardation.

Schizophrenia—chronic undifferentiated type

The term "chronic undifferentiated" has been used to describe the disorder in patients who show mixed schizophrenic symptoms and definite schizophrenic thought, affect, and behavior but who cannot be clearly classified under one of the other types of schizophrenia.

Schizophrenia—other types

It is not unusual in a disease group as complex as schizophrenia that a variety of terms have been used as various workers emphasize different aspects of the multiple symptom pattern. Thus the term *periodic relapsing schizophrenia* has been applied to a group of cases originally studied by Gjessing. These patients are subject to exacerbations of the disease, occurring at more or less regular intervals and accompanied by alterations in nitrogen balance. Some of these cases have been reported to respond to treatment with thyroxin.

Another term widely used is *pseudoneurotic schizophrenia*. This concept was introduced by Hoch and Polatin to identify a large group of patients who frequently are misidentified as psychoneurotic but who in reality show the autistic and dereistic approach to life that is characteristic of schizophrenia. A diffuse withdrawal from life and an ambivalence are seen. These patients have an all-pervading anxiety, with many hysterical and bodily or vegetative symptoms. Phobias are often present. The patient may have psychotic episodes, between which the personality is well integrated; in such intervals diagnosis is difficult. The Rorschach test is reported to be of help in pointing out the thinking disorder in these cases. A sodium Amytal interview may release unexpected psychotic material.

Examination. There appears *behaviorally* to be a defect in the patient's awareness of social or interpersonal realities. It is helpful to think of the symptom picture as composed of (1) fundamental and (2) accessory symptoms.

1. Fundamentally, the disease process shows a defect in *associative* function: Associations lose their continuity; two ideas

are combined into one (condensation); there are clang associations, blocking, dearth of ideas, and pressure of thoughts;
paralogical thinking occurs in which ideas are linked by mere
grammatical form, similarity, habit, etc., rather than by logical
ordering. There is stereotypy, a clinging to one idea, senseless
naming or touching of all visible objects, and echolalia (repeating over and over what someone else has said). In the
realm of *affectivity* there may be marked emotional indifference, even to a complete imperviousness to pain and discomfort in severe cases; in milder cases there is seeming oversen-
sitivity of emotion but a lack of depth. Affective expression
may be inconsistent with thought or action or may alter rapidly because of haphazard accidental associations. Emotional
deterioration is apparent rather than real, as after decades of
emotional indifference affect can be produced in all its original vividness, even to long-past events. *Ambivalence* is commonly seen, often as the simultaneous appearance of thought
and counterthought. The simple functions of sensation, perception, memory, orientation, consciousness, and motility are
intact. Apparent alteration of these functions is based upon
negativism, indifference, reluctance to think, or randomness
of responses. Activity and behavior are marked by lack of interest, initiative, and definite goals and by inadequate adaptation to the environment. Stereotypy is characteristic and
unpleasant stubbornness frequent. There is a limitation of
contacts with the outside world, often with an apparently
complete absorption with autistic fantasy. Despite the latter,
outside events may register in memory with remarkable clarity, and patients may later answer questions which they did
not seem to comprehend when asked.

2. It is the accessory symptoms that usually lead to social
difficulties and give the disease its external stamp. *Hallucinations* are most frequently auditory and of a persecutory nature. Hallucinations of body sensations, taste, and smell are
common but tactile and visual uncommon. *Delusions* are usually persecutory, but commonly seen too are those of grandeur,
of inferiority, or of being loved or defiled or diseased. These
are rarely well systematized. Mutually contradictory beliefs
can be held and, although the self remains alien to the delusion, they are impervious to logic. *Memory disturbances* may

include amnesias, hyperesthesia, and déjà vu type phenomena. The patient may act as two persons, either simultaneously or alternately, or may incorporate all or part of the behavior of some other person. *Speech* and *writing* show abnormalities such as blocking, poverty of ideas, incoherence, clouding, delusional content, and emotional anomalies. Mutism may last for decades. Speech may show affected mannerisms. There may be verbigeration, distortions similar to dreams, with fusion of ideas (condensation), substitutions, distortions, accidental associations, and word salad. Writing shows bizarre changing of margins, random repetition of words, letters, and sentences, queer designs, shapes, and curliques. The so-called *catatonic symptoms* of behavior can occur in any type of schizophrenia and consist of catalepsy (rigidity and waxy flexibility of psychic quality); stupor (intense inhibition, blocking, lack of interest, loss into own autisms); hyperkinesis; stereotypies of speech, movement, expression, and even of hallucinations (all of which tend to become abbreviated with time); mannerisms (stilted, pompous, mocking, etc.); negativism (which may be passive, active, or a denial of own inner striving and functions); and echopraxia and command automatism (in which patient feels his thoughts, actions, etc. are being forced by someone else).

The findings of the *physical* examination are nonspecific, but it is not uncommon that schizophrenics have an asthenic habitus, with pale blotchy skin, and poor oily complexion. They are unkempt and frequently underweight but may show either anorexia or bulimia. There is not infrequently autonomic instability shown by cardiovascular variations and hyper- or hypoactivity of sweat glands. Impotence and menstrual irregularities are common. There are poor motor coordination, awkward gait, laughing and crying spells, and fits of rigidity. *Laboratory* evidence of mild thyroid, adrenal, or liver dysfunction is variable. *Psychological* tests, when confirmed clinically, are of great assistance. Disturbances in abstract thinking with a tendency to overgeneralization may be noted on intelligence tests. Projective tests may speed thorough clinical understanding by uncovering bizarre or contaminated (e.g., "moss growing on a dog") associations, delusions, fears, motivations, and ways of handling sexual or aggressive feelings toward specific individuals in the patient's life. Psychological testing may clearly bring out the highly symbolic nature of the patient's mental productions as well as the failure to distinguish between what is self and not self (loss of ego boundaries).

Prognosis. Langfeld has proposed that there are two types of schizophrenia: *process schizophrenia,* in which the illness progresses inevitably toward a final state of deterioration, and *reactive schizophrenia,* with onset in temporal relationship to a traumatic event in persons with better premorbid adjustment and with more favorable outcome of the illness. In patients ill less than 1 year, most clinicians believe that a history of an acute onset, the presence of catatonic symptoms, or the presence of much affective disturbance augurs a good deal of hope for the future. On the other hand, a sickness beginning at a young age and progressing slowly without much overt anxiety bodes ill for the future. The following data are illustrative.

	Remissions
Hospitalized less than 3 months, first illness	75%
Hospitalized less than 1 year, first illness	50%
Hospitalized 1 to 2 years	10%
Hospitalized over 2 years	1% to 2%

Treatment. As the etiology of schizophrenia is not known, so the treatment must remain empirical. Experience has demonstrated, however, that many patients will improve with a combined approach utilizing organic, psychological, and environmental treatments tailored carefully to the individual needs of each patient. No truly satisfactory remedy exists to repair the devastating personality damage encountered in many of these individuals. With the exception of those hospitalized schizophrenics who make a rapid improvement with nursing care, pharmacological treatment, electroshock, or insulin and those ambulatory schizophrenics who happily discover a properly supportive environment, these patients require long supportive care. Great skill is often needed to establish and maintain the close doctor-patient relationship necessary for successful management of these patients. Many a psychiatrist becomes discouraged, however, by the slow progress, deep hostility, and strong self-punishing tendencies seen in schizophrenics. There is impressive evidence that highly structured psychotherapy is of very little use with schizophrenic patients. At times when the schizophrenic is freely communicative, the psychotherapist must beware lest fascination with deciphering the intricate and emotionally rich implications of his patient's words distract attention from the often more important interpersonal feelings being masked by the delusions.

In evaluating disturbed psychiatric patients, too much weight must not be placed upon any single symptom. Thorough anamnestic study of the case with attention to special personality assets as well as liabilities will lead to a more successful therapeutic plan than will rules of thumb.

General agreement exists in regard to the importance of therapy as a "growing up" experience during which the patient gains a firmer grasp of the real nature of human relationships, gives up his severe distortions of the world about him, and achieves a more honest appreciation of his own latent capacities. Throughout months of therapy, frightening sexual or aggressive fantasies may form the main content of interviews. Opinions vary as to the proper technique for dealing with this material. Followers of Rosen advocate active participation in the patient's delusional system, forming an immediate intimacy with the patient and using schizophrenic symbolic language in disagreeing, questioning, or interpreting. Fromm-Reichmann advocated a more conservative, patient approach, in which the therapist attempts to understand the changing meanings and goals of the patient's pathological behavior as the latter tests whether the therapist will abandon him, show disrespect, or confirm his fears in other ways. Interpretation with schizophrenics focuses heavily upon the genetics of symptomatic behavior rather than its meaning. Unlike neurotics, these patients tend not to repress the meaning of their symptoms. Still another approach is to view the patient's distorted behaviors and fantasies as products of the disease, to be forgotten as soon as possible. In this role the therapist, while empathizing with and accepting the patient's bizarre feelings, takes a very down-to-earth attitude about them and continually encourages the patient in a supportive manner to begin to deal more directly with the world around him.

An aspect of therapy which many a time determines success or failure is the way the patient's environment is handled. Where indicated, the physician should not fail to help friends, relatives, or employers to react with understanding to the patient's behavior; more often than not, thorough treatment will involve at some time social case work with an important member of the schizophrenic's own family.

Aid should be provided toward an increasingly healthy schedule of living. In keeping with the patient's capacities, some type of supervised activity and socialization program should be instituted. Occupational therapy and group therapy aimed at actively working through the behavior aberrations at the moment they occur are valuable.

The phenothiazine tranquilizers and other ataractics have produced as marked a change in the management of schizophrenic patients as did ECT with psychotic depression. Although these drugs seem to have some antipsychotic action, in the main, they act as nonsedative tranquilizers. With relief from agitation and anxiety, the disturbing secondary symptoms of the illness become less prominent and patients are able to better adapt their behavior to the demands of the environment. In some reported cases the quieting effect has permitted the patient to live a sheltered life in the community despite the continued presence of delusions and hallucinations. In other cases as the patient becomes less agitated, delusions and hallucinations seem to diminish in importance and even disappear. Due to the fluctuant nature of the illness control studies of drug therapy are difficult, but they are at this point a necessity if a rational approach to chemotherapy is to develop. Certainly today, however, every schizophrenic patient should be given an adequate trial on pharmacological treatment before such measures as regressive shock treatment are considered. For example, chlorpromazine may be given in doses of 600 to 2000 mg. daily, later tapered off to 600 to 800 mg., and continued for several months or years, as need be. Other phrenotropic drugs are used in similar fashion. (See tables, pp. 308 to 319.

Although there is considerable talk about target symptoms and the therapeutic merits of one phenothiazine over another, there is little to guide one in selecting from among the various phenothiazines for the specific symptom picture of any given patient. Usually the drug preference is the physician's, and a change is made only if untoward complications arise. The usual error is failure to give a sufficiently large dose for a sufficient length of time. Another common mistake is to add a similar drug to one inadequately administered and another to that, etc. ("polypharmacy").

During periods when the disorder is aggravated, somatic therapies are often of value. Electroconvulsive therapy (10 to 20 treatments), regressive shock treatments (1 to 3 convulsions daily until the desired state of regression is achieved), electronarcosis, or insulin coma therapy (40 to 100 comas) may be used.

Electroconvulsive therapy has the greatest hope of success in recent illnesses which display depressive or catatonic symptoms. It is reported that about 40% of patients who have failed to respond to electroconvulsive therapy will improve with a course of insulin comas. Lobotomy is occasionally tried in patients incapacitated over 2 years who have failed to respond to other techniques. Such surgery, however, has for the most part fallen out of favor and, in any case, should not be used in the absence of facilities for thorough rehabilitation.

SUGGESTED READINGS

Arieti, S.: Interpretation of schizophrenia, New York, 1955, Basic Books, Inc., Publishers.

Artiss, K. L.: Milieu therapy in schizophrenia, New York, 1962, Grune & Stratton, Inc.

Astrup, C.: Schizophrenia—conditional reflex studies, Springfield, Ill., 1962, Charles C Thomas, Publisher.

Astrup, C., Fossum, A., and Holmboe, R.: Prognosis in functional psychoses, Springfield, Ill., 1962, Charles C Thomas, Publisher.

Bellak, L.: Schizophrenia, New York, 1958, Grune & Stratton, Inc.

Betz, B.: Strategic conditions in the psychotherapy of persons with schizophrenia, Amer. J. Psychiat. 107:203, 1950.

Bleuler, E.: Dementia praecox or the group of schizophrenias, New York, 1951, International Universities Press, Inc.

Brown, G. W., Bone, M., Dalison, B., and Wing, J. K.: Schizophrenia and social care, London, 1966, Oxford University Press.

Burton, A., editor: Psychotherapy of the psychoses, New York, 1961, Basic Books, Inc., Publishers.

Cole, J.: A unique study which may never be repeated. In May, P. R. A.: Treatment of schizophrenia—a comparative study of five treatment methods, New York, 1968, Science House, Inc.

Cumming, J., and Cumming, E.: Ego and milieu: theory and practice of environmental therapy, Chicago, 1966, Aldine Press.

Danziger, L., and Kindwall, J. A.: Treatment of periodic relapsing catatonia, Dis. Nerv. Syst. 15:35, 1954.

Davis, J. M.: Efficacy of tranquilizing and antidepressant drugs, Arch. Gen. Psychiat. 13:552, 1965.

Ekstein, R., and Wallerstein, J.: Observations on the psychotherapy of borderline and psychotic children. The psychoanalytic study of the child, New York, 1956, International Universities Press, Inc., vol. 2.

Engelhardt, D. M., and Freedman, N.: Maintenance drug therapy: the schizophrenic patient in the community, Int. Psychiat. Clin. 2: 933, 1965.

Essen-Mollere, I.: Twin research in psychiatry, Int. J. Psychiat. 1:466, 1965.

Fish, B., Shapiro, T., Halpern, F., and Wile, R.: The prediction of schizophrenia in infancy: a ten year follow-up report of neurological and psychological development, Amer. J. Psychiat. 121:68, 1965.

Fish, F. J.: Schizophrenia, Bristol, 1962, John Wright & Sons.

Frosch, J.: The psychotic character: clinical psychiatric considerations, Psychiat. Quart. 38:81, 1964.

Gjessing, R.: Disturbances of somatic function in catatonia with a periodic course and their compensation, J. Ment. Sci. 84:608, 1938.

Goldberg, S. C.: Prediction of improvement in schizophrenics under four phenothiazines, Arch. Gen. Psychiat. 16:107, 1967.

Hamilton, D., and Wall, J.: The hospital treatment of dementia praecox, Amer. J. Psychiat. 105:346, 1948.

Heston, L. L., and Denney, D.: Interactions between early life experience and biological factors in schizophrenia, J. Psychiat. Res. 6:363, 1968.

Hoch, P. H., and Cattell, J. P.: The diagnosis of pseudoneurotic schizophrenia, Psychiat. Quart. 33:17, 1959.

Itil, T. M.: Elektroencephalographische Studien bei psychosen und psychotropen Medikamenten, Istanbul, 1964, Ahmet Sait Matbaasi.

Jackson, D. D., editor: The etiology of schizophrenia, New York, 1960, Basic Books, Inc., Publishers.

Jacobson, E.: The self and the object world, New York, 1964, International Universities Press, Inc.

Kalinowsky, L. B., and Hoch, P. H.: Somatic treatments in psychiatry, New York, 1961, Grune & Stratton, Inc.

Kety, S.: Biochemical theories of schizophrenia, I and II, Science 129:1528, 1590, 1959.

Kraepelin, E.: Psychiatrie, ein Lehrbuch für Studierende und Arzte, ed. 8, Leipzig, 1913, Barth, vol. 3.

Lindelius, R.: A study of schizophrenia, Acta Psychiat. Scand. (Supp. 216): 1, 1970.

Mandell, A. J.: Impasse resolution with the schizophrenic patient, Arch. Gen. Psychiat. 8:486, 1963.

May, P. R. A.: Treatment of schizophrenia, New York, 1968, Science House, Inc.

Mayer-Gross, W.: Diagnostic significance of certain tests of carbohydrate metabolism in psychiatric patients and the question of "oneirophrenia," J. Ment. Sci. 98:683, 1952.

Mednick, S. A.: Breakdown in individuals at high risk for schizophrenia: possible pre-dispositional paranatal factors, Ment. Hyg. 54:50, 1970.

Mednick, S. A., Mora, E., Schulsinger, F., and Mednick, B.: Paranatal conditions and infant development in children with schizophrenic parents, Soc. Biol. 18:S-103, 1971.

Pasamanick, B., Scarpitti, F. R., and Dinitz, S.: Schizophrenics in the community, New York, 1967, Appleton-Century-Crofts.

Pollin, W., Allen, M. G., Hoffer, A., Stabenau, J. R., and Hrubec, Z.: Psychopathology in 15,900 pairs of Veteran twins: evidence for a genetic factor in the pathogenesis of schizophrenia and its relative absence in psychoneurosis, Amer. J. Psychiat. **126:**597, 1969.

Robins, E., and Guze, S. B.: Establishment of diagnostic validity in psychiatric illness: its application to schizophrenia, Amer. J. Psychiat. **126:**983, 1970.

Rosenthal, D.: Sex distribution and the severity of illness among samples of schizophrenic twins, J. Psychiat. Res. **1:**26, 1961.

Sargant, W., and Slater, E.: An introduction to physical methods of treatment in psychiatry, ed. 4, Baltimore, 1964, The Williams & Wilkins Co.

Shakow, D.: Segmental set—a theory of the formal psychological deficit in schizophrenia, Arch. Gen. Psychiat. **61:**1, 1962.

Shakow, D.: Psychological deficit in schizophrenia, Behav. Sci. **8:**275, 1963.

Smith, K., Pumphrey, M., and Hall, J. C.: The "last straw": the decisive incident resulting in the request for hospitalization in 100 schizophrenic patients, Amer. J. Psychiat. **120:**228, 1963.

Smith, K., Thompson, G. F., and Koster, H. D.: Sweat in schizophrenic patients: identification of the odorous substance, Science **166:**398, 1969.

Spandoni, A. J., and Smith, J. A.: Milieu therapy in schizophrenia, Arch. Gen. Psychiat. **20:**547, 1969.

Stabenau, J. R., Pollin, W., and Allen, M. G.: Twin studies in schizophrenia and neurosis, Seminars Psychiat. **2:**65, 1970.

Sullivan, H. S.: Schizophrenia as a human process, New York, 1962, W. W. Norton & Co., Inc.

Vaillant, G. E.: Prospective prediction of schizophrenia remission, Arch. Gen. Psychiat. **11:**509, 1964.

Vetter, H. J.: Language behavior in schizophrenia: selected readings in research and theory, Springfield, Ill., 1968, Charles C Thomas, Publisher.

Wing, J. K.: Early childhood autism; clinical, educational and social aspects, New York, 1966, Pergamon Press, Inc.

Paranoid states

The paranoid conditions are disorders of thinking characterized by suspiciousness, blaming others (projection), and paralogical reasoning to the point of delusion formation. Such thinking is seen at times in many persons (paranoid personalities) and may occur as a prominent symptom in all of the major psychoses and occasionally in the psychoneuroses and character disorders. When paranoid symptoms occur in the course of some other psychosis (senile psychosis, paranoid type; schizophrenia, paranoid type; alcoholic psychosis, paranoid type; etc.) the symptoms of the accompanying psychosis blend with the paranoid features. In the schizophrenic and organic types of paranoid conditions derogatory hallucinations may be an outstanding feature. To designate those paranoid schizophrenics who fail to show diffuse personality dilapidation, the term "paraphrenia" was used by Kraepelin.

Paranoia. True paranoia (monomania or litigious paranoia) designates only those rare cases in which highly systematized delusions of insidious onset exist along with the preservation of other personality functions. The intricate and elaborate paranoid system of these patients often develops insidiously, proceeding at first logically from the misinterpretation of an actual event. Individual patients may exhibit both persecutory and grandiose traits and often believe themselves to be endowed with superior abilities. In spite of the chronic course, the condition does not seem to interfere with the rest of the patient's thinking.

Involutional paranoid state. This term is used to designate delusion formation having its onset in the involutional period. The characteristic thought disorders of schizophrenia are lacking although depressive content may indicate that it is in reality only a paranoid variety of the involutional psychosis.

Other paranoid states. Characterized by paranoid delusions, these may occur lacking the logical nature of systematization seen in paranoia and yet not manifesting the bizarre fragmentation and deterioration of the schizophrenic reactions. Such states are likely to be of relatively short duration although they may become persistent and chronic.

Etiology. The etiology of the paranoid reactions is not known, although constitutional factors have been believed to be important. In Freudian theory, developed from the famous Schreber case, paranoid reactions have been considered to be defenses against unconscious homosexuality. Recent studies have not supported this point of view. Freud has hypothesized a mechanism in which "I love him" is denied by "No, I hate him" and the projective accompaniment "He hates me." More recently others have conjectured that paranoid symptoms may be a defense against the wish to kill, the wish to receive passively oral or anal pleasures, the fear of being damaged, or a variety of other such unconscious attitudes.

These syndromes occur more frequently in males than females, having an onset usually during or after the third decade of life. They make up no more than 10% of mental hospital admissions.

Prognosis. In early cases prognosis is guarded; in long-standing cases it is poor.

Treatment. These patients in general are resistant to psychotherapy although in cases of mild degree remissions may apparently follow an explanatory supportive type of psychotherapy by a physician who can engage the patient's trust. Hospitalization is necessary for those who become intensely litigious, assaultive, or homicidal. Treatment with tranquilizers may be of use in relieving anxiety, agitation, and the drive to assaultiveness.

SUGGESTED READINGS

Arthur, A. Z.: Theories and explanations of delusions: a review, Amer. J. Psychiat. 121:105, 1964.

Bieber, I., et al.: Homosexuality: a psychoanalytic study of male homosexuals, New York, 1962, Basic Books, Inc., Publishers.

Bonner, H.: The problem of diagnosis in paranoic disorder, Amer. J. Psychiat. 107:677, 1951.

Burton, A., editor: Psychotherapy of the psychoses, New York, 1961, Basic Books, Inc., Publishers.

Cameron, N.: Personality development in psychopathology, Boston, 1963, Houghton Mifflin Co.

Freedman, N., Cutler, R., Engelhardt, D. M., and Margolis, R.: On the modification of paranoid symptomatology, J. Nerv. Ment. Dis. 144:29, 1967.

Freud, S.: Psychoanalytic notes upon an autobiographical account of a case of paranoia. In Collected papers, London, 1950, Hogarth Press, Ltd., vol. 3.

Kitay, P. M.: Symposium on reinterpretations of the Schreber case: for its theory of paranoia, Int. J. Psychoanal. 44:191, 1963.

Klaf, F. S.: Female homosexuality and paranoid schizophrenia, Arch. Gen. Psychiat. 4:84, 1961.

Liber, B.: Elusive mental cases—slight paranoia, New York J. Med. 50:435, 1950.

Ovesey, L.: Pseudohomosexuality, the paranoid mechanism, and paranoia, Psychiatry 18:163, 1955.

Retterstol, N.: Paranoid and paranoiac psychoses, Springfield, Ill., 1966, Charles C Thomas, Publisher.

Revitch, E.: The problem of conjugal paranoia, Dis. Nerv. Syst. 15:271, 1954.

Rosen, H., and Kiene, H.: Paranoia and paranoiac reaction type, Dis. Nerv. Syst. 11:330, 1946.

Rosen, H., and Kiene, H.: Early reversible paranoic reaction, J. Nerv. Ment. Dis. 109:291, 1949.

14
Neuroses

Definition. Psychoneuroses are personality disturbances which show neither gross disturbances of reality testing nor severely antisocial behavior and which seem determined mostly by environmental factors. These factors may be separated for convenience into two categories: those environmental influences acting on the infant or child, which produce a defect in personality development, and those influences immediately preceding an exacerbation of psychoneurotic symptoms, i.e., the precipitating stress.

With onset often in early adult life, these conditions tend to be chronic, the patient usually from very early life presenting evidence of periodic or constant maladjustment of varying degree. Symptoms are at their peak in the period of active reproductive activity and social responsibility. Men and women are affected about equally, although, for specific psychoneurotic syndromes, sex differences exist. Disturbances related to interpersonal conflict or sexual functioning are common. Many of the symptoms seen in this group are expressed through the autonomic nervous system. The degree to which symptoms interfere with activities varies. Some patients retreat into complete invalidism; others lead an outwardly healthy existence, successfully concealing their illness from acquaintances. Although most never require hospitalization, at times a stay within the hospital may be advisable to alleviate severe tensional crises.

Although Sigmund Freud, father of dynamic psychiatry, postulated constitutional and biological factors underlying neurotic illness, the nature and importance of such organic neurotic predisposition have only recently been investigated. It is now known from both animal and human studies that genetic and fetal conditions can influence later tension level, irritability, and other behaviors, such as degree of persistence in overcoming obstacles, related to adaptation. For the present, therapy of these conditions is based almost entirely upon attempts to modify neurotic behavior patterns through psychotherapy founded upon theoretical notions of the importance of previous life experience and current social stress as the etiological determinants. These postulations concern the psychiatrist with modifying learned patterns of feelings, attitudes, defenses against anxiety, and modes of problem solving which developed during infancy and childhood and which appear inappropriately as neurotic or immature adjustments to the demands of adult life.

Classification. There is considerable variance in the classification systems used to describe psychoneurotic disorders, although a dozen or more separate categories have found some acceptance. Anxiety neurosis, hysteria, obsessive-compulsive neurosis, and neurotic depression seem to be the most universally accepted forms in practice; even these may at times have sufficient symptoms in common to warrant a more general term. Formerly the label *mixed psychoneurosis* was utilized, qualified by additional terms such as "with hysterical features," "with obsessive features," or "with depression and anxiety," etc. Somewhat more recently the A. P. A. used the concept of neurotic reactions to life stress and specified a classification based upon (1) anxiety reaction, (2) phobic reaction, (3) dissociative reaction and conversion reaction, (4) obsessive-compulsive reaction, and (5) depressive reaction. Currently the A. P. A. nomenclature has reverted to the classical notion of neurosis, specifying eight major types with two subtypes within hysterical neurosis.

The defense mechanisms serve as a basis for symptom formation. For, although anxiety may be dispelled in this manner, the mechanism of defense itself now forms a means by which the conflict is expressed and neurotic symptoms develop.

The subject of neurosis is usually discussed within the framework of psychoanalytic theory. In this view, *anxiety re-*

action (in Freud's original thinking "anxiety hysteria") is the simplest kind of psychoneurosis, in which uncomfortable inner tension appears in the presence of certain objects, places, persons, or animals. It is seen in childhood as the first neurotic reaction that children experience. It has been postulated that unclear or partial memories of events which arouse intense emotion but are not understood, as, for example, the sexual act between the parents (the primal scene), observation that girls lack a penis (the castration fears), etc., form permanent unconscious fixations which lie at the basis of these displacements.

The concept of "actual neurosis," now very rarely used, refers to Freud's early oversimplified notion—later discarded—that some cases of anxiety reaction are caused by lack of sexual gratification or other meaningful emotional outlets.

Conversion hysteria is felt to have its origin in the childhood Oedipal conflict (child's love fixated on one parent, with jealousy toward parent of opposite sex). It differs from anxiety hysteria in that the anxiety is "converted" into a dysfunction that symbolically represents the conflicts; for example, a paralyzed limb may act as a defense against feared or secretly desired hostile aggressive action. Hysterics may also experience episodes of *dissociation,* in which confusion, amnesia, or multiple personality serves to defend against awareness of the anxiety-laden conflicts.

Closely related to hysteria is the *phobic neurosis,* in which the anxiety, instead of being converted into a physical symptom, is experienced as fear but as fear removed (displaced) in space and time and related to apparently innocuous objects or places. Although similar to anxiety hysterics, phobic patients are distinguished by their prominent use of avoidance (avoidance of the feared objects or places) as a way of escaping the experience of anxiety.

Obsessive-compulsive neuroses arise as an outcome of fixation in the anal stage of development. The anal character traits of orderliness, frugality, and obstinacy are clearly seen.

In patients with psychoneurotic *depression,* deeply helpless and dependent feelings are common, although hysterical or obsessive-compulsive dynamisms—or both—may be observed also. The diagnosis is based primarily upon the prominence of depressive symptoms.

SUGGESTED READINGS

Alvarez, W. C.: The neuroses, Philadelphia, 1951, W. B. Saunders Co.

Cameron, N., and Margaret, A.: Behavior pathology, Boston, 1951, Houghton Mifflin Co.

Denker, P. G.: Results of treatment of psychoneuroses by the general practitioner. A follow-up study of 500 patients, Arch. Neurol. Psychiat. **57:**504, 1947, including the discussion.

English, O., and Pearson, G.: Emotional problems of living, ed. 3, New York, 1963, W. W. Norton & Co., Inc.

Eysenck, H. J., editor: Behavior therapy and the neuroses, New York, 1960, Pergamon Press, Inc.

Fenichel, O.: The psychoanalytic theory of neurosis, New York, 1945, W. W. Norton & Co., Inc.

Freud, S.: The basic writings of Sigmund Freud (translated by A. A. Brill), New York, 1938, Modern Library, Inc., p. 1001.

Freud, S.: Collected papers, London, 1924-1952, Hogarth Press, Ltd., vols. 1 to 5.

Hoch, P. H., and Zubin, J.: Depression, New York, 1954, Grune & Stratton, Inc.

Horney, K.: Neurosis and human growth, New York, 1950, W. W. Norton & Co., Inc.

Knight, R. P.: Evaluation of the results of psychoanalytic therapy, Amer. J. Psychiat. **98:**434, 1941.

Laughlin, H. P.: The neuroses in clinical practice, Philadelphia, 1956, W. B. Saunders Co.

McNair, D. M., and Lorr, M.: An analysis of mood in neurotics, J. Abnorm. Soc. Psychol. **69:**620, 1964.

Ross, T. A.: The common neuroses, Baltimore, 1937, The Williams & Wilkins Co.

Thorpe, J. G., Schmidt, E., Brown, P. T., and Castell, D.: Aversion relief therapy: a new method for general application, Behav. Res. Ther. **2:**71, 1964.

Ulett, P. C., and Gildea, E. F.: Survey of surgical procedures in psychoneurotic women, J.A.M.A. **143:**960, 1950.

Anxiety neurosis

Symptoms of anxiety occur when the subject is faced with real or symbolic danger. This apprehension is expressed through widespread autonomic discharge. Although it occurs from time to time in all human beings, a diffuse free-floating anxiety or readiness for anxiety may in some patients lead to the syndrome of continuous tension or recurrent exacerbations. This is usually seen in young adults and is known as anxiety neurosis. Beginning with Beard's description of nervous exhaustion in 1869, over the years various terms have been applied to the symptom complex: "neurocirculatory asthenia," "hyperventilation syndrome," "effort syndrome," "vasomotor neurosis," and "anxiety tension state."

It is usual to discover that these patients early learned to fear intense affects of anger, hate, love, or erotic attraction. In the course of daily living when these feelings would tend to be aroused the substitutes of intense confusion and a sense of loss of self-control, as well as autonomic discharge phenomena, were utilized.

Anamnesis. The patient comes to the doctor with the *chief complaint* being spells of dyspnea, palpitation, irritability, dizziness, insomnia, faintness, weakness, chest pain, trembling, headache, or "attacks." *Past history* reveals that first symptoms usually appear in the second decade of life and may be of dramatic onset associated with stress situations, muscular exertion, pregnancy, or military service. Often beginning with a choking sensation, these attacks precede fears of fainting, dying, or "losing the mind." Crowded busses, movies, or public gatherings are often the setting for the attacks. Increasing irritability and intolerance for noises and for children and wife may precipitate the need for hospitalization. *Family history* may reveal a high incidence of this disorder in the immediate family. It is important to differentiate anxiety neurosis from acute reactions to intense life stress in otherwise well-adapted persons as well as from schizoid or borderline schizophrenic patients. In the former condition, an acute onset close in time to severe trauma (death of a loved one, wartime fear, exposure to tornado or other sudden unanticipated natural disaster) in a previously adequate personality is characteristic. An anxious schizoid personality, on the other hand, may require careful study over an extended period to distinguish it from anxiety neurosis.

Examination. The patient, *behaviorally,* is fidgety and apprehensive and often mildly depressed. His conversation is filled with worries and concerns over heart, lungs, inability to concentrate, and other symptoms. *Physically,* slight inconstant tachycardia, tachypnea, flushed face and neck, moist cool palms, tremor of fingers, and brisk tendon reflexes are seen.

Laboratory examination shows that basal metabolic rate is normal or raised due to motor restlessness; sighing respirations may be visualized on a breathing tracing.

Prognosis. In only a small percentage does the neurosis interfere with general life pursuits. The illness may be of brief duration or proceed for many years with exacerbations or remissions.

Treatment. Complete medical work-up to reassure the patient and physician at the beginning of the treatment.

Explain the nature of the disease and symptoms to the patient.

Encourage the patient to return to a regular balance of work and play.

Provide psychotherapy with the working through of anxiety-provoking conflicts in the context of present meaningful relationships.

Make judicious use of sedatives and such psychopharmacological agents as meprobamate (Miltown, Equanil), chlordiazepoxide (Librium), diazepam (Valium), and others.

SUGGESTED READINGS

DiMascio, A., and Barrett, J.: Comparative effects of oxazepam in "high" and "low" anxious student volunteers, Psychosomatics 6:298, 1965.

Freud, S.: The problem of anxiety, Albany, N. Y., 1936, The Psychoanalytic Quarterly Press, and New York, 1936, W. W. Norton & Co., Inc.

Gellhorn, E.: The neurophysiological basis of anxiety. A hypothesis, Perspect. Biol. Med. 8:488, 1965.

Hoch, P., and Zubin, J.: Anxiety, New York, 1950, Grune & Stratton, Inc.

Lehmann, H. E., and Ban, T. A.: Pharmacotherapy of tension and anxiety, Springfield, Ill., 1970, Charles C Thomas, Publisher.

Leighton, D., et al.: The character of danger, New York, 1963, Basic Books, Inc., Publishers.

Levitt, E., Persky, H., and Brady, J.: Hypnotic induction of anxiety, Springfield, Ill., 1964, Charles C Thomas, Publisher.

Masserman, J. H.: Anxiety: protean source of communication. In Masserman, J. H., editor: Science and psychoanalysis, New York, 1965, Grune & Stratton, Inc., vol. 8.

Meares, A.: The management of the anxious patient, Philadelphia, 1963, W. B. Saunders Co.

Uhlenhuth, E. H., Covi, L., and Lipman, R. S.: Indications for minor tranquilizers in anxious outpatients. In Black, P., editor: Drugs and the brain, Baltimore, 1969, The Johns Hopkins Press.

Wheeler, E. O., White, P. D., Reed, E. W., and Cohen, M. E.: Neurocirculatory asthenia (anxiety neurosis, effort syndrome, neurasthenia): a twenty-year follow-up study of 173 patients, J.A.M.A. 142:878, 1950.

Wittenborn, J. R.: The clinical psychopharmacology of anxiety, Springfield, Ill., 1969, Charles C Thomas, Publisher.

Hysterical neurosis

Hysteria is the name applied to a disease or personality disorder characterized by an involuntary psychogenic loss or disorder of function. Symptoms characteristically begin and end suddenly in emotionally charged situations and are symbolic of the underlying conflicts. Often they can be modified by suggestion alone. It apparently occurs more frequently in women and the symptoms are limited typically to impairment of motor or sensory functions (blindness, paresthesia, paralysis, etc.) but may also include psychological dysfunction (dissociation) and autonomic disturbance. The term "hysterical" is not uncommonly applied to describe the occurrence of isolated conversion symptoms appearing either alone or in company with other types of psychiatric disorder.

Types. The major types of hysterical neurosis include *hysterical neurosis, conversion type,* and *hysterical neurosis, dissociative type.* In the conversion type special senses or voluntary nervous system are affected, causing such symptoms as blindness, deafness, anosmia, anesthesias, paresthesias, paralyses, ataxias, akinesias, and dyskinesias. The patient often shows an inappropriate lack of concern about these symptoms which may actually provide secondary gains by winning him sympathy or relieving him of unpleasant responsibilities. This type of hysterical neurosis must be distinguished from psychophysiological disorders, which are mediated by the autonomic nervous system, from malingering, which is done consciously, and from neurological lesions, which cause anatomically circumscribed symptoms. In the other major type of hysterical neurosis, the dissociative type, the alterations may occur in the patient's state of consciousness or in his identity, with production of such symptoms as amnesia, somnambulism, fugue, and multiple personality.

Hysterical disorders in which elements of injury and compensation seem to play a role in producing and maintaining the symptoms have been termed "compensation neurosis" by some authors. In these patients the symptoms seem to be maintained or exaggerated by the fact that the social environment rewards the symptoms. They are found in Veterans Hospitals and among Workmen's Compensation cases.

Anamnesis. Despite the fact that the *complaints* elicited by a careful history are extremely numerous, paradoxically the patient may come to the clinic only under the pressure of relatives and frequently shows a strange indifference ("la belle indifférence") to her usually dramatic handicaps. The *history* is one of recurrent accidents, illnesses, operations, sexual and menstrual difficulties, as well as gross interpersonal abnormalities. A majority suffer from frigidity, dyspareunia, and difficulties during pregnancy. A previously conditioned sensitivity to illness often leads to prolonged convalescence and tendency to invalidism. Unlike obsessional patients, hysterics tend to be unaware of the ideas underlying their feelings and actions. Symptoms usually have onset in early adolescence or soon after marriage although history of sexual misunderstanding and conflict arising before the age of 7 years may be eventually elicited during psychotherapy.

The overt interpersonal difficulties and sexual symptoms of the hysteric stem from defensive manipulation of others, which is experienced as safer (more under control by the patient) than free expression of feelings directly. Underlying these difficulties, it is usual to discover a type of basic distrust of friendship, love relations, or comfortable intimacy with another. This deep distrust of closeness, while somewhat similar to that observed in the borderline or schizophrenic patient, is accompanied by less disorganization of the personality.

Examination. In *behavioral* terms in the doctor's interview these patients (usually young girls) tend to dress in a naively seductive fashion; in conversation they seem to escape the experience of anxiety by avoidance mechanisms such as amnesia and dissociation of ideas. In these patients the mood, popularly known as "hysterical," is characterized by lability and poor emotional control. In addition to conversion symptoms, there may occur anxiety attacks, periods of indifference, or depressive episodes accompanied by suicidal gestures. Hysterical attacks may vary from episodic histrionic loss of emotional control to motor seizures which are differentiated from epilepsy only with difficulty. In *physical* examination certain diagnostic tricks may be found useful in distinguishing conversion symptoms. In hysterical blindness visual fields remain the same when tested at varying distances from the eyes and the patient does not collide with the furniture. Anesthetic areas are frequently of stocking and glove type, not coinciding with sensory nerve distribution. Paralyses may be shown to alter in degree when the patient's attention is directed elsewhere. The Rorschach *psychological* test may show overemphasis on color responses, with "blood" seen in card II, and the content shows excessive preoccupation with the body.

Prognosis. Prognosis for the relief of presenting complaints through dramatic suggestion or patient psychotherapy is good; psychotherapeutic efforts at modifying the hysterical character are believed well worthwhile by most psychotherapists but long-term follow-up studies are few and difficult to carry out in a valid manner.

Treatment. Medical concern directed toward the symptoms tend to fix them more firmly and impede therapy. Therefore, repeated examination of the affected part and hospitalization are to be avoided.

Removal of presenting symptoms in the emergency room can sometimes be effected by such means as suggestion and persuasion, hypnotism, and intravenous sodium Amytal (particularly good for amnesia).

Psychotherapy must overcome resistances through the development of a positive relationship. Analysis of blocks to affectional feelings and broad reeducation of interpersonal attitudes are of value. In the psychoanalytic approach, material stemming from unresolved Oedipal and oral feelings is found to be genetically important and appears prominently in the transference. Basic distrust of self and others and deep inadequacy feelings tend to underlie severe hysteria.

SUGGESTED READINGS

Abse, D. W.: Hysteria and related mental disorders: an orientation to psychological medicine, Bristol, 1966, John Wright & Sons, Ltd.

Breuer, J., and Freud, S.: Studies in hysteria, New York, 1936, Nervous & Mental Diseases Publishing Co.

Deckert, G. H., and West, L. J.: Hypnosis and experimental psychopathology, Amer. J. Clin. Hypn. 5:256, 1963.

Farber, L.: Will and willfulness in hysteria. In The ways of the will, New York, 1968, Basic Books, Inc., Publishers.

Guze, S. B., and Perley, M. J.: Observations on natural history of hysteria, Amer. J. Psychiat. **119**:960, 1963.

Halleck, S. L.: Hysterical personality traits, Arch. Gen. Psychiat. **16**:750, 1967.

Janet, P.: The major symptoms of hysteria, ed. 2, New York, 1920, The Macmillan Co.

Lindemann, E.: Hysteria as a problem in a general hospital, Medical Clinics of North America, Philadelphia, 1938, W. B. Saunders Co.

Ljungberg, L.: Hysteria, a clinical prognostic and genetic study, Acta Psychiat. Neurol. Scand. **32** (supp. 112):1, 1957.

Marmar, J.: Orality in the hysterical personality, J. Amer. Psychoanal. Ass. **1**:656, 1953.

McGill, V. J., and Welch, L.: Hysteria as a conditioning process, Amer. J. Psychother. **1**:253, 1947.

Purtell, J. J., Robins, E., and Cohen, M. E.: Observations on the clinical aspects of hysteria. A quantitative study of 50 patients and 156 control subjects, J.A.M.A. **146**:902, 1951.

Rabkin, R.: Conversion hysteria as social maladaptation, Psychiatry **27**:349, 1964.

Seitz, P. F. D.: Symbolism and organ choice in conversion reactions, Psychosom. Med. **13**:254, 1951.

Slater, E.: The thirty-fifth Maudsley lecture: "Hysteria 311," J. Ment. Sci. **107**:359, 1961.

Vieth, I.: Hysteria, the history of a disease, Chicago, 1965, University of Chicago Press.

Woerner, P. I., and Guze, S.: Family and marital study of hysteria, Brit. J. Psychiat. **114**:161, 1968.

Ziegler, F. J., and Imboden, J.: Contemporary conversion reactions; II. A conceptual model, Arch. Gen. Psychiat. **6**:279, 1962.

Ziegler, F. J., Imboden, J., and Meyer, E.: Contemporary conversion reactions: a clinical study, Amer. J. Psychiat. **116**:901, 1960.

Ziegler, F. J., Imboden, J., and Rodgers, D.: Contemporary conversion reactions; II. Diagnostic considerations, J.A.M.A. **186**:307, 1963.

Phobic neurosis

Phobic neurosis (anxiety hysteria) is a concept initiated by Freud to refer to cases where the anxiety is connected with a particular object or situation which symbolically represents the neurotic conflict. Neurotic reactions in children are frequently of this kind and involve the appearance of anxiety attacks associated with phobic objects, castration fears, and other symbols of danger. The phobic syndrome was classified by Janet with obsessive-compulsive neurosis under the term "psychasthenia."

Phobias occur in many psychoneuroses but only in a very small percentage of cases predominate the symptom picture. In these patients anxiety appears when the patient finds himself in places which tend to threaten the sense of self-control. The patient thus must avoid such distressing situations, and his life becomes increasingly sequestered. Types of phobias encountered include acrophobia (high places), agoraphobia (open places), algophobia (pain), astraphobia (thunder and lightning), claustrophobia (closed places), coprophobia (excreta), hematophobia (blood), hydrophobia (water), lalophobia (speaking), mysophobia (dirt), necrophobia (dead bodies), nyctophobia (darkness), pathophobia (disease), peccatiphobia (sinning), phonophobia (speaking aloud), photophobia (strong light), sitophobia (eating), taphephobia (being buried alive), thanatophobia (death), toxiphobia (being poisoned), xenophobia (strangers), zoophobia (animals).

Treatment. Although traditional psychotherapeutic techniques are often used, more recently there appears greater promise of favorable outcome with the technique of reciprocal inhibition. Presumably the successful outcome of short-term psychotherapy depends upon whether the phobic neurosis is mild and of recent origin in a personality with many areas of competence. In patients having chronic, multiple progressively worsening phobias, the symptoms often represent an attempt to reduce intense disorganizing inner conflict by participating in only a few life situations. Removing through reeducation and conditioning this simple defensive life strategy may bring a measure of relief while other serious life conflicts are being resolved.

SUGGESTED READINGS

Arieti, S. A.: A re-examination of the phobic symptom and of symbolism in psychopathology, Amer. J. Psychiat. **118:**106, 1961.

Freud, S.: Analysis of a phobia in a five-year-old boy. In Collected papers, London, 1950, Hogarth Press, Ltd., vol. 3.

Rachman, S.: Phobias: their nature and control, Springfield, Ill., 1968, Charles C Thomas, Publisher.

Terhune, W.: The phobic syndrome, Arch. Neurol. Psychiat. **62:**162, 1949.

Wolpe, J.: The experimental foundations of some new psychotherapeutic methods. In Abracha, C. H., editor: Experimental foundations of clinical psychology, New York, 1962, Basic Books, Inc., Publishers, p. 554.

Wolpe, J.: Psychotherapy by reciprocal inhibition, Stanford, Calif., 1958, Stanford University Press.

Obsessive-compulsive neurosis

Obsessive or anancastic thoughts are those which perseverate and cannot be put out of consciousness. When translated into action they are known as compulsions. These symptoms may occur in the course of psychotic illness but alone may be the most noticeable symptom of an incapacitating neurosis.

Anamnesis. Indecisiveness may prevent an early visit to the physician by a patient who as his *chief complaint* constantly ruminates about avoiding dirt or germs, has recurring sexual thoughts, and spends his time in such elaborate rituals as hand washing, object touching, and prolonged dressing. *Past history* is that of a rigid, orderly person, perhaps of superior intellectual capacity. Maternal overconcern about bowel training, table manners, and cleanliness is felt to be a conditioning factor. Traits such as penuriousness and stubbornness are believed to develop in the anal sadistic (retentive) phase of childhood as a defense against open or implied parental threats. When present in mild degree, conscientiousness and adherence to strict ethical codes may be valuable character traits of these individuals. This form of neurosis usually appears in adolescence and advances during adult life, but obsessional rituals may occasionally be seen as early as 2 years of age in children of disturbed families.

Examination. The individual, *behaviorally,* is clean, neat, and overly polite and speaks in a guarded way about his symptoms rather than his personal feelings. Often indecisive, these patients show a striving for perfection and superiority with symptoms expressive of guilt. Anxiety and depression may be present in various degrees, particularly if rituals are prevented. Unjustified fear of their own dangerous impulses may be admitted. The compulsive rituals have been said to represent a caricature of masturbation which expresses a variety of psychological urges. In contrast to the visual daydreams of the hysteric, the fantasies of the compulsion neurotic tend to be verbalized and bring back the archaic attitudes that accompanied the first use of words. The compulsion neurotic, being afraid of his emotions, is afraid of things that arouse emotions. His defenses are intellectual and verbal. *Psychological* tests reveal paucity of imaginative productions, great attention to detail and a tendency toward a stereotyped, overcontrolled approach to the solution of tasks. These patients may conventionalize responses excessively and deny disturbing feelings aroused by the test.

Treatment. Problems in therapy arise from the patient's overintellectualizations and inability to experience feelings and to free-associate. Countertransference problems may result from the patient's inability to accept formulations other than his own and from the ambivalence and stubbornness of this character type. Some therapists advise gradual prohibition of compulsions as a means of producing anxiety, which in turn leads to new behavior. In mild cases psychotherapy may be of value, and techniques of reciprocal inhibition should be considered. Long-term psychotherapy may be recommended if feasible for the patient. In chronic severe cases, lobotomy has been used combined with an active postoperative rehabilitation program. Insulin and electroshock therapy are not indicated.

SUGGESTED READINGS

Goodwin, D. W., Guze, S. B., and Robins, E.: Follow-up studies in obsessional neuroses, Arch. Gen. Psychiat. **20:**182, 1969.

Ingram, I. M.: The obsessional personality and obsessional illness, Amer. J. Psychiat. **117:**1016, 1961.

Ingram, I. M.: Obsessional illness in mental hospital patients, J. Ment. Sci. **107:**382, 1961.

Pollitt, J. D.: Natural history studies in mental illness: a discussion based on a pilot study of obsessional state, J. Ment. Sci. **106:**93, 1960.

Wolpe, J.: Pychotherapy by reciprocal inhibition, Stanford, Calif., 1958, Stanford University Press.

Depressive neurosis

Depression as a symptom is seen in varying degree in nearly all psychoneurotics, but in some it is the predominant symptom. With complaints including insomnia, anorexia, decreased sexual drive, weight loss, constipation, fatigue, and menstrual disturbances, the entity somewhat resembles manic-depressive psychosis but differs from it in the depth of guilt and depression, degree of retardation, and in the absence of delusions or hallucinations. It is important to keep in mind that suicide can occur.

As in all psychoneuroses, psychotherapy is the usual mode of treatment. Electroshock, however, may be used to dispel the depression, but, in the usual case, it does not affect the other psychoneurotic symptoms favorably, and anxiety may even be increased. Antidepressant drugs are often of benefit and both the iminodibenzyl derivatives and the monoamine oxidase inhibitors have been advocated.

The terms "neurotic depression," "neurotic depressive reaction," and "mixed psychoneurosis with depression" have been used to describe the above condition. The term "reactive depression" is often used synonymously with these. Actually "reactive depression" is a purely descriptive term, implying that the symptoms of depression, whether in a neurosis or psychosis, have arisen in response to a known environmental problem (loss of loved ones, financial difficulty, marital discord, etc.). The use of this term usually implies an illness of short duration that is amenable to psychotherapy. The term does not accurately define a distinct disease entity, for in modern dynamic psychiatry every depression is reactive in the sense that it is a reactivation of infantile mood disturbances, in response to current life stresses which symbolically resemble earlier traumatic relationships. Actually one can think in terms of a continuum from a minor to a grossly traumatic precipitating factor—from one detectable only after careful analysis of mental content to a precipitating factor evident to all. The former is classed as endogenous depression, the latter exogenous or reactive. It is apparent that the better prognosis of the latter (i.e., reactive depression) should but emphasize the fact that the personality that succumbs with depression only to a maximum trauma must be better adjusted than one developing symptoms to a minimal or hidden stress.

SUGGESTED READINGS

Ascher, E.: A criticism of the concept of neurotic depression, Amer. J. Psychiat. **108**:901, 1952.

Ayd, F. J.: Recognizing the depressed patient, New York, 1961, Grune & Stratton, Inc.

Clayton, P., Desmarais, L., and Winokur, G.: A study of normal bereavement, Amer. J. Psychiat. **125**:168, 1968.

Hoch, P. H., and Zubin, J.: Depression, New York, 1954, Grune & Stratton, Inc.

Kay, D. W. K., Garside, R. F., Beamish, P., and Roy, J. R.: Endogenous and neurotic syndromes of depression: a factor analytic study of 104 cases: clinical features, Brit. J. Psychiat. **115**:377, 1969.

Kendell, R. E.: The classification of depressive illness, London, 1968, Oxford University Press.

Kiloh, L. G., and Garside, R. F.: The independence of neurotic depression and endogeneous depression, Brit. J. Psychiat. **109**:451, 1963.

Mendels, J.: Depression: the distinction between syndrome and symptom, Brit. J. Psychiat. **114:**1549, 1968.

Mendelson, M.: Psychoanalytic concepts of depression, Springfield, Ill., 1960, Charles C Thomas, Publisher.

Neurasthenic neurosis

The term *neurasthenia* (neurasthenic neurosis) predates psychoanalytic theory and refers to a severe chronic anxiety neurosis, often accompanied by obsessive or depressive features, which seems fixed and less labile or responsive to changes in life situation than is true of most anxiety neurosis. Fatigue is a prominent symptom accompanied by an inability to participate in active work and social relationships.

Depersonalization neurosis

When inner conflicts are not being adequately defended against by neurotic mechanisms, a patient may begin to exhibit anxiety and markedly disruptive changes in personality. One such symptom, however, which in many cases never leads on to any more severe symptoms, is depersonalization.

Depersonalization neurosis is a term for individuals who experience parts of their bodies as not belonging or as suddenly expanding greatly or changing in size or shape. Face, hands, head, or genitals are commonly selected, and the experience is usually transient and uncanny and may be identifiably in response to a meaningful event or encounter. This condition illustrates the fact that, as any neurosis increases in severity, experiences and symptoms resembling pyschotic behavior may be reported. Nevertheless, it is not usual for neuroses to transmute into true psychoses. Rather the borderline or schizoid neurotic tends to be more difficult to treat than other psychoneurotic patients. Although such symptoms may occur either alone or as part of some other primary mental disorder, such as an acute situational reaction, brief experiences of depersonalization are not necessarily a symptom of illness.

Hypochondriacal neurosis

The term *hypochondriacal neurosis* refers to individuals chronically and obsessively preoccupied with fancied bodily sensations and dysfunctions. Depending upon the particular case, elements of hysterical neurosis, obsessive-compulsive neurosis, depressive neurosis, or even psychosis may be identified. In addition to these standard diagnostic categories, several others may be mentioned because of their past common usage.

The term *traumatic neurosis* refers to those cases in which symptoms emerge immediately following a violently disturbing life experience. Fenichel states that probably many individuals classified under this heading are really psychoneurotics in whom the neurotic predisposition was unrecognized and the trauma actually only a contributory cause.

15

Personality disorders and certain other nonpsychotic mental disorders

Personality disorders

Every person exhibits certain habitual attitudes and reaction patterns in human relationships which have existed since early years and may be designated as his character structure. When these ways of behaving become inappropriately exaggerated, the individual may be said to suffer a character disorder. In most cases these patterns of behavior cause the individual little or no anxiety or sense of distress. These disorders are manifested by lifelong patterns of action or behavior rather than by mental or emotional symptoms.

Attempts at classifying these disorders have resulted in no acceptable scheme. Yet the outworn, all-inclusive, wastebasket category *psychopath* is no longer considered useful, since it referred to *all* deviate behavior patterns not frankly psychotic or psychoneurotic. Persons with character disorders tend to create in a stereotyped fashion particular interpersonal conflicts which arise from the individual's own style of thinking, valuing, and feeling about specific life situations. An adequate scheme for categorizing character disorders will have to consider systematically multivariate verbal, motor, and physiological pathways for emotional release and also diverse but highly influential structural aspects of situations and relationships. Former attempts at classification have included such types as the following: excitable, explosive, irritable, quarrelsome, anxious, depressive, phlegmatic, artistic, egocentric, schizoid, hysterical, impulsive, litigious, etc.—terms which may describe the behavior of any of us at some time or other. Perhaps in the broadest sense we all have personality disturbances, in that we overwork some defense or reactive mechanism. The transient and not the prolonged and incapacitating nature of these idiosyncracies, however, spells the difference between a normal person and one showing a character disorder.

Formerly in the American Psychiatric Association terminology, the term "personality trait disturbance" was used to describe individuals unable to maintain their emotional equilibrium and independence under minor or major stress, because of disturbances in emotional development. The term "personality pattern disturbance" was applied to persons who function in a disturbed fashion rigidly in all situations and in whom the core personality type could rarely be altered by any kind of therapy.

In the 1968 A.P.A. classification, 10 *personality disorders* are designated: paranoid, cyclothymic, schizoid, explosive, obsessive-compulsive, hysterical, asthenic, antisocial, passive-aggressive, and inadequate.

Paranoid personality. Individuals of this type show a propensity for projection mechanisms expressed by suspiciousness, envy, irritability, extreme jealousy, and stubbornness. Reality-testing, however, is not grossly impaired, and stable, well-formulated delusions are absent.

Cyclothymic personality (affective personality). These persons are characterized by outgoing adjustment to life situations, with apparent warmth and friendliness and ready enthusiasm for competition. They are frequently alternating between moods of elation and sadness without obvious relation to external events or with a grossly exaggerated intensity of emotion.

Schizoid personality. Showing avoidance of close interpersonal relationships and lack of aggressiveness, with inability to express hostility and with autistic thinking, these cold, aloof, fearful individuals exhibit emotional detachment and avoidance of competition with consequent solution of problems in daydreaming. They are described in childhood as quiet, shy, obedient, sensitive, and retiring and at adolescence receive the appellation of introvert.

Explosive personality (epileptoid personality disturbance). These persons have periodic outbursts of rage with verbal and/or physical aggressiveness. They differ from normals in the unexpectedness and intensity of such behavior and their inability for control. At times they may be regretful and repentant. Such persons are excitable and overresponsive to environmental pressures. If the patient is amnesic for the outburst, a diagnosis of hysteria or convulsive disorder should be considered.

Obsessive-compulsive personality (anankastic personality). Characterized by chronic excessive or obsessive concern with adherence to standards of rationalism, conscience, or conformity, these individuals are rigid, overconscientious, and have an inordinate capacity for work. There is a reduced capacity for relaxation and for experiencing emotions. The self is experienced as being monitored and directed rigidly by a set of inner directives or moral principles.

Hysterical personality (histrionic personality disorder). These persons demonstrate excitability and emotional instability. They tend to overreact and to dramatize. Their behavior is attention getting and seductive. Immature, self-centered, and often vain, such persons may appear entertaining but are willfully manipulative and dependent on others.

Asthenic personality. These persons are of low energy level and show an incapacity for enjoyment. They are easily fatigued, lack enthusiasm, and are oversensitive to physical and emotional stress.

Antisocial personality (sociopathic personality disturbance). The group with this problem includes those individuals with chronic or lifelong disturbance who are ill primarily in forms of behavior which conflict with the customs, rules, and laws of society. The failure to conform to the rules of prevailing cultural milieu may often be symptomatic of other severe personality disorder, neurosis, psychosis, organic brain injury, or other disease, and so the likelihood of such conditions should also be considered. One subgroup of such disorders has been referred to in psychoanalytic parlance as *impulse neurosis.*

The inability of these patients to deny themselves wished-for pleasures or to inhibit aggressive impulses has been understood as a means of avoiding severe depression or anxiety. The inability of many of these patients to form an adult sexual relationship has led to studies relating symptoms to primitive sexual expression. Such formulations have been developed for kleptomania (doing forbidden things secretly, often with sexual coloring), gambling (sexual excitement with need for punishment), and pyromania (sadistic drive to destroy).

Under this category fall persons who are chronically in trouble with society. They seem to suffer a defect in concept of time relating to self, with no concern for either past or future; hence, they show concern only with the present and have been called hedonistic. They have no concern for the consequences of their actions and profit neither from experience nor from punishment, maintaining no real loyalties to any person, group, or code. They are often chronic liars, show marked emotional immaturity with poor judgment, and lack any sense of responsibility. Their manner is frequently disarming, they have the ability to ingratiate themselves with others, and they may appear likable although superficial. They often have an ability to rationalize their behavior so that it appears reasonable and justified. The group intended here includes individuals often referred to by such terms as "psychopath," "psychopathic personality," or "constitutional psychopathic inferior."

Some individuals manifest disregard for the usual social codes and come into conflict with them as a result of having all their lives lived in an abnormal environment. They may be capable of strong loyalties. These individuals typically do not show significant personality deviations other than those implied by adherence to the values or codes of their own predatory, criminal, or other social group.

Passive-aggressive personality. In this type the picture may be characterized predominantly by helplessness and indecisiveness (with a tendency to clinging, pouting, stubbornness, and passive obstructionism) or by oscillation from this to a persistent reaction to frustration with irritability, temper tantrums, and destructive behavior. These persons may be adept at covertly and "innocently" fomenting crises between others.

Inadequate personality. This type is one in which the individuals show inadequate response to intellectual, emotional, social, and physical demands. Grossly they are neither physically nor mentally deficient on examination but show lack of adaptability, ineptness, poor judgment, social incompatibility, and lack of stamina.

SUGGESTED READINGS

Aichorn, A.: Wayward youth, New York, 1955, Meridian Books, Inc.

Brody, F. B.: Borderline states, character disorders and psychotic manifestations—some conceptual formulations, Psychiatry 23:75, 1960.

Bromberg, W.: The treatability of the psychopath, Amer. J. Psychiat. 110:604, 1954.

Cleckley, H.: The mask of sanity, ed. 4, St. Louis, 1964, The C. V. Mosby Co.

Craft, M., et al.: 100 admissions to a psychopathic unit, J. Ment. Sci. 108:564, 1962.

Gibbens, T. C. N., Pond, D. A., and Stafford-Clark, D. A.: A follow-up study of criminal psychopaths, J. Ment. Sci. 105:108, 1959.

Gurr, T. R.: Why men rebel, Princeton, N. J., 1970, Princeton University Press.

Guze, S. B.: A study of recidivism based upon a follow-up of 217 consecutive criminals, J. Nerv. Ment. Dis. 138:575, 1964.

Jenkins, R. L.: The psychopathic or antisocial personality, J. Nerv. Ment. Dis. 131:318, 1960.

Maughs, S.: The psychopathic personality—review of the literature, progress in neurology and psychiatry, New York, 1956, Grune & Stratton, Inc., vol. II.

O'Neal, P., Robins, L. N., King, L. J., and Schafer, J.: Parental deviance and the genesis of sociopathic personality, Amer. J. Psychiat. 118:1114, 1962.

Redl, F., and Wineman, D.: Children who hate, Glencoe, Ill., 1951, The Free Press.

Reich, W.: Character analysis, ed. 3, New York, 1949, Orgone Institute Press.

Robins, L. N.: Deviant children grown up: a sociological and psychiatric study of sociopathic personality, Baltimore, 1966, The Williams & Wilkins Co.

Schneider, K.: Psychopathic personalities, Springfield, Ill., 1958, Charles C Thomas, Publisher.

Thompson, G. N.: Sociopathic personality, its neurophysiology and treatment. In Rinkel, M., editor: Biological treatment of mental illness, New York, 1966, L. C. Page & Co.

Tooth, G.: The aggressive psychopathic offender, Lancet 1:42, 1969.

Williams, D.: Cerebral basis of temperament and personality, Lancet 2:1, 1954.

Sexual deviations

Deviant sexual behavior may be a symptom of other fundamental psychiatric disorder, such as schizophrenia, psychoneurosis, or senile psychosis, or it may occur as a predominant behavior aberration of a disordered personality. The term "deviation" suggests behavior counter to custom or accepted cultural mores. In the light of studies by Kinsey and others, however, much that we have formerly termed aberrant is found to be rather common behavior. Therefore, we must evaluate symptoms of sexual deviation in the light of current and regional social approval as well as potential danger to society and the production of discomfort in the patient. Freud has defined *perversion* as a reaction to castration fear, with regression to infantile sexuality as the only possible sexual outlet.

Sexual perversions most commonly considered include *homosexuality,* attraction for or sexual relations with persons of the same sex, which may be either passive or active in character; *fetishism,* in which some object substitutes for the genitals; and *transvestitism,* in which the subject wears clothes of persons of the opposite sex. In *exhibitionism* sexual pleasure is obtained by exposing one's genitals; *voyeurism* (scoptophilia) is a perversion in which the individual enjoys sexual excitement from watching naked men, naked women, and naked children, normal or perverse sexual acts, or excretory acts; sometimes the subject watches himself in a mirror during sexual intercourse. *Bestiality* (erotic zoophilia) involves use of an animal as a sex object. This may be partly determined by the environment and is common among persons brought up on farms. *Pedophilia* is an attraction to children as sex objects and *pederasty* refers to anal intercourse with small children. In the oral acts of *fellatio* and *cunnilingus* the mouth becomes a substitute for the genitals. *Sadism* (active algolagnia) is a perversion in which cruelty to others is substituted for the sex act or in which cruelty may accompany the sex act, as in *flagellation,* where satisfaction is achieved through whipping the partner; in *masochism* (passive algolagnia) the patient must experience pain himself in order to enjoy the sex act, or he seeks out suffering as a substitute for sexual enjoyment. Patients with *gerontophilia* need an elderly sexual partner, and this can be regarded as a displacement of incestuous wishes. *Necrophilia* is defined as sexual intercourse with the dead. Some authors have suggested that the choice of a chronically sick or crippled partner is really a modified form of necrophilia. *Transexualism* is a type of abnormality in which patients believe that they have the mind of the opposite sex in the wrong body. Male patients, for example, claim they are changing their sex and are frightened of all male activity, including erections. *Masturbation* is one form of autoerotism; practically all men masturbate to some degree during adolescence, and although it creates no physical harm, it may produce much guilt and shame.

SUGGESTED READINGS

Baittle, B., and Kobrin, S.: On the relationship of a characterological type of delinquent to the milieu, Psychiatry **27**:6, 1964.

Baker, H. J., and Stoller, R. J.: Sexual psychopathology in the hypogonadal male, Arch. Gen. Psychiat. **18**:631, 1968.

Becker, H. S.: Outsiders: studies in the sociology of deviance, New York, 1964, The Free Press of Glencoe, Inc.

Becker, H. S., editor: The other side: perspectives on deviance, New York, 1964, The Free Press of Glencoe, Inc.

Belleau, T., and Arsenian, J.: Homicide and hospitalization: a case report, Psychiatry **30**:73, 1967.

Bieber, I., et al.: Homosexuality, a psychoanalytic study, New York, 1962, Basic Books, Inc., Publishers.

Karpman, B.: The sexual offender and his offenses; etiology, pathology, psychodynamics and treatment, New York, 1954, Julian Press, Inc.

Kenyon, F. E.: Studies in female homosexuality, Brit. J. Psychiat. **114**:1337, 1968.

Kinsey, A., Pomeroy, W., Martin, C., and Gebbard, P. H.: Sexual behavior in the human female, Philadelphia, 1953, W. B. Saunders Co.

Kinsey, A., Pomeroy, W., and Martin, C.: Sexual behavior in the human male, Philadelphia, 1948, W. B. Saunders Co.

Masters, W. H., and Johnson, B. E.: Human sexual response, Boston, 1966, Little, Brown & Co.

Masters, W. H., and Johnson, B. E.: Human sexual inadequacy, Boston, 1970, Little, Brown & Co.

Rosen, I., editor: The pathology and treatment of sexual deviation, London, 1964, Oxford University Press.

Alcoholism

"Alcoholism" is the general term to designate the condition in which alcohol intake is great enough to damage physical health and personal or social functioning or when it has become a prerequisite to normal functioning. The term *episodic excessive drinking* is used when alcoholism is present and the individual becomes intoxicated as frequently as four times a year. *Intoxication* is defined as a state in which the individual's coordination or speech is definitely impaired or his behavior is clearly altered. Persons who become intoxicated more than twelve times a year or are recognizably under the influence of alcohol more than once a week, even though not intoxicated, are classified under the term *habitual excessive drinking.* The term *alcohol addiction* is used when there is direct or strong presumptive evidence that the patient is dependent upon alcohol. This may be demonstrated either by withdrawal symptoms or by an inability to go 1 day without drinking. When heavy drinking continues for 3 months or more, it is reasonable to presume addiction to alcohol.

Alcoholism affects nearly 5 million persons in the United States today and is a major social, economic, and medical problem in many countries throughout the globe. It is found as part of the symptom complex in character disorders or borderline psychotic individuals as well as in neurotic and other psychiatric disorders. The search for a common etiology has not been entirely rewarding. A marked sense of inferiority and helplessness with strong dependency needs may be combined with fantasies of self-importance and belief in a right to be taken care of. Alcohol can temporarily drown the frustration of inferiority feelings and the conflict of impossible ambitions.

The World Health Organization has defined alcoholism as a chronic behavioral disorder manifested by repeated drinking of alcoholic beverages in excess of the dietary and social uses of the community and to an extent that interferes with the drinker's health or his social or economic function. Dr. Ebbe Hoff states that in alcoholism there is: (1) loss of controlled alcohol intake—the victim finds himself drinking when he intends not to drink or drinking more than he has planned; (2) functional or structural damage—physiological, psychological, domestic, economic, or social; (3) use of alcohol as a kind of universal therapy—a psychopharmacological substance by which the problem drinker attempts to keep his life from disintegrating.

Despite common belief, alcoholism is not a skid row problem. More than 70% of alcoholics reside in respectable neighborhoods. The risk rate among drinkers in the United States is approximately 1 in 18. The estimated ratio of female to male alcoholics is 1 to 4. The life expectancy of an alcoholic is approximately 10 to 12 years less than average life expectancy. The estimated cost to industry runs into the billions of dollars. Alcoholism contributes heavily to crime and to at least 50% of traffic accidents.

Diagnosis. The warning signs of alcoholism include frequent drinking sprees, a steady increase in intake, solitary drinking, early morning drinking, Monday morning absenteeism, frequent disputes about drinking, and the occurrence of blackouts (a period of time in which, while remaining otherwise fully conscious, the person undergoes a loss of memory). An individual may probably be considered an alcoholic if he continues to drink despite the fact that his drinking causes physical illness, headache, gastric distress, or hangover and repeatedly causes trouble with his wife, his employer, or the police.

Treatment. The successful therapeutic approach is often a multifaceted one involving psychotherapeutic, social, and medical methods in both hospital and community settings. Countertransference problems in the psychotherapist are often major. The psychotherapist may be tricked or provoked by the patient into retaliatory or rejecting responses or may in a contagious fashion begin to feel as hopeless about the patient as the patient does about himself. These patients tend to be experts in self-destructive acting out as a defense against experiencing tension or disappointment. The conditioned reflex treatment of alcoholism (which develops an aversion to drink by negative conditioning) and or disulfiram (Antabuse, 0.5 Gm. daily for 1 to 3 weeks, then maintenance on 0.25 to 0.5 Gm. daily) serves only to help the patient resist alcohol during ongoing psychotherapy. The goals of psychotherapy should be consistent with the resources of the patient and his environment and must be tailored to the needs of the individual. Denial is a major mental mechanism seen in most alcoholics and should be dealt with in therapy.

The A. A. (Alcoholics Anonymous) is reputed to be helpful to about 50% of its members. Its "12-step" program is built around principles of comradeship, self-help, and a Good Samaritan attitude toward other alcoholics. It combines the therapeutic principles of activity groups with a revival type of religious identification and a service club appeal. It helps to elevate the patient's self-esteem by making him useful to other alcoholics, as well as to strengthen his resistance to temptation by moral suasion and group pressure. It requires the self-admission of the individual that he is powerless over alcohol and that his life has become unmanageable. Al-Anon and Ala-Teens are parallel organizations developed to help the spouse and children of alcoholics.

SUGGESTED READINGS

Alcoholics Anonymous: The story of how many thousands of men and women have recovered from alcoholism, New York, 1955, Works Library Publications.

Alcoholics Anonymous: Twelve steps and twelve traditions, New York, 1953, Alcoholics Anonymous Publishing Co.

A.M.A. Committee on Alcoholism and Addiction and Council on Mental Health: Dependence on barbiturates and other sedative drugs, J.A.M.A. **193:**673, 1965.

Catanzaro, R. J.: Alcoholism—the total treatment approach, Springfield, Ill., 1968, Charles C Thomas, Publisher.

Chafetz, M. E.: Liquor: the servant of man, Boston, 1965, Little, Brown & Co.

Chafetz, M. E., and Demone, H. W., Jr.: Alcoholism and society, New York, 1962, Oxford University Press, Inc.

Gordon, J. E.: The epidemiology of alcoholism. In Kruse, H. D., editor: Alcoholism as a medical problem, New York, 1956, Paul B. Hoeber, Inc.

Hart, W. T.: A comparison of promazine and paraldehyde in 175 cases of alcohol withdrawal, Amer. J. Psychiat. **118:**323, 1961.

Himwich, H. E.: Alcohol and brain physiology and alcoholism, Springfield, Ill., 1956, Charles C Thomas, Publisher.

Jellinek, E. M.: The disease concept of alcoholism, New Haven, Conn., 1960, Hill House Press.

Kaim, S. C., Klett, C. J., and Rothfeld, B.: Treatment of the acute alcohol withdrawal state: a comparison of four drugs, Amer. J. Psychiat. **125:**1640, 1969.

Kissin, B., Rosenblatt, S. M., and Machover, S.: Prognostic factors in alcoholism, Psychiat. Res. Rep. Amer. Psychiat. Ass. 24:22, March, 1968.

McCord, W., and McCord, J.: Origins of alcoholism, Palo Alto, Calif., 1960, Stanford University Press.

Pittman, D. J., and Gordon, C. W.: Revolving door: a study of the chronic police case inebriate, Yale University Center of Alcohol Studies, monograph no. 2, Glencoe, Ill., 1958, The Free Press.

Tamerin, J. S., and Mendelson, J. H.: Psychodynamics of chronic inebriation: observations of alcoholics during process of drinking in experimental group setting, Amer. J. Psychiat. **125:**886, 1969.

Thomas, D. W., and Freedman, D. X.: Treatment of alcohol withdrawal syndrome: comparison of promazine and paraldehyde, J.A.M.A. **188:**316, 1964.

Wilson, W. P., and Wolk, M.: The treatment of delirium tremens, N. Carolina Med. J. 26:552, 1965.

Drug dependence

Drug abuse is the term generally employed to refer to the use, usually by self-administration, of any drug in a manner that deviates from approved medical and social patterns. The term *drug dependence* refers to a *physical* dependence on drugs other than alcohol, tobacco, and ordinary caffeine-containing beverages. Dependence on medically prescribed drugs is also excluded as long as the drug's use is indicated and the intake is proportionate to the medical need. *Habituation (psychic dependence)* refers to the situation in which a person desires and becomes accustomed to a drug but is not physically dependent upon it. *Tolerance* refers to that state in which the body's tissues become accustomed to the presence of the drug and fail to respond to concentrations ordinarily effective; thus increasingly large quantities are required to produce the desired effect. *Addiction* is a condition of physical dependence, habituation, and tolerance.

The abuse of and addiction to different drugs varies from time to time and from country to country. At this time in the United States, it is estimated that perhaps 10 million individuals have used marihuana, although only one tenth of this number are heavy users. There are an estimated 250,000 to 500,000 nonnarcotic drug abusers and perhaps 100,000 hard narcotics addicts. Although drug abuse occurs in all strata of society, it is most prevalent in the slum districts of large highly urbanized areas. Seventy percent of all narcotics addicts in the United States live in ten big cities.

The reason given for taking drugs by nearly half of the addicts is to obtain the desired euphoria, to feel "normal," and to overcome a state of depression. Other reasons cited are curiosity and the influence of friends or the environment. Narcotics addicts have a wide range of personality characteristics, with perhaps 10% having psychopathic personality disorders. The majority are described as emotionally unstable, immature, impulsive, unreliable, angry against society, and unable to establish long-range goals or meet the demands of the environment. Four out of five narcotics addicts are male, with

Table 5. Drug dependence

Class of drug	Psychic dependence	Physical dependence	Tolerance	Characteristics of intoxication	Characteristics of withdrawal
Cannabis sativa (marihuana, hashish)	Moderate to strong	No	Not demonstrated	Milder preparations induce drowsy, euphoric state with inappropriate laughter and disturbances in perception of space and time; stronger preparations (hashish) induce psychotic reaction with hallucinations; pupils normal, conjunctivae injected	No specific withdrawal symptoms
Psychostimulants (amphetamines)	Variable	Mild to absent	Slowly developed, not equal for all components of central nervous system	Agitation, tachycardia, paranoid thought disturbances with high doses; pupils dilated and sluggishly reactive with high doses; acute brain syndrome common; convulsive seizures may occur	Lethargy, somnolence, general malaise, psychic depression, often with suicidal tendency; acute brain syndrome may persist for weeks
Opiates (morphine, heroin, etc.)	Strong	Develops early	Yes	Pinpoint pupils; analgesia with or without depressed sensorium; patient may be alert and appear normal; respiratory depression with overdose	Dilated and reactive pupils, gastrointestinal disturbances, low back pain, rhinorrhea, lacrimation, gooseflesh

	Varies greatly, usually not intense	No	High degree, develops rapidly	Unpredictable psychic disturbance, extreme lability of affect, chaotic disruption of thought, danger of uncontrolled behavior; pupils dilated and reactive to light	No specific symptoms; effects may persist for indefinite period after discontinuation of drug
Hallucinogens (psychostimulants, psychomimetics); (LSD, mescaline, morning glory seed, etc.)	Yes	Yes	Yes	Drowsiness, with nystagmus on lateral gaze; ataxia; slurred speech; respiratory depression with overdose; pupil size and reaction appear normal	General agitation, tremulousness, insomnia, gastrointestinal disturbances, blepharoclonus, hyperpyrexia, acute brain syndrome, convulsive seizures
Barbiturates	Yes	No	Moderate	Apprehension, tremulousness, tachycardia, hyperventilation, mydriasis; large doses produce toxic psychosis with visual, auditory, and tactile (formication) hallucinations; paranoid delusions and resistant behavior may occur	Should be immediately withdrawn; depression and delusions may persist for weeks
Cocaine					

Negroes and Caucasians being about equal in number. Eighty percent of narcotic drug users are between 20 and 40 years of age with an increasingly large number of teenagers involved with marihuana and hallucinogens. In the last few years deaths associated with drug addiction, most often from acute reaction or overdosage, have markedly increased.

The argot of the addict is colorful and includes such phrases as the following: *acid,* LSD; *bennies,* amphetamines; *blow a stick,* to smoke a marihuana cigarette; *cold turkey,* abrupt withdrawal from narcotics without medication; *fix,* an injection of narcotics; *goofballs,* barbiturates; *grass,* marihuana; *head (acid head, pothead),* one high on LSD, marihuana, or hashish; *hooked,* to be dependent on drugs; *joypot,* the intermittent use of heroin by a nonaddict; *junkie,* a narcotics addict; *kick the habit,* to stop using the drugs; *mainline,* to take drugs intravenously; *nod,* to behave in a lethargic or somnolent manner, or, when under the influence of drugs; *O.D.,* overdose of drugs, often lethal; *pusher,* a seller of drugs; *score,* to obtain drugs; *skin pop,* to inject drugs under the skin; *stoned,* to be high on drugs; *trip,* a hallucinogenic experience; *turned on,* excitement or sensory experience after taking drugs; *weed,* marihuana.

Opium, opium alkaloids, or their derivatives. Addiction to opium is a chronic physiological intoxication in which the drug injection is maintained by an individual suffering from personality disòrder. The particular difficulties of an addict are determined not only by physiological and psychological factors but also by cultural attitudes toward the addict who, after his funds are gone, may be led to criminal means of obtaining the drug. Opiate addiction occurs most frequently in persons who are immature or self-centered, or in dependent persons who tend to have a psychoneurotic or psychopathic life pattern. In general, it should be looked upon as a symptom of these disorders; it is noteworthy that psychotics are rarely attracted to opiates.

Therapeutic introduction to opiate addiction in the United States occurs in less than 5% of cases; most begin opiates experimentally through association with addicts (although those who handle the drug—medics and nurses—may also be tempted). Regular administration of opiates produces tolerance, leading to steadily increasing dosage, with withdrawal symptoms if the drug is stopped. The drug is taken for its effect of "false euphoria" which includes a sexual-like pleasure experienced over the whole body, not accompanied by any diminution of intellectual functions or disturbance of behavior. Side effects of nausea, itching, miosis, anorexia, and constipation are borne willingly, and the addict's life becomes one of nonproductivity, socioeconomic and family problems, apathy, lowered sex drive, and frequently criminal activities to support a costly habit.

EXAMINATION. Because of legal restrictions, the problem of obtaining opiates is a difficult one for the addict, who may become adept at feigning acute medical conditions, such as coronary occlusion, kidney stone, or acute abdomen, to receive morphine. Because of this unreliability, close examination is important. Scars from unsterile hypo abscesses may have a black tinge from sterilization of the needle by matches. Objective signs of the *morphine abstinence syndrome* include yawning ("the yaps"), lacrimation, rhinorrhea, and perspiration; these appear in 10 to 15 hours, followed by gooseflesh, mydriasis, and tremors. In more severe cases there are insomnia, restlessness, hyperpnea, and a rise in systolic blood pressure followed by the appearance of vomiting, diarrhea, and weight loss (as much as 5 pounds per day).

PROGNOSIS. With an adequate rehabilitation and follow-up program, about 20% of addicts remain abstinent; many others obtain a worthwhile remission lasting several years.

TREATMENT. The treatment of addiction to drugs is far from satisfactory. Traditional commitment of narcotics users to Federal Prison Hospitals resulted in an increasingly high rate of relapse. In fact, a lasting cure was the rare exception with many addicts using such periods of hospitalization merely to reduce the cost of their habit by a decrease in the level of drug tolerance. More recently treatment of the drug abuser and addict in his home community has given greater promise of success. *Medical-psychiatric* hospital-based programs admit heroin and other addicts on a voluntary basis for detoxification, attention to medical problems, and psychiatric treatment. Other programs (of the *Synanon type*) use group pressure, interpersonal confrontation, and a therapeutic community to help drug abusers change their behavior. *Addicts Anonymous* is a voluntary program modeled after Alcoholics Anonymous, providing group meetings and interpersonal support. *Periodic testing* with nalorphine (Nalline) injections, plus thin-layer chromatography and other methods of urine examination, may be used to test for evidence of readdiction. *Substitute programs* in which methadone (cyclazocine or dolophine-*dl*-4,4-diphenylamino-3-heptanol) is substituted for heroin are now widely used but still on an experimental basis. In the methadone treatment programs, 1 mg. of methadone has an abstinence-suppressing potency of 3 to 4 mg. of morphine or 1 mg. of heroin. Ordinarily 10 to 20 mg. of methadone orally twice daily is sufficient. When the patient is psychologically ready for participation in the total rehabilitation program, methadone may be gradually withdrawn.

Barbiturates. The conservative employment of barbiturates as a temporary relief from tensional symptoms is a blessing to many so afflicted, but persons suffering from insomnia, tension headaches, anxiety attacks, or other manifestations of anxiety may gradually become *physiologically dependent upon* these drugs. *Tolerance* to the drugs may develop, but it is less noticeable than with opiates.

EXAMINATION. Regular ingestion of large doses leads to *intoxication,* marked by signs of cortical and cerebral dysfunction, such as increased emotional lability, impairment of intellect, disorientation, dysarthria, ataxia, and nystagmus. Abrupt withdrawal of barbiturate or a marked reduction of dosage in a chronically intoxicated individual leads to an *abstinence syndrome.* More threatening to life than the opiate abstinence syndrome, this condition is characterized by weakness, tremors, feelings of intense panic, increase in pulse, respiration, temperature, and blood pressure accompanied by nausea, vomiting, and rapid weight loss. After about 30 hours grand mal convulsions may appear. This phase may be followed in 3 to 7 days by delirium similar to delirium tremens with agitation, confusion, and hallucinations. The total syndrome may last 2 to 3 weeks, and recovery can occur with no permanent changes.

TREATMENT. Gradual withdrawal of the addicting barbiturates is indicated, with the substitution of short-acting pentobarbital in place of the longer-acting barbiturate to which the patient has become addicted. Once the patient's tolerance level has been determined, the pentobarbital can be withdrawn at the rate of about 10% of total dosage per day.

Prescribe Dilantin, 0.1 Gm. t.i.d., for 2 weeks.

Provide vigilant therapeutic attention to nutrition, fluid balance and prevention of infection. After 2 to 4 weeks a well-rounded psychological, social, and occupational rehabilitation program is indicated and preferably is commenced within a closed ward where the patient's activities can be supervised.

Other hypnotics, sedatives, or tranquilizers. Addiction to a variety of chemical agents comes about through a complex interaction of physiological, pharmacological, socioenvironmental, and personality factors. This dependence may be in the form of addiction (physiological and psychological dependence) or habit formation (mostly psychological dependence). Agents involved include meprobamate (Miltown and Equanil), chlordiazepoxide (Librium), paraldehyde, chloral hydrate, ethchlorvynol (Placidyl), glutethimide (Doriden), methyprylon (Noludar), methaqualone (Revonal), diazepam (Valium), dextropropoxyphene (Darvon), or ethinamate (Valmid).

Cocaine. This drug produces habituation. Continued stimulation leads not only to euphoric excitement and pleasant hallucinations but also to dangerous paranoid delusions, digestive disorders, emaciation, and even convulsions. Perforation of the nasal septum can occur from snuffing cocaine powder ("snow").

Cannabis sativa (hashish, marihuana). This drug is also known as pot, hemp, charge, gear, kef, Mary Jane, stuff, tea, weed, and grass. It is widely taken by teen-agers and others in search of an escape from reality. The World Health Organization—Expert Committee on Addiction-Producing Drugs has pointed out that physical dependence on this drug does not occur. Temporary psychoses have been reported. The major danger seems to be that the use of this drug frequently leads to use of other addicting and more dangerous agents.

Other psychostimulants. The excessive intake of amphetamines for their exhilarating effects has become a major problem. Such drugs may be inhaled or taken orally ("pep pills," "goofballs") or by injection ("mainlining").

Hallucinogens, etc. A variety of psychedelic drugs, including lysergic acid diethylamide (LSD), mescaline, stramonium, nutmeg, and banana peels, have been used to produce hallucinatory and psychotic-like states. Similar "jags," consisting of euphoria and excitement, have been produced by the sniffing of glue, gasoline vapors, lacquers, paint thinners, ether, catnip, and lighter fluid.

TREATMENT. The treatment of these conditions involves not only hospitalization with immediate removal of the offending agent but also a thorough exploration of the personaltiy problems leading to the use of such agents, with therapy aimed at the underlying characterological and environmental problems.

SUGGESTED READINGS

Cameron, D. C.: Addiction, current issues, Amer. J. Psychiat. **120**:313, 1963.

Chein, I., Gerard, D., Lee, R., and Rosenfeld, E.: The road to H., New York, 1964, Basic Books, Inc., Publishers.

Cole, J. O.: Report on the treatment of drug addiction. In President's Commission on Law Enforcement and the Administration of Justice Task Force report: Narcotics and drug abuse, Washington, D. C., 1967, U. S. Government Printing Office.

Cole, J. O., and Wittenborn, J. R.: Drug abuse: social and psychopharmacological aspects, Springfield, Ill., 1969, Charles C Thomas, Publisher.

Connell, P. H.: Amphetamine psychosis, London, 1958, Chapman & Hall, Ltd.

Essig, C. H.: Addiction to non-barbiturate sedative and tranquilizing drugs, Clin. Pharmacol. Ther. **5**:334, 1964.

Ewing, J. A., and Grant, W. J.: The bromide hazard, Southern Med. J. **58**:148, 1965.

Farnsworth, D. L.: Hallucinogenic agents, J.A.M.A. **185**:878, 1963.

A Federal Source Book: Answers to the most frequently asked questions about drug abuse. Produced jointly by the Defense Department, Health, Education, and Welfare Department, Justice Department, Labor Department, and Office of Economic Opportunity, Washington, D. C., 1970, U. S. Government Printing Office.

Freedman, A. M.: Treatment of drug addiction in a community general hospital, Comp. Psychiat. **4**:199, 1963.

Freedman, A. M., Fink, M., Sharoff, R., et al.: Cyclazocine and methadone in narcotic addiction, J.A.M.A. **202**:191, 1967.

Glatt, M., Pittman, D., Gillespie, E., and Hills, D.: The drug scene in Great Britain, London, 1967, Edward Arnold (Publishers) Ltd.

Isbell, H.: Addiction to barbiturates and the barbiturate abstinence syndrome, Ann. Intern. Med. **33**:108, 1950.

Isbell, H.: Historical development of attitudes towards opiate addiction in the United States. In Farber, F. M., and Wilson, R. H. L., editors: Control of the mind, New York, 1963, McGraw-Hill Book Co., vol. 2.

Jaffe, J. H., Zaks, M. S., and Washington, E. N.: Experience with the use of Methadone in a multimodality program for the treatment of narcotics users, Int. J. Addict. 4:481, 1969.

Keeler, M. H.: Adverse reaction to marihuana, Amer. J. Psychiat. 124: 674, 1967.

Kolb, L.: Drug addiction a medical problem, Springfield, Ill., 1962, Charles C Thomas, Publisher.

Massengale, O. N., et al.: Physical and psychologic factors in glue sniffing, New Eng. J. Med. 269:130, 1963.

Maurer, D. W., and Vogel, V. H.: Narcotics and narcotic addiction, ed. 3, Springfield, Ill., 1967, Charles C Thomas, Publisher.

McGlothlin, W. H., and West, L. J.: The marihuana problem, an overview, Amer. J. Psychiat. 125:126, 1968.

Nyswander, M. E.: The methadone treatment of heroin addiction, Hosp. Practice 2:27, 1967.

Rockwell, D. A., and Ostwald, P.: Amphetamine use and abuse in psychiatric patients, Arch. Gen. Psychiat. 18:612, 1968.

Ungerleider, J. F., et al.: "The bad trip"— the etiology of the adverse LSD reaction, Amer. J. Psychiat. 124:1483, 1968.

Wikler, A.: Opioid addiction. In Friedman, A., and Kaplan, H., editors: Comprehensive textbook of psychiatry, Baltimore, 1967, The Williams & Wilkins Co.

Wikler, A.: Diagnosis and treatment of drug dependence of the barbiturate type, Amer. J. Psychiat. 125:758, 1968.

Wilner, D. L., and Kassebaum, G. G., editors: Narcotics, New York, 1965, McGraw-Hill Book Co.

Wittenborn, J. R., Brill, H., Smith, J. P., and Wittenborn, S. A.: Drugs and youth, Proceedings of the Rutgers Symposium on Drug Abuse, Springfield, Ill., 1969, Charles C Thomas, Publisher.

World Health Organization—Expert Committee on Addiction-Producing Drugs: Thirteenth report, WHO Techn. Rep. Ser. no. 273, 1964.

16
Miscellaneous—psychiatric conditions not in standard nomenclature

Munchausen's syndrome (chronic factitious illness). This term is used for patients who consciously distort their medical history, produce misleading physical findings and laboratory results through self-inflicted lesions, and wander from one hospital and one city to another seeking medical care. Sometimes the motive is simply the desire for free board or haven from the police, some patients are drug addicts using the method to satisfy their craving, and in others psychological motives include a grudge against physicians or desire to be the center of attention.

Ganser's syndrome (prison psychosis). This rare illness, most frequently observed in prisoners, has been referred to as "hysterical pseudostupidity." Characteristically, these patients give utterly incorrect and often ridiculous replies to questions, although there is usually no doubt that they are alert and not confused in the usual sense; they behave, other than verbally, as persons oriented to their environment. It has been described as a dissociative state, intermediate between psychosis and psychoneurosis, and between malingering and disease. The patient usually recovers within a few days or weeks.

Gilles de la Tourette's disease (tic convulsif). Symptoms begin in childhood with an increasing display of motor tics, from spasmodic grimacing to violent movements of the body; pathognomonic is the compulsive coprolalia in which the patients are compelled to utter obscenities, accompanied by compulsive coughing, spitting, blowing, and barking sounds.

Physical examinations, including neurological tests and EEG, are usually negative and strong elements of self-punishment may be present. Although previously reported to have a poor outcome, recent therapy with Haloperidol has given promising results.

Folie à deux (double insanity). This term coined by La-sèque and Falret in 1873 refers to the transfer of delusions from one partner to another by association. When the active partner imposes his delusions on the passive one, the term "folie imposée" is used. When the passive partner resists the influence of suggestions but later develops a full-fledged psychosis, including delusions and hallucinations and perhaps eventually showing a psychotic picture totally different from that of the dominant partner, the term used is "folie communiquée. "Folie simultanée" develops when transmission and suggestibilty are negligible and the delusions occur simultaneously. The terms "folie à trois," "folie à quatre," and "folie à cinq" have also been reported. Care should be taken in diagnosis to determine whether there is a genetic factor involved, for the term should be used only in cases where the partners are not consanguineous, there is no history of schizophrenia on either side, and there is a definite alleviation of symptoms in at least one partner in a longitudinal study.

Capgras syndrome. The Capgras syndrome is a rare condition characterized by the delusional conviction that certain persons in the environment are not their real selves but instead are doubles, impersonating and behaving like persons known to the patient.

Amok. In sudden unprovoked outbursts of rage occurring in natives of the Malay peninsula the afflicted person, usually armed with a knife, attacks, maims, or kills indiscriminately all who come within his path. Although originally considered a reaction due to frustration and humiliation, in recent reports this behavior has been associated with toxic conditions and delusional psychoses.

Latah. Also seen among Malaysians is a state of suspension of all normal activity and with mimetic or echo reactions provoked by startle. The condition may exist for years.

Malingering. Simulation of disability or illness is sometimes used consciously with the motive of some secondary gain (e.g., by soldiers and prisoners). Some authors state that normal individuals do not malinger and that the condition is either a forerunner of some more serious mental illness or else a symptom of some disorder of personality. Differential diagnosis includes consideration of various neurotic conditions in which secondary gain is often a feature but on a level beyond the conscious control of the patient. Proof of malingering may require a bit of detective work.

SUGGESTED READINGS

Challas, G., Chapel, J. L., and Jenkins, R. L.: Tourette's disease: control of symptoms and its clinical course, Int. J. Neuropsychiat. **3** (supp. 1):95, 1967.

Goldin, S., and MacDonald, J. E.: The Ganser state, J. Ment. Sci. **101**:267, 1955.

Herzl, R. A.: Chronic factitious illness: Munchausen's syndrome, Arch. Gen. Psychiat. **18**:569, 1968.

Kallman, F. J., and Mickey, J. S.: Genetic concepts and folie à deux: a re-examination of "induced insanity" in family units, J. Hered. **37**:298, 1946.

Kamal, A.: Folie à cinq, Brit. J. Psychiat. **111**:583, 1965.

Lennox, W.: Amnesia, real or feigned, Amer. J. Psychiat. **99**:732, 1943.

Todd, J.: The syndrome of Capgras, Psychiat. Quart. **31**:250, 1957.

Yap, P. M.: Mental disease peculiar to certain cultures, a survey of comparative psychiatry, J. Ment. Sci. **97**:313, 1951.

17
Psychophysiological disorders

To understand and treat psychosomatic disorders requires a comprehensive approach to the patient. The physician's attitude toward the illness is based on the fact that disturbances of organs, thinking, emotions, and social adjustment may result from the interaction of many qualitative factors within a total life pattern. For an individual with a psychosomatic disorder, it is common to observe a bodily dysfunction related to a special way of responding to difficulties in living. Indeed for asthma, neurodermatitis, peptic ulcer, rheumatoid arthritis, ulcerative colitis, hypertension, and for a number of other disorders, quite specific patterns of personality maladjustment have been postulated. Franz Alexander stated that, for each of these conditions, differences in childhood experience, interpersonal attitudes, and precipitating stress can be distinguished.

Cannon first demonstrated that an *acute reaction to stress* includes rising blood pressure, tachycardia, deepening respiration, tachypnea, and changes in gastrointestinal motility. Subsequent research upon the autonomic nervous system, hypothalamus, and cortex has demonstrated pathways related to emotion. In *chronic reactions to stress,* neurogenic mechanisms become less important and hormonal regulations gain in importance. As Selye states in describing "the adaptation syndrome," defective hormonal mechanisms produced by prolonged and excessive environmental stress may lead to tissue pathology.

Where emotional conflicts seem to be symbolically expressed through bodily dysfunction, "organ language" is often a key to the symptom's meaning. It has long been recognized in our daily speech that such terms as "pain in the neck," "he gripes me," "I can't stomach that," and "you broke my heart" refer to physical expression of feelings derived from interpersonal friction.

An organ predisposed through heredity, through constitution, through infection, through trauma, or through physiological imbalance may become conditioned to give a disordered response to specific emotional or social stimuli. In the psychoanalytic literature, psychophysiological disorders have been referred to as *organ neuroses.* Psychoanalysts focusing upon the symbolic significance of symptoms have thought of psychosomatic conditions as *affect equivalents,* in which symptoms represent the expression of a powerful inner emotion or in which symptoms are the physical result of unconscious attitudes. Upper gastrointestinal disturbances may occur in chronically frustrated, oral-receptive persons, cardiac arrhythmias in those with repressed impulses to fight or flee, respiratory difficulties as the result of emotional trauma at separation from mother, etc.

Successful diagnosis and therapy of psychophysiological disorders demand cooperation among internist, surgeon, and psychiatrist; teamwork among nurses, social workers, occupational therapists, and physiotherapists is frequently important. Initial understanding of symptoms may be attained by a careful history which seeks temporal correlations between the appearance of symptoms and life crises, or symbols of such crises.

The physician does well to bear in mind that many patients have initial difficulty in comprehending that emotional and social forces do contribute to their illness. For this reason thorough physical and laboratory work-up is best completed early, the findings and their interpretation presented frankly, and adequate time spent with the patient to help him understand his illness sufficiently to cooperate in treatment.

When patients doubt the role of important causative factors, it is often helpful to gain intimate grasp of the patient's own private formulation to explain his symptoms. Then, as the patient begins to feel that the physician is really interested in *his* point of view, he will more freely divulge those hidden feelings and attitudes which provide valuable diagnostic and psychotherapeutic clues.

A flexible, supportive type of psychotherapy is useful in these disorders. The frequency, length, and number of interviews can be varied to suit the circumstances. When symptoms are severe, several brief interviews may be held in a single day. Under other conditions widely spread contacts held at the time of return visits for medical treatment may suffice. Interviews held in a private room, although desirable, may be replaced by bedside chats in the case of hospitalized ward patients.

SUGGESTED READINGS

Alexander, F.: Psychosomatic medicine, New York, 1950, W. W. Norton & Co., Inc.

Dunbar, F.: Emotions and bodily changes, New York, 1954, Columbia University Press.

Gildea, E. F.: Special features of personality which are common to certain psychosomatic disorders, Psychosom. Med. **11:**273, 1949.

Goldman, D., and Ulett, G. A.: Practical psychiatry for the internist, St. Louis, 1968, The C. V. Mosby Co.

Kissen, D. M.: The significance of syndrome shift and late syndrome association in pychosomatic medicine, J. Nerv. Ment. Dis. **136:**34, 1963.

Lacey, J. I., and Lacey, B. C.: The law of initial value in the longitudinal study of autonomic constitution: reproducibility of autonomic responses and response patterns over a four-year interval, Ann. N. Y. Acad. Sci. **98:**1257, 1962.

Life stress and bodily disease; formulation, Proc. Ass. Res. Nerv. Ment. Dis. **29:**1059, 1950.

Malmo, R. B.: Activation. In Bachrach, A. J., editor: Experimental foundations of clinical psychology, New York, 1962, Basic Books, Inc., Publishers.

Roessler, R., and Greenfield, N. S.: Incidence of somatic disease in psychiatric patients, Psychosom. Med. **23:**413, 1961.

Saslow, G., and Buchmueller, A. D.: Flexible psychotherapy in psychosomatic disorders, Hum. Organization **8:**673, 1949.

Selye, H.: The physiology and pathology of exposure to stress, Montreal, 1950, Acta, Inc., annual supplements 1951, 1952, 1953, 1954.

Silverman, S.: Psychological cues in forecasting physical illness, New York, 1970, Appleton-Century-Crofts.

Spielberger, C. V., editor: Anxiety and behavior, New York, 1966, Academic Press, Inc.

Wenger, M. A., et al.: Autonomic response specificity, Psychosom. Med. **23:**185, 1961.

Wolf, S., and Goodell, H.: Harold G. Wolff's stress and disease, ed. 2, Springfield, Ill., 1968, Charles C Thomas, Publisher.

Ziskind, E.: Psychophysiologic medicine, Philadelphia, 1954, Lea & Febiger.

Skin disorder

Embryologically the skin and central nervous system arise from ectoderm, and, like the nervous system, the skin serves as a means of communication between a person's inner and outer worlds (for example, blushing). Yet in view of much current uncertainty about the role of psychic factors in skin disorders, it is well to evaluate each new case with an unprejudiced observant eye. In patients with *dermatitis factitia, pruritus, neurodermatitis,* and *trichotillomania* psychic factors predominate. For example, history of pleasure in physical exhibitionism has been reported in cases of neurodermatitis. In such conditions as *hyperhidrosis, urticaria, rosacea, psoriasis, herpes, warts, lichen planus,* and *alopecia* psychic factors may or may not be significant. Some reports have correlated urticaria with suppressed weeping, pruritus with inhibited or vicariously gratified sexual excitement, and neurodermatitis with obsessive-compulsive traits. Endocrine imbalance, disturbance in autonomic regulation of skin physiology, and—at the cortical level—conversion mechanisms may all play a part in producing these disorders.

SUGGESTED READINGS

Barchilon, J., and Engel, G. L.: Dermatitis: an hysterical conversion symptom, Psychosom. Med. 14:295, 1952.

Graham, D. T., Kabler, J. D., and Graham, F. K.: Physiological response to the suggestion of attitudes specific for hives and hypertension, Psychosom. Med. 24:159, 1962.

Greenhill, M. H., and Finesinger, J. E.: Neurotic symptoms and emotional factors in atopic dermatitis, Arch. Derm. Syph. 46:187, 1942.

Kaneko, Z., and Takaishi, N.: Psychometric studies on chronic urticaria, Folia Psychiat. Neurol. Jap. 17:16, 1963.

Kepecs, J. G., Robin, M., and Brunner, M.: Relationship between certain emotional states and exudation into the skin, Psychosom. Med. 13:10, 1951.

Kroger, W. S.: Current studies of hypnosis in allergy, Ann. Allerg. 22:123, 1964.

Lester, E. P., Wittkower, E. D., Kalz, F., and Azima, H.: Phenotropic drugs in psychosomatic disorders (skin), Amer. J. Psychiat. 119:136, 1962.

Musaph, H.: Itching and scratching, Philadelphia, 1964, F. A. Davis Co.

Musaph, H.: Psychodynamics of itching, Int. J. Psychoanal. 49:336, 1968.

Wittkower, E. D.: Studies of the personality of patients suffering from urticaria, Psychosom. Med. 15:116, 1953.

Musculoskeletal disorder

That anxiety and fear often are accompanied by increase in muscle tone is commonly recognized. Increased muscle tone becomes especially important as an aggravating factor in various forms of arthritis, backache, tension headache, or any other condition in which muscle irritation or spasm may play a role.

Tension headache is usually described as a dull constant pain or "pressure feeling" beginning gradually and lasting from a few minutes to days, weeks, or even years. The headache may be occipital, frontal, or over the top of the head and it is often associated with noticeable muscular tension. This type of headache may be relieved by treating the underlying emotional disorder, although temporary relief usually is attained by combination doses of sedatives and mild analgesics.

Attempting to elucidate the common observation that exacerbations of *rheumatoid arthritis* follow emotional stress, a number of psychoanalytic studies have discovered a history of development as a child under excessively restricting parental attitudes. An important mode of discharging tension and relieving frustration is muscle activity (e.g., hard work, sports, gardening). Before development of disease, the patients apparently restrict this physical freedom. Under more severe life stress, these patients tend to seek a passive, dependent status and channel all aggression into increased muscle tone and—in some way now poorly understood—into arthritis.

SUGGESTED READINGS

Brenner, C., Friedman, A. P., and Carter, S.: Psychologic factors in the etiology and treatment of chronic headache, Psychosom. Med. **11**:53, 1949.

Cleveland, S. E., and Fisher, S.: Behavior and unconscious fantasies of patients with rheumatoid arthritis, Psychosom. Med. **16**:327, 1954.

Gottschalk, L. A., Serota, H. M., and Shapiro, L. B.: Psychological conflict and neuromuscular tension; I, Preliminary report and method as applied to rheumatoid arthritis, Proc. Ass. Res. Nerv. Ment. Dis. **29**:735, 1950.

Holmes, T. H., and Wolff, H. G.: Life situations, emotions and backache, Psychosom. Med. **14**:18, 1952.

Moos, R. H.: Personality factors associated with rheumatoid arthritis: a review, J. Chronic Dis. **17**:41, 1964.

Scotch, N. A., and Gieger, H.: The epidemiology of rheumatoid arthritis:

a review with special attention to social factors, J. Chronic Dis. 15:1037, 1962.

Respiratory disorder

Hyperventilation syndrome. Hyperventilation (panting) is a basic physiological accompaniment of excitement. Such forced respiration, even when unnoticed by the patient, can produce biochemical changes in the blood, resulting in reflex alterations of cerebral circulation; reduction of consciousness or syncope may follow. Clinically this phenomenon is used as a test to induce slowing and abnormal discharge in the EEG. Prolonged hyperventilation can result in shifts in CO_2 and $H+$ ion concentration, alkalosis, tingling and coldness of the extremities, tachycardia, palpitation, carpopedal spasm, and tetany.

Tense, anxious, or depressed patients may hyperventilate without realizing it when placed in difficult situations; frequently they report some or all of the signs noted above without mentioning overbreathing. Voluntary hyperventilation can be used to demonstrate to patients the origin of their symptoms.

Bronchial asthma. Psychophysiological correlations have been seen clinically in many asthmatics and, in a few studies, increased secretions and changes (constriction and dilatation) in the bronchi related to stressful topics have been observed directly. A strong desire for protection by and dependence upon a maternal figure, which is met by actual or fantasied rejection, is believed to be commonplace in asthmatics. Inhibited urges to confess and to weep have been correlated with the attacks. Immaturity in the sexual area with failure to marry successfully is also frequent. Nevertheless, as with most psychophysiological reactions, it is important to define the relationship of the psychic to the allergic, infectious, and endocrine factors specifically in each case.

Vasomotor rhinitis. Since the nasal mucous membrane is continuous with that of the bronchi, significant functional changes can appear here with any type of respiratory disorder. Altered morphology can occur during stressful interviews; like changes also can be produced by pollen in allergic individuals, and sufficient pollen can produce this reaction in any subject.

Experiments have shown that during exposure to emotional conflict, relatively low concentrations of pollen for short periods of time can lead to rhinitis.

SUGGESTED READINGS

Doust, J. W. L., and Leigh, D.: Studies on the physiology of awareness. The interrelationships of emotions, life situations, and anoxemia in patients with bronchial asthma, Psychosom. Med. 15:292, 1953.

Groen, J. J., and Pelser, H. E.: Experience with and results of group psychotherapy in patients with bronchial asthma, J. Psychosom. Res. 4:191, 1960.

Guze, S. B., Gabbard, J., Roos, A., and Saslow, G.: Chronic psychogenic hyperventilation, Arch. Neurol. Psychiat. 67:434, 1952.

Knapp, P. H., and Nemitz, I. S.: Personality variations in asthma, Psychosom. Med. 19:443, 1957.

Schiavi, R. C., Stein, M., and Sethi, B. B.: Respiratory variables in response to a pain-fear stimulus and in experimental asthma, Psychosom. Med. 23:485, 1961.

Cardiovascular disorder

Vasomotor instability and disturbances of heart action. Many psychiatric disorders manifest one or more symptoms of cardiovascular instability (e.g., spontaneous vasodepressor syncope, paroxysmal auricular tachycardia). Although few psychological generalizations can be made about these ubiquitous symptoms, such individuals tend to give a history of childhood neurotic traits and as adults often experience severe anxiety attacks and nightmares. The patient's equating of cardiac sensations with danger of imminent death may lead to a vicious circle (anxiety—vasomotor disturbance—cardiac sensation—anxiety), which can threaten medical management of true heart lesions.

Essential hypertension. Essential hypertension is the end result of a still incompletely defined group of physiological and psychological dysfunctions. A commonly accepted formulation holds that emotional conflict leads to chronic vasoconstriction by release of a pressor agent from the kidney. It is known that the blood vessels of the kidney are very reactive to both emotional and physical stimuli and that neurogenic impulses mediated by sympathetic ganglia may lead to this release.

Psychiatric investigation of hypertension has revealed difficulty in handling hostile feelings, subnormal assertiveness, and obsessive-compulsive traits. Hypertension may be considered a state of chronically inhibited rage (similar to Cannon's rage reactions in animals) arising from conflict between passive dependent longings and competitive feelings. Careful histories may reveal an earlier period in which chronic aggressiveness was suddenly controlled by much interpersonal acquiescence. In most cases psychotherapy can do little but aid medical management, perhaps because case finding techniques now are difficult to apply sufficiently early in the disease to recommend psychotherapy.

Angina and coronary occlusion. It is a frequent observation that attacks of coronary insufficiency follow prolonged periods of fatigue and worry and may immediately follow a threat to vocational security. Investigation of life patterns reveals an unusually high value placed on work achievements, a tendency to work long hours, and depressed feelings when forced to be inactive. Characteristics of perfectionism and a tendency to brood may extend back to childhood.

As is well known, coronary insufficiency is a common disorder among men of high income, administrators, and physicians. Often they have a poor prognosis because of their need to deny emotional factors and their tendency to react to the illness itself as an intense frustration.

Other changes in vascular tone. Reports of vasospasm or vasodilatation symptomatic of personality difficulty have appeared with reference to Raynaud's disease, migraine, and other conditions.

An illustration of this type of malady is *migraine,* an excruciating, pulsating, recurrent headache often presaged or accompanied by visual disturbances, vomiting, and transient sensorimotor changes. Migraine attacks lasting a few minutes to two or three days occur in 5% of the population (higher incidence in women than in men). The discomfort arises from extreme dilatation of the external carotid artery branches and may localize and progress in a characteristic manner; transient neurological signs are thought due to cerebral vasoconstriction. Migraine patients are usually overconscientious and ambitious persons who tend to experience guilt in reaction to genuine enjoyment. Many tend to remain overattached to parents or parent surrogates. Overt expression of rage has been known to terminate an attack suddenly.

Once commenced, the attack may be relieved in 8 out of 10 patients by administering, parenterally, ergotamine tartrate. Caffeine 0.5 mg. combined with ergotamine tartrate is available in tablet form and two tablets taken at the earliest premonition, one to four times as necessary, at half-hour intervals, may abort an attack. This medication is also available in suppository form for cases in which nausea and vomiting are severe. Psychotherapy which aims at helping the patient to identify situations that stir resentment and to express himself more freely prevents further attacks. More intensive psychotherapy should be urged where this fails.

SUGGESTED READINGS

Chambers, W. N., and Reiser, M. F.: Emotional stress in the precipitation of congestive heart failure, Psychosom. Med. 15:38, 1953.

Fischer, H. K.: Hypertension and the psyche. In Brest, A. N., and Moyer, J. H., editors: Hypertension, Philadelphia, 1961, Lea & Febiger, pp. 110-117.

Gressel, G. C., et al.: Personality factors in arterial hypertension, J.A.M.A. 140:265-271, 1949.

Millet, J. A. P., Lief, H., and Mittelman, B.: Raynaud's disease: psychogenic factors and psychotherapy, Psychosom. Med. 15:61, 1953.

Sacks, O.: Migraine: the evolution of a common disorder, New York, 1970, American University Press Services, Inc.

Weiss, E.: Emotional factors in cardiovascular disease, Springfield, Ill., 1951, Charles C Thomas, Publisher.

Wolff, H. G.: Headache and other head pain, ed. 2, London, 1963, Oxford University Press.

Hemic and lymphatic disorder

A few studies and case reports have linked certain blood responses and blood dyscrasias with psychological stress. For example, men recently exposed to battle in Korea, but in whom no strictly organic explanation could be entertained, demonstrated a marked transitory fall in neutrophil count. Decrease in clotting time, rise in erythrocyte sedimentation, rise in relative blood viscosity, purpura, hemolytic crises, and changes in eosinophil and lymphocyte levels have been reported to follow emotional stress in certain cases. At the present time, however, the nature of these relationships remains speculative and controversial.

SUGGESTED READING

Benedict, R. B.: Psychosomatic correlations in certain blood dyscrasias. Psychosom. Med. 16:41, 1954.

Gastrointestinal disorder

In early life, feeding activities are the all-important source of relief from physical discomfort. They provide security and emotional satisfaction. Early successes and failures of parents in meeting their infant's physical and psychological needs influence the first feelings a child develops about himself and about his own oral and anal activities. In later years as other sources of pleasure and relief from tension become available, these early patterns may persist and influence behavior in a wide variety of situations.

Anorexia. This symptom is common with both neurotic and psychotic disorders. Perhaps most frequently it is associated with depressive feelings.

Anorexia nervosa. Occurring particularly in fragile, immature girls, the triad of anorexia, emaciation, and amenorrhea may resemble initially an adolescent dietary fad. A developmental history of family overconcern with feeding problems and a confusion between sexual activities and feeding activities may be observed. In a few patients who find the demands of adulthood impossible to deal with, psychotic episodes, death by starvation, or suicide may take place. In cases where the patient shows little self-concern or desire for treatment, hospitalization on a closed ward, with psychotherapy, frequent small feedings, isolation from the family, and a planned daily program are required.

Bulimia. An intense craving for food which substitutes for emotional drives is symptomatic of a wider personality disturbance; commonly, bulimia may be a defense against disappointment or depression.

Cardiospasm. Constriction of the middle and lower portions of the esophagus in reaction to a situation the patient "can't swallow" tends to be a conversion* type of symptom. Diagnosis is confirmed by x-ray examination. Dilatations and surgical

---

*Certain authorities prefer to make a clear separation between conversion reactions and psychophysiological disorders (see A.P.A. Diagnostic and Statistical Manual, 1952, p. 29).

procedures should be a last resort since combined medicinal and psychotherapeutic efforts often produce complete relief.

Nervous vomiting. This occurs in psychoneurotics and often during pregnancy. Where nausea and vomiting since infancy have habitually accompanied interpersonal conflict, these physiological reactions may become conditioned to a variety of life stimuli of which the patient may be only dimly aware. Symbolically, vomiting may express an unconscious desire (e.g., the wish to get rid of what is inside) or may deny an unconscious desire (e.g., the wish to swallow or incorporate).

Peptic ulcer. Clinical experience indicates that ulceration with gastric hyperactivity, hypersecretion, engorgement of the mucosa, and hyperacidity is usually (about 80%) related to life situations. It tends to occur in a person who experiences frustration and resentment within the context of strong dependent attachments. Most psychiatric investigations have reported conflicts between passivity and aggressiveness, with reaction formation (the opposite type of behavior) a prominent defense mechanism which covers up a strong irrational need to achieve security from others.

Elimination disturbances. Toilet training by those mothers who demand that the child "give to them" in terms of obedience, punctuality, excessive neatness, and regular production of feces may create strong functional associations between interpersonal giving-and-taking conflicts and bowel regulation. Thus feces may be viewed symbolically as something of value, a gift or a possession; in such cases constipation may express the wish to keep or retain, and diarrhea (irritable colon or mucous colitis) expresses resentful giving.

Ulcerative colitis. This physiological dysfunction apparently involves parasympathetic stimulation of the lower bowel with production of the mucolytic enzyme lysozyme, which deprives the bowel of its protective coating of mucin. In certain personalities this dysfunction may occur as a reaction to a variety of stresses, but it is reputed to occur particularly in situations which demand independent accomplishment or arouse fear of not being capable of doing something. There is little agreement among psychiatrists as to personality type although ulcerative colitis as a suicide equivalent or as part of a grief reaction has been reported. Strong desires to be taken care of by others (oral dependent longings), reaction to frustration with bottled-up aggressive feelings, and attempted restitution through "anal giving" (diarrhea) have been formulated by some. It is generally agreed that many of these patients are immature and frequently do not permit successful psychotherapeutic intervention. When psychotherapy is attempted during a relapse, extreme care may have to be practiced around situations which may threaten the patient's infantile dependence on the therapist, to avoid worsening the disorder.

SUGGESTED READINGS

Alexander, F., French, T. M., and Pollock, G.: Psychosomatic specificity, Chicago, 1968, University of Chicago Press, vol. 1.

Anthony, E. J.: An experimental approach to the psychopathology of childhood encopresis, Brit. J. Med. Psychol. **30**:146, 1957.

Beaumont, W.: Experiments and observations on the gastric juice and the physiology of digestion, Plattsburgh, N. Y., 1833, F. P. Allan.

Bliss, E. L., and Branch, C. H.: Anorexia nervosa, its history, psychology and biology, New York, 1960, Paul B. Hoeber, Inc., Medical Book Department of Harper & Bros.

Cannon, W. B.: The wisdom of the body, New York, 1939, W. W. Norton & Co., Inc.

Engel, J. L.: Studies of ulcerative colitis; V, Psychological aspects and their implications for treatment, Amer. J. Dig. Dis. **3**:315, 1958.

Feinstein, A. R.: The treatment of obesity. An analysis of methods, results and factors which influence success, J. Chronic Dis. **11**:349, 1960.

Goldblatt, P. B., Moore, M. E., and Stunkard, A. J.: Social factors in obesity, J.A.M.A. **192**:1039, 1965.

Karush, A., and Daniels, G.: Ulcerative colitis, Psychosom. Med. **15**:140, 1953.

Moore, M. E., Stunkard, A. J., and Srole, L.: Obesity, social class and mental illness, J.A.M.A. **181**:962, 1962.

Pilot, M. L., Muggia, A., and Spiro, H. M.: Duodenal ulcer in women, Psychosom. Med. **29**:586, 1967.

Sullivan, A. J., and McKell, T. E.: Personality in peptic ulcer, Springfield, Ill., 1950, Charles C Thomas, Publisher.

Thoroughman, J. C., et al.: Psychological factors predictive of surgical success in patients with intractable duodenal ulcer: a study of male veterans, Psychosom. Med. **26**:618, 1964.

Wolf, S., and Wolff, H. G.: Human gastric function, New York, 1943, Oxford University Press, Inc.

Zigler, R., and Sours, J. A.: A naturalistic study of patients with anorexia nervosa admitted to a medical center, Comp. Psychiat. **9**:644, 1968.

Genitourinary disorder

Disturbances of genital and urinary functions may occur under stress in normal persons and also in a wide variety of psychopathological states. It is generally accepted that enuresis, amenorrhea, dyspareunia, frigidity, impotence, and premature ejaculation are, in most cases, strongly determined by psychological factors. Considerable evidence also exists that dysmenorrhea, infertility, chronic leukorrhea, urinary frequency, polyuria, oliguria, urinary retention, and urgency may, in certain persons, be produced or aggravated by life conflict. Individual case studies suggest that depressed or helpless feelings may lead more commonly to urinary retention while feelings of fear may choose expression by urgency or frequency. Urgency as a response to stress is said to be experienced in the urethra while urgency as a cue to bladder distention is sensed suprapubically. There is a growing body of observations to document the fact that many disturbed renal and sexual functions may express or accompany psychological conflicts; nevertheless, these relationships are as yet unclear.

SUGGESTED READINGS

Beach, F. A.: "Psychosomatic" phenomena in animals, Psychosom. Med. **14:**261, 1952.

Ferenczi, S.: Sex in psychoanalysis, New York, 1952, Basic Books, Inc., Publishers.

Hastings, D. W.: Impotence and frigidity, Boston, 1963, Little, Brown & Co.

Life stress and genital disorders; part 12. In Wolff, H. G.: Life stress and bodily disease, Ass. Res. Nerv. Ment. Dis. Proc. **29:**1059, 1950.

Masters, W. H., and Johnson, D. E.: Human sexual response, Boston, 1966, Little, Brown & Co.

Schwartz, M. S., and Stanton, A. H.: A social psychological study of incontinence, Psychiatry **13:**399, 1950.

Endocrine disorder

Diabetes mellitus. Long-term medical-psychiatric studies have shown close correlations between time of onset of diabetes mellitus or times of exacerbation of the disease (indicated by the appearance of ketonuria without changes in diet, activity, dosage of insulin, trauma, or infection) and times of life stress. The phenomenon of overeating in reaction to emotional conflict is also commonly reported in diabetics and provides a ready mechanism for metabolic decompensation. In addition in some cases a period of emotional tranquility may lead to a remission in diabetes. Certain investigators report a low marriage rate (47% of males between 25 and 55 years old are married), poor grading of all emotional responses, strong feelings of shyness, and a need to rely on others. Exacerbations are believed often to follow events which lead the patient further to devalue himself. Patients are said to react to the illness with exaggerated feelings of helplessness and may blame others for their condition.

Hyperthyroidism. Apparently in this condition psychic dysfunctions are partly etiological and partly a result of metabolic disturbance. The behavioral symptoms that occur with hyperthyroidism are overactivity, emotional lability, anxiety, and overt fear. It has been stated that persons who are sensitive and impressionable and who react keenly to life, with marked feeling of insecurity and an unusual sense of responsibility, are those in whom an undue emotional stress may serve to precipitate hyperthyroidism. Counterphobic behavior (doing repetitively what one most fears) is reported to be frequent. Psychotic episodes are not uncommon and may take the form of a manic excitement, a depression, or a paranoid illness. The psychosis can disappear with correction of the thyroid disturbance but this is by no means the rule.

Myxedema. In cases of myxedema the slowness and difficulty in thought and action may be confused with a depression. A small number of psychoses with varied symptomatology have been reported to accompany this condition. Disappearance of the mental disorder with administration of thyroid preparation has been demonstrated.

Chronic obesity. An increase in adipose tissue of 15% or more over the norm for a given height and physiological age has been called obesity. A morbid increase in hunger (bulimia), resulting either from brain damage (rare), from cultural conditioning, or (most commonly) from an abnormal emotional dependence upon eating pleasures for security and self-esteem produces this positive energy balance. Endocrine and constitutional factors are usually important in determining metabolic efficiency as well as the distribution of fat in the body.

Therapy limited to drugs and reducing diets frequently fails in chronic cases. With such patients, too forceful or rapid reducing regimes have been known to be attended by psychiatric illness. Because of these patients' craving for love and esteem, their sensitivity to criticism, and underlying loneliness, they are often difficult to keep in individual therapy. Group therapy is believed by many to be particularly helpful.

SUGGESTED READINGS

Bruch, H.: Physiologic and psychologic interrelationships in diabetes in children, Psychosom. Med. **11**:200, 1949.

Burdon, A. P., and Paul, L.: Obesity, Psychiat. Quart. **25**:568, 1951.

Crowley, R. M.: Psychoses with myxedema, Amer. J. Psychiat. **96**:1105, 1940.

Hinkle, L. E., Evans, F. M., and Wolf, S.: Studies in diabetes mellitus, Psychosom. Med. **13**:160, 1951.

Lidz, T., and Whitehorn, J. C.: Life situations, emotions and Graves' disease, Psychosom. Med. **12**:184, 1950.

Pitts, F. N., and Guze, S. B.: Psychiatric disorders and myxedema, Amer. J. Psychiat. **118**:142, 1961.

Wyden, P.: The overweight society, New York, 1965, William Morrow & Co., Inc.

Disorder of an organ of special sense

The diagnosis of a disorder of a special sense organ is applied to any disturbance of any organs of special sense in which emotional factors play a role. Ordinarily such disturbances are seen as one symptom of hysterical neurosis (conversion reaction). On the other hand, there is some evidence, as with primary *atypical facial neuralgia,* that neurological disturbance may occasionally be related to the emotions.

SUGGESTED READINGS

Engel, G. L.: Primary atypical facial neuralgia, Psychosom. Med. **13**:375, 1951.

Fowler, E. P., and Zeckel, A.: Psychophysiological factors in Ménière's disease, Psychosom. Med. **15**:127, 1953.

Ulett, G. A.: Flicker sickness, Arch. Ophthal. (Chicago) **50**:685, 1953.

Weil, A., and Nosik, W.: Some electrophysiological and clinical observations in hemifacial spasms, Proceedings of the American EEG Society, J. EEG Clin. Neurophysiol. **7**:470, 1955.

18
Transient situational disturbances and conditions without manifest psychiatric disorder

The term *transient situational disturbance* is used to refer to a variety of behavioral-emotional disturbances which can occur as acute reactions (adjustment reactions) to overwhelming environmental stress. In daily life situations one faces frequently the problems of illness, accident, disappointments in interpersonal relationships, and failure to achieve hoped-for goals. Major disasters differ from the above only in degree, unexpectedness, longer duration, unfamiliarity, lack of opportunity for escape or for effective action, and the absence of important support by others. The sudden death, loss, or illness of another valued family member would be an example of life trauma often precipitating an *adjustment reaction*. Healthy persons have a variety of conscious and unconscious mechanisms for effectively coping with such situations. If the patient has good adaptive capacity, his symptoms usually recede as the stress diminishes.

The immediate symptoms of stress are fear, anxiety, grief, annoyance, or anger, which can result in more or less appropriate reaction or, at the height of the stress, in paralysis of all action or in purposeless hyperactivity. From prolonged stress (as in combat reaction) there may be a residuum of restlessness, tremor, anorexia, asthenia, fatigue, insomnia, reaction to startle, phobias, nightmares, etc. that can last for months. Physical symptoms from chronic stress include tachycardia, precipitation of coronary attacks, and aggravation of peptic ulcer. Irrational behavior, drinking, and promiscuity can also result. Later symptoms too can include shame, guilt, depression, and loss of self-esteem from memories of one's inefficiency at the time of crisis. Symptoms from reaction to stress are often contagious: panic can spread through an audience, an anxious mother upset her children, or the unhappy home life of the boss increase the consumption of headache pills by the office force. In fortunate, healthy individuals the period of recovery from symptoms of stress may be brief and for some a good night's sleep is the best tonic. After prolonged stress the rebound may be less complete and the patient's life may not be characterized by quite the same vigor.

In differential diagnosis and in assessment of the patient's ability to manage stress, one must weigh the magnitude of the stress in terms of how it would be seen by others; also in terms of the stress tolerance of the individual, his life style and current life situation, his preparation to meet stress through past experiences ("sheltered life, etc."), the number of other stresses at this time ("last straw"); and the possible solutions available to him.

In preparing for treatment one must decide whether it is possible to change the situation, to change the patient, or to permit escape from that which is intolerable. One must judge the coping mechanisms of the patient and decide whether he perseverates in using coping mechanisms that are inappropriate or unworkable or whether he may be guided to use of better coping mechanisms. Reassurance, encouragement, and involvement in constructive activity are essential with the early return to duty or work situation. Adequate nutrition, sleep, and mild sedation are useful.

The prevention of situational maladjustments begins in early home training for the gradual responsibilities of growing up through shared responsibilities at home, preparation through wholesome, adequate adult interpersonal relationships, with good support at times of crisis in childhood and adolescence. A knowledge of life's traumata and emotional interplay is readily learned from one's peers and the communications media. A proper preparation for dealing with strong emotions and health matters is a responsibility of home and school as in the development of a personal supporting life philosophy. The balance of adequate support without the development of too much protection and dependence is a difficult parental task. In an enlightened employment situation the prevention of situational maladjustment is aided by clear lines of authority, good channels of communication, assignment of tasks within the range of the worker's competence, and personnel policies that enhance employment security. Continuing support from family, friends, and peers is of great importance.

Transient situational disturbances are classified as follows:

Adjustment reaction of infancy. Crying spells and appetite disturbance may occur at separation from the mother.

Adjustment reaction of childhood. Attention-getting behavior and nocturnal enuresis may occur with jealousy over a new sibling. The first day at school with its presentation of new and strange relationships, tasks, and situations may create intense temporary anxiety.

Adjustment reaction of adolescence. At puberty the incidence of psychosis rises sharply. It is held by many that schizophrenic and manic-depressive psychoses which have their onset after the age of 20 years actually begin in this period of life. Signs and symptoms of such incipient psychoses are difficult, however, to distinguish from the normal vicissitudes of adolescence. Conflicts involving urges of self-expression, attempts at emancipation from parental control, emotional hypersensitivities, exaggerated self-assertiveness or regressive timidity, and tendencies toward intense or dereistic fantasies lead at times to fleeting psychoneurotic or psychotic disorganization which has been characterized by the general term "adolescent turmoil."

The symptom pictures presented in these patients—frequently similar to those of a schizoaffective psychosis—may indicate the necessity for physical methods of therapy such as phenothiazine medication or electroshock therapy. One should apply such methods with caution because prognosis with hospitalization and brief psychotherapy alone is often good.

Adjustment reaction of adult life. The adjustment reaction may revolve around difficulties of the marital relationship, stress or fear of military combat, pregnancy and child rearing, unwanted pregnancy, bereavement, and the like. If the symptoms are of sufficient gravity or tend to persist, the appropriate diagnosis of psychotic disturbance is used.

Adjustment reaction of later life. In aging persons major adjustment reactions occur not only with awareness of the problems of the climacteric and an increasing number of physical disturbances but also as a result of retirement from work, attendant loss of goal drive and motivation, decreasing daily activity, and a reduction in financial income. Breakup of the family through separation or death and loss of old friends are additional factors. Attention must be given to orderly planning for retirement with proper scheduling of preventive physical examinations and medical procedures, attention to diet, physical exercise, and the involvement in group interaction (golden age clubs, etc.) together with emotional support from family and friends.

SUGGESTED READINGS

Ausubel, D. P.: Theory and problems of adolescent development, New York, 1958, Grune & Stratton, Inc.

Both, H. M., Modlin, H. C., and Orth, M. H.: Situational variables in the assessment of psychotherapeutic results, Bull. Menninger Clin. **26:**2, 1962.

Eaton, M. T., Jr.: Executive stresses do exist but they can be controlled, Personnel **8:**18, March-April, 1963.

Eaton, M. T., Jr., and Livingston, D.: Marriage counseling by the family doctor, New Zeal. Med. J. **61:**359, 1962.

Holmes, A. J.: The adolescent in psychotherapy, Boston, 1964, Little, Brown & Co.

Horney, K.: The neurotic personality of our time, New York, 1937, W. W. Norton & Co.

Raush, H. L., Goodrich, W., and Campbell, J. C.: Adaptation to the first years of marriage, Psychiatry **26:**4, 1963.

Reinhardt, R. F.: The flyer who failed, an adult situational reaction, Amer. J. Psychiat. **6:**740, 1924.

Social maladjustment without manifest psychiatric disorder

Current psychiatric terminology permits the use of diagnostic classification for individuals who are without diagnosable psychosis, or other classic psychiatric illness, but who nevertheless have problems severe enough to warrant examination by a psychiatrist. For them the term "social maladjustment without manifest psychiatric disorder" has been suggested. Under this category would fall persons with *"marital maladjustment"* who appear psychologically normal but who are unable to adapt to meaningful situations and demonstrate significant conflict and maladjustments therein, yet for whom life is otherwise normal. The term *"social maladjustment"* is used to describe persons unable to adjust when thrown into a new culture, whereas *"occupational maladjustment"* is used to describe persons with significant and handicapping conflicts within the work situation. *"Dyssocial behavior"* describes persons who are not classifiable as antisocial personalities yet who manifest disregard for the usual social codes and often come into conflict with them as a result of living their lives in an abnormal environment. Here we find persons who are predators and who follow more or less *criminal tendencies*, such as racketeers, gamblers, prostitutes, and dope peddlers. These persons may be capable of strong loyalties. They usually do not show significant personality deviations other than those implied by adherence to the values or codes of their own predatory, criminal or other social group.

These categories clearly are of direct interest to psychiatrists, since preventive psychiatry depends largely upon interventions during normal life crises which assist the individual to master potentially disorganizing experiences and thus prevent them from becoming fixed as behavioral disorders. Potentially disruptive stresses tend to occur in relation to specific developmental stages or life situations. These include early changes in child adaptation which require new learning such as weaning, toilet training, the first experience of leaving the family to attend school, and in adolescence the experience of graduation and the first intense heterosexual commitment. Later in life marriage or parental relationships as well as certain job situations may provide intense stress. Marital and occupational stresses tend to arise when the original bases for initial marital or job choice have modified with time. A marriage which may have been satisfactory before the arrival of children may not be well-adapted to parenthood. Certain occupational roles develop new personality functions or interests which then lead to alteration in values which can affect marital or parental adaptation. In all of these situations the task of a psychiatrist is first of all to differentiate between chronic established psychiatric disorder and transient social maladjustment. This can be done by examining the duration of the symptoms, the temporal proximity of symptoms to the particular social stress, and the appropriateness of the intensity to the stress. The nature of the symptoms occurring with social maladjustment are limited to anxiety, depression, insomnia, mild psychosomatic disturbances, and the like. More serious symptoms such as phobia, delusion formation, obsessional symptoms are indications of psychiatric illness rather than an isolated problem of social maladjustment. Previous levels of intellectual and affective and social functioning achieved by the patient also contribute to the differentiation.

Treatment. Brief psychotherapy carried on in close proximity to the stress involved, with a focus on the present situation, can be useful in instances of social maladjustment. Within several weeks a follow-up should be planned to be sure that the pathological responses to stress do not become fixed.

SUGGESTED READINGS

Ackerman, N. W., Beatman, S., and Sherman, S. N., editors: Exploring the base of family therapy, New York, 1961, Family Service Association of America.

Ackerman, W.: The psychodynamics of family life, New York, 1958, Basic Books, Inc., Publishers.

Birren, J. W.: The psychology of aging, Englewood Cliffs, N. J., 1964, Prentice-Hall, Inc.

Boszormeny-Nagy, I., and Framo, S., editors: Intensive family therapy, New York, 1965, Hoeber Medical Division, Harper & Row, Publishers.

Burgess, E. W., editor: Aging in Western societies, Chicago, 1960, University of Chicago Press.

Erickson, E.: Childhood and society, ed. 2, New York, 1964, W. W. Norton & Co., Inc.

Farber, S. M., et al., editors: Man and civilization: the family's search for survival; a symposium, New York, 1964, McGraw-Hill Book Co.

Group for the Advancement of Psychiatry: Death and dying: attitudes of patient and doctor, symposium no. 11, New York, 1965, The Group.

Group for the Advancement of Psychiatry: Psychiatry and the aged: an introductory approach, symposium no. 59, New York, 1965, The Group.

Lidz, T.: The family in human adaptation, New York, 1963, International Universities Press, Inc.

McCord, W., and McCord, J.: Psychopathy and delinquency, New York, 1956, Grune & Stratton, Inc.

Post, F.: The clinical psychiatry of late life, New York, 1965, Pergamon Press, Inc.

Schneider, K.: Psychopathic personalities, Springfield, Ill., 1968, Charles C Thomas, Publisher.

19
Behavior disorders of childhood and adolescence

Interest in child psychiatry has developed rapidly during the past quarter of a century. Within this time the management of disturbed children has shifted from the juvenile courts, schools, and churches into the psychiatric setting of child guidance clinics. In 1909 William Healy initiated a 5-year study of juvenile delinquents, and in 1912 the Boston Psychopathic Hospital had the first mental hospital outpatient clinic to accept children as patients. Great inspiration has come from the mental hygiene movement wherein it has been hoped that early attention to the disorders of childhood would prevent major neuroses and psychoses in later adult life. For example, Melanie Klein taught that psychoanalysis at the age of 2 to 4 years may promote healthier adult ego integration and prevent later pathogenic defenses against disruptive aggressive drives. The verity of such an assumption as yet awaits conclusive data, but it is now recognized that the emotional disorders of childhood form, within their own right, a medical specialty in which the child psychiatrist devotes his attention not only to the child patient but also to the child's family.

The general principles underlying etiology, diagnosis, and therapy of adult psychiatric disorders apply also in child psychiatry. A number of problems, however, assume special importance.

Case finding. Although no easily administered screening tests exist for the early detection of child psychiatric disorders, nevertheless certain general principles guide the pediatrician, the schoolteacher, or the parent in defining such problems. Only rarely is the behavior disorder identified as a clear-cut new entity. Usually the problem is more confusing, being an exaggeration of established behavior patterns in the child. For adequate evaluation such a shift in adaptation usually requires repeated observations of the child and of his family and must be carried out by a clinician with considerable experience.

In well-baby clinics, pediatricians' offices, and nursery schools the infant's slow development of walking, talking, or socialization requires a differential diagnosis between constitutional defect, prenatal brain damage, environmental understimulation, or early emotional trauma. It has been shown that mild brain damage is associated with poor prenatal and obstetrical care and is one cause contributing to some emotional disorders. This factor being present does not diminish the importance of a thorough study of the child's and the family's psychological processes, which often determine the outcome of treatment. After the child's problems have been clarified, special psychotherapeutic skill and tact are necessary to bring this unwelcome possibility to the parents' awareness without creating an avoidance of the problem but, instead, instilling a desire to cooperate in further diagnostic study. This is a particularly difficult situation when the child is a victim of parental rejection, overprotection, overstimulation, overpermissiveness, overindulgence, or overcontrol—situations in which the parent's own needs serve to blind her or him to the child's real nature.

The *diagnostic study* aims to assess psychopathology—a particularly difficult task because of the normal disturbances that attend growth—and also to evaluate the developmental state as compared to the development expected at a given age in the child's social milieu. The treatment plan depends upon an evaluation of the problems for further personality growth imposed (1) by the disorder itself and previous distorted development and (2) by socioenvironmental forces such as parental personalities, influence of other family members or people at school, cultural values held by adults about this particular symptomatic behavior, and the motivation of those responsible for the child to help the child and to face their own part in the disturbance. A complete diagnosis may include investigation of possible constitutional, medical, psychological, and social factors in etiology, a description of the child's methods of dealing with anxiety and of his capacities for interpersonal relatedness, as well as a prediction of potential assets within the child and within his psychological habitat. Obviously, gathering this information requires an extensive intake evaluation sometimes involving contacts with parents, teachers, family physician, neighbors, etc., as well as with the child. A trial period of case work with a parent and exploratory psychotherapy with the child are often required before the problem becomes clear.

The new classification by the A. P. A. refers to the behavior disorders of childhood and adolescence as being divided into six major categories: *hyperkinetic reaction, withdrawal reaction, overanxious reaction, run away reaction, unsocialized aggressive reaction,* and *group delinquent reaction.* The *hyperkinetic reaction* is one observed frequently in males and consists of restlessness in the classroom, impulsive action, and a difficulty in concentration and intellectual development. Frequently the referral is by the teacher who has difficulty in controlling the child's focus of attention and the child's tendency to distract others in the classroom. In some cases there is evidence of minimal organic brain damage, and this may occur in the absence of intellectual deficit. In these cases amphetamines as well as psychotherapy can be useful. In other instances such behavior may be an aspect of a childhood neurosis. Like the *withdrawal reaction,* the *overanxious reaction* and the *run away reaction* are symptomatic of either neurotic or transient situational personality disorders. The *unsocialized aggressive reaction* has been seen in children described by F. Redl and others and should be considered as a personality growth disturbance. These children have extremely poor control over their aggressive and sexual impulses, and usually they have been poorly socialized by their parents and even subtly encouraged by the pleasure of their parents in their expressions of aggression. Finally, the *group delinquent reaction* is a subculture-specific condition, found particularly in the slums of our large cities, where groups of late childhood or early adolescent children find security in anti-social acts supported by mutual peer identifications.

The present classification is behavioristic in orientation and does not fit with the classification used to describe adult disorders. Therefore, we shall also present the more traditional categories of childhood syndromes here.

Transient situational personality disorders. Because of the almost unlimited variety of disorders, there seems to be even less unanimity about nomenclature among child psychiatrists than among those who work with adults. A child may be easily influenced by environmental changes of all kinds, and the behavior disorders of childhood have been classified as adjustment reactions of infancy and childhood under the general heading given above. This grouping includes (1) *habit disturbance* such as nail biting, thumb sucking, enuresis, soiling, masturbation, and tantrums; (2) *conduct disturbance* such as truancy, stealing, destructiveness, cruelty, sexual offenses, and use of alcohol; and (3) *neurotic traits,* including tics or habit spasms, somnambulism, stammering, overactivity, and phobias. Often underlying these symptoms are rather severely disturbed self-expectations and perceptions of others as having hostile, rejecting motives.

Personality growth disturbances. Somewhat analogous to adult personality pattern disturbances are those problems in personality growth which interfere with school or social adjustment. Here may be mentioned as illustrations the over-conforming, pseudomature child, who cannot relate childishly to other children, the child with a reading or other educational disability, and the pseudofeebleminded child.

Psychophysiological disorders. The commonly encountered disorders in this group include feeding difficulties (chronic anorexia, food faddism, recurrent vomiting, obesity), difficulties of coordination (writing dysfunctions), respiratory dysfunctions (asthma, rhinitis), neurodermatitis, enuresis, lower bowel dysfunctions (colitis, constipation), etc.

Since physical handicaps and diseases with their possibly frightening accompaniments (medical examinations, hospitalizations, temporary separation from home) involve particular emotional stress for the child, the psychological reactions and social retardations resulting therefrom are an important part of pediatric psychiatry. In managing such situations, as Pearson has stated, pediatric psychiatry may be only common sense, but it is surprising how little the average person knows about this kind of common sense.

Psychoneuroses. The classic psychoneuroses are diagnosed in children but not with the frequency that such disorders occur in adults. Phobias, anxiety states, hysterical symptoms, and depressive states are seen. In addition, neurotic symptoms unique to childhood occur. For example, Spitz has described "anaclitic depression" and chronic withdrawal states resulting from the institutional environment in infants, and Bowlby has described a similar withdrawal phenomenon in children 1½ to 4 years old, following placement in a general hospital for brief periods.

Psychoses. Psychoses are comparatively rare in the period of childhood but increase as adolescence is approached. Marked disorganization of affect and thinking, bizarre, reversible sensory or motor dysfunctions, inhibitions of learning, and severe interpersonal difficulties are seen. Kanner has presented the concept of the "autistic child" as a contribution to the study of schizophrenia in childhood. Goldfarb has shown that about 50% of autistic children have "soft" neurological signs and less severe family psychopathology. These mildly organic types of autistic children can sometimes be helped with special education for the child and with family or individual psychotherapy for the parents, who may be withdrawn and confused about a child who can actually be handled more effectively if the parents are given understanding. It has been found that these children and some of their mothers have speech disorders; there is a disorder in perception of time, space, and causality. Most of the children with autism have severe language disorder and a significant group are mute. The disorder presumably arises during the first year of life as a failure of attachment to the mother and a failure, therefore, to develop a self-concept as a human being. These children tend to orient toward inanimate objects in a very stereotyped, repetitive way and to demonstrate active withdrawal from relationships which apparently make them quite anxious. Although Eisenberg reports a poor outcome with outpatient psychotherapy, Bettlheim has reported two fifths of these patients as markedly improved when given intensive long-term residential treatment. Presumably the most effective approach to autism lies in the prevention of disturbed early mother infant relationships and in the prevention of organic brain disorder in fetal or early infant development. The differential diagnosis between psychoses and neurological disorders is frequently difficult; in fact, some autistic children have been misdiagnosed as deaf or brain-damaged patients.

Treatment. Psychotherapy with children must be adapted to the communication skills of each developmental stage. Treatment of infants is in terms of substitute mothering. With young children, in play therapy, interchange occurs largely at a symbolic or purely emotional level. With somewhat older children, the therapist still communicates via play but can also make interpretations and encourage verbal understanding of important issues. With the young adolescent (perhaps the most challenging therapeutic relationship) at certain times an adult type of interview may be possible, and at other times communications may be smoother if supported by a card game or other recreation which does not prevent sensitive discussion of feelings; at still other times a pal type of companionship, perhaps taking a walk together, is what can be accepted. No matter what the child's age, the psychotherapist becomes more emotionally involved than is the case in work with most adult patients. For the child, the therapist usually becomes a supportive, identification figure, as well as one who uncovers, interprets, or confronts with preconscious or unconscious elements. Because of the child's immaturity and great dependence, the therapist must take pains not to evoke more intense affect or guilt than can be borne without panic, withdrawal, or further regression.

In recent years clinicians have increasingly recognized that for many child disorders the focus of work should be the family rather than the child alone. The child's psychopathology in these cases is not simply an internalized structure but is rather an expression of an active family interaction process. For these cases the clinician must try to ascertain what relationships within the family represent the core conflict. Many times the child's symptoms serve to uncover a much more significant marital conflict; in these cases the treatment of choice may be group or individual therapy with the parents. In situations in which each member of the family seems to make a significant contribution to the conflicts, family therapy is indicated. Particularly with certain kinds of chronic handicaps such as infantile autism or mild brain damage in a child, it may be useful to form a group of parents, all of whom have the same type of problem child, to assist each other in managing the particular difficulties of that disorder and in accepting the child's limitations. With middle-class verbal families therapy tends to identify pathological types of communication and interaction, including the double bind, chronic power alignments as of mother and son against father and daughter, family myths which serve as rationalizations for disturbed behavior, and special family roles such as the helpless one or the scapegoat. With poor slum families the therapist may initially have to visit the home and will be required to give more of himself emotionally and to face the practical survival problems of the family with them in order that a psychotherapeutically useful process can be initiated. These families tend to use violence rather than verbalized principles for influencing each other. This violence in the families of delinquent children has no predictability but fosters constant vigilance and a sense of helplessness. These families lack sufficient sense of the past and the future and need models for identification. Often the parents, being occupationally and economically as well as psychologically helpless, abdicate parental responsibility to one of the older children so that family power is vested much more in the children than is true in middle-class families.

The problem of whether to provide institutional treatment, always a difficult one, is particularly so here. On the one hand, institutional treatment is an especially powerful tool because of the child's psychological dependence upon the environment; on the other hand, removal from the family may do violence to normal identifications and the development of a "me-feeling" based upon family tradition. Institutional treatment is indicated where the family and social circumstances are unusually malignant and where the child's disorder is severe and chronic. In addition to psychotherapy and other medical treatment where indicated, the institution provides a therapeutic group-living milieu designed to encourage his interpersonal adaptiveness and also provides parental surrogates, usually by the device of "cottage parents" who sleep and eat with a fixed group of children.

In conclusion, then, the specialty of child psychiatry is really a multidisciplinary one. While the rationale for treatment grows out of the child's problem, most frequently the child is treated in conjunction with the family or larger social grouping. The psychiatric team approach is particularly indicated. Therefore, the basic clinical staff of a child guidance clinic is made up of pediatrician, psychologist, psychiatrist, and psychiatric social worker.

SUGGESTED READINGS

Aries, P.: Centuries of childhood, New York, 1962, Alfred A. Knopf, Inc.

Bakwin, H., and Bakwin, R. M.: Clinical management of behavior disorders in children, ed. 3, Philadelphia, 1966, W. B. Saunders Co.

Beller, E. K.: Clinical process, New York, 1962, The Free Press of Glencoe, Inc.

Burks, H. I.: Effects of amphetamine therapy on hyperkinetic children, Arch. Gen. Psychiat. 11:604, 1964.

Chess, S.: Diagnosis and treatment of hyperactive child, New York J. Med. 60:2379, 1960.

Conners, C. K., and Eisenberg, L.: The effects of methylphenidate on symptomatology and learning in disturbed children, Amer. J. Psychiat. 120:458, 1963.

Eisenberg, L.: The management of the hyperkinetic child, Develop. Med. Child Neurol. 8:593, 1966.

Erikson, E. H.: Childhood and society, ed. 2, New York, 1963, W. W. Norton & Co., Inc.

Fish, B.: Drug use in psychiatric disorders of children, Amer. J. Psychiat. 124:31, 1968.

Freud, A.: Concept of developmental lines, Psychoanal. Stud. Child 18:245, 1963.

Freud, A.: Psychoanalytical treatment of children, London, 1946, Imago Publishing Co., Ltd.

Glover, E.: Psychoanalysis and child psychiatry, London, 1953, Imago Publishing Co., Ltd.

Jenkins, R. L.: Classification of behavior problems of children, Amer. J. Psychiat. 125:68, 1969.

Jessner, L., and Pavenstedt, E.: Dynamic psychopathology in childhood, New York, 1959, Grune & Stratton, Inc.

Kanner, L.: Child psychiatry, ed. 4, Springfield, Ill., 1971, Charles C Thomas, Publisher.

Kraft, I. A.: The use of psychoactive drugs in the out-patient treatment of psychiatric disorders of children, Amer. J. Psychiat. 124:1401, 1968.

Krug, O., et al.: Diagnostic process in child psychiatry, report no. 38, New York, 1957, Group for the Advancement of Psychiatry.

Meyer, R.: Essentials of pediatric psychiatry, New York, 1962, Appleton-Century-Crofts.

Minuchin, S.: Families of the slums, New York, 1968, Basic Books, Inc., Publishers.

O'Neal, P., and Robins, L. N.: The relation of childhood behavior problems to adult psychiatric status: a thirty-year follow-up study of 150 subjects, Amer. J. Psychiat. 114:961, 1958.

Pincus, J. H., and Glaser, G. H.: The syndrome of minimal brain damage in childhood, New Eng. J. Med. 275:27, 1966.

Rexford, E. N.: A developmental approach to problems of acting out, a symposium, New York, 1966, International Universities Press, Inc.

Robins, L. N.: Deviant children grow up; a sociological and psychiatric study of sociopathic personality, Baltimore, 1966, The Williams & Wilkins Co.

Shaw, C. R.: Psychiatric disorders of childhood, ed. 2, New York, 1970, Appleton-Century-Crofts.

Shirley, H. F.: Pediatric psychiatry, Cambridge, Mass., 1963, Harvard University Press.

Werry, J. S., Weiss, G., Douglas, V., and Martin, J.: Studies on the hyperactive child. III. The effect of chlorpromazine upon behavior and learning ability, J. Amer. Acad. Child Psychiat. 5:292, 1966.

20
Mental retardation

Mental deficiency is a disorder defined by incomplete maturation of attention, perception, and cognition as well as of social adaptability. Psychological tests are particularly important in establishing the diagnosis, whereas neurological, psychiatric, and social service studies help to evaluate and form an appropriate treatment plan. About 3% of school-age children are sufficiently retarded to require special classes or other services to promote their development.

Since 1961, patients with mental retardation have been classified into eight etiological patterns, and the degree of deficiency in adaptive behavior is specified as part of the diagnosis.* Their classification and recommended coding as given at the end of this chapter clearly demonstrates that there are many different kinds of mentally retarded patients. Only a few of the classical varieties will be discussed here.

Patients with milder cases of mental retardation may not be diagnosed before reaching school, where they manifest difficulty in learning but may attain sixth-grade performance level toward the end of adolescence. Although they are not capable of a high-school education, with special help those patients with mild impairment can become self-supporting. They require supervision as adults only in serious stress situations. Moderately severe retardates can talk but lack social awareness and usually can accomplish only a fourth-grade level in

---

*See A Manual on Terminology and Classification in Mental Retardation, Willimantic, Conn., 1961, American Association on Mental Deficiency.

school. Under careful supervision and with special adult help, many of these patients can eventually undertake an unskilled or semiskilled occupation. Severe retardates, so-called levels III and IV in degree of retardation, require hospitals or other special care environments throughout their lives. Various degrees of guidance, support, and control are indicated, depending upon whether the patient has learned speech, mastery of bodily functions, and ways to protect himself. With those who do learn to communicate one tries to inculcate simple health habits.

The psychiatrist's job in diagnosis is a complex one and places special emphasis upon the maturation level of the patient's motor, auditory, visual, and speech functions. Educability depends on the patient's potentials for conforming to his culture and for responsive interpersonal relationships. Such a complex diagnosis is necessary in order to make a prognosis and proceed with a treatment plan.

The etiology of mental deficiency is varied. Some 30% of patients show no other symptoms but may have a family history of mental defect. Prenatal infections (especially viral) or childhood encephalitides apparently cause about 20% of cases. Asphyxia, anoxia, and cerebral hemorrhage resulting from prolonged labor or from brain damage associated with prematurity account for perhaps another 20% (cerebral palsy, cerebral diplegia, choreoathetosis). In mild form in children, the syndrome may be difficult to distinguish from incipient schizophrenia.

An undetermined number of patients show a mild or moderately severe retardation apparently associated with loss of interest and curiosity about the world around them which begins within the first year or year and a half of life as a result of parental neglect. Commonly this syndrome occurs in large cities in very poor families who leave their infants and young children to be cared for in situations in which there is very little activity, social stimulation, or contact of any kind with other adults or children. The child's interest in learning becomes so muted that the developmental process is disrupted.

Mongolism. Less than 10% of defectives suffer from mongolism. In one study such children occurred once in every 688 births. This form of amentia is said to occur more frequently when mothers are past 40 years of age. Although first described by Down in 1860, it was not until 100 years later (1960) that cytologists succeeded in numbering the chromosomes of afflicted patients, thus permitting a major breakthrough toward understanding etiology. A chromosomal abnormality (trisomy) was found as an extra forty-seventh chromosome in the twenty-first and twenty-second pair of chromosomes. Such chromosomal nondysjunction was present, particularly when the patient was the offspring of an older mother. The defect appeared as a deformed chromosome, because of translocation, in one of a pair of 46 chromosomes in the offspring of younger mothers, and here there appears to be some hereditary predisposition. Defects occur in the skull, eyes, tongue, hands, and feet. A narrow, sloped palpebral fold and frequent epicanthus give the patient an oriental appearance. Usually these patients are placid and inert and show considerable variation in the degree of mental defect.

Cretinism. Cretinism occurs sporadically as a result of congenital aplasia of the thyroid gland. It is endemic to some areas of the world. The child appears normal at birth but by the sixth month shows signs of the illness. There are retardation of growth and bone development and a general lethargy. The skin is often yellowish in color, loose, and wrinkled. There may be puffiness of the features with thickening of the eyelids, nostrils, and lips. Myxedematous swelling of the hands, feet, and back of the neck is common. The abdomen may be prominent, with umbilical hernia. Hair on scalp and eyebrows is scanty, temperature subnormal. Breathing may be sonorous and the child has a dry, "leathery" cry.

All degrees of mental impairment are found, but usually the patient is an imbecile. Usually he is weak and often placid, good tempered, and affectionate.

Treatment should be begun immediately with whole thyroid (dried gland). Begin in children 3 to 6 months of age with $\frac{1}{4}$ grain daily. This may be increased with age. Tredgold recommends $\frac{1}{2}$ grain per day for each year of the child's age. Maximum dose is 5 grains daily. Treatment must be continued after the symptoms have disappeared or they will return. Maintenance medication one to two times weekly is often sufficient. If treatment is delayed until the patient is an adult, little or no improvement will be seen.

• • •

There exist also in any large hospital for the mentally deficient a number of patients whose conditions are hereditary in nature and are associated with signs and symptoms apart from those of mental deficiency. The following conditions are included.

Phenylpyruvic oligophrenia. Phenylketonuria characterizes this rare, recessive, inherited biochemical defect. Clinical imbecility may be accompanied by dwarfing, seizures, dermatitis, kyphosis, and accentuated reflexes. Fair hair and blue eyes are common features. These patients excrete phenylpyruvic acid in the urine, which may be detected by the development of a transient, deep bluish green color upon the addition of a few drops of 5% ferric chloride solution.

Treatment of these patients by phenylalanine-restricted diets has produced definite improvement in the EEG's and some promising clinical results. Hemocysteinuria is a similar syndrome recently defined, and it would appear likely that additional defects specific to the metabolism of single essential amines may yet explain other cases of retardation.

Huntington's chorea. In the majority of cases this has its onset in middle life as a chronic, progressive psychosis with dementia, and it is accompanied by chronic movements, wasting, and rigidity. In a number of cases, however, the onset occurs in childhood and so this illness is then classified as a mental deficiency.

Epiloia. This is a syndrome of tuberous sclerosis, sebaceous adenoma, and epilepsy. The mental symptoms range from idiocy to the level of a high-grade moron.

Neurofibromatosis. In this condition, also known as von Recklinghausen's disease, multiple nerve tumors are found covering the whole body. Pigmented patches of skin and mental defect are variable accompaniments.

Oxycephaly. Oxycephaly, or acrocephaly. is an anomaly in which a high or pointed head is accompanied by mental defect. A similar defect is also found with *hypertelorism,* in which the head is too wide, or with *microcephaly,* in which the skull is smaller than normal size, both conditions being due to premature synostosis of the cranium.

Arachnodactyly. This is a condition in which long spidery fingers and toes, combined with long limbs, occur with mental defect and often with coloboma, dislocation of the lens of the eye, and cardiac defect.

Nevoid amentia. This condition, known also as Sturge's or Weber's or Kalischer's disease, shows a combination of mental impairment and meningeal and facial angioma.

Friedreich's ataxia, Laurence-Moon-Biedl syndrome, retinitis pigmentosa, polydactyly, and *pituitary dystrophy* are found among the mentally deficient.

Amaurotic idiocy. Both the juvenile type and the infantile type (Tay-Sachs disease) show progressive cerebromacular degeneration with severe mental deficiency.

Treatment. In the treatment of conditions of limited brain capacity, the patient's actual performance will depend to a considerable extent upon his motivation to train himself and upon the skill and persistence of those who are helping him to develop. Initially, it is the physician's responsibility to assess the severity of presumed cortical deficiency. With level III or IV patients the parents need to recognize the real situation and to consider institutional placement. Involved in this decision are not only the availability of special schools and clinics but also an evaluation of how much emotional and physical strain the parents and siblings could withstand were the child to remain in the family. With children who score over 20 to 30 I.Q. points, more serious consideration may be given to the possibility of maintaining the child in the home, provided the mother has the energy and personal resources to work intensively, under professional guidance, to train the child. Many communities now have special educational counselors and clinics to advise parents about special home training techniques and to evaluate at regular intervals the child's readiness for more complex tasks. Public schools often maintain special classes for the retarded. During his childhood years, daily routines should avoid complexity and stress personal hygiene, social amenities, punctuality, and understandable speech. As the child grows older, vocational guidance becomes important and the social worker acts as interpreter of the illness to the family or to the employer. The rate of development, although much slower than in normal persons, need not be inconsequential. Recently psychologists skilled in conditioning and reinforcement learning schedules have developed new methods of programmed education which break down learning to read and learning to count skills into smaller units more manageable by the patient. By skillful repetitive use of principles of reinforcement and associative learning, some formerly uneducable retardates have been able to obtain simple schooling. With an adequate educational program, it may be that even level II and level III patients could become more self-sufficient in the future than has been true in the past. Hospital programs not infrequently discharge such patients in their twenties or thirties to begin a semi-independent life.

The psychiatrist can assist in evaluating attitudes and symptoms which interfere with attainable educational or job achievements. Commonly, for example, these patients experience conflict around dependence-independence problems and may react by either exaggerating or denying their handicaps. Parents of these patients, as with parents of any chronically helpless child, commonly show intrusiveness and an overcontrolling attitude because of their deep concern to be helpful and push the child to accomplishments beyond his capacity. This common parental syndrome often leads to a lack of self-confidence and various types of neurotic responses.

CLASSIFICATION OF MENTAL RETARDATION
1. Mental retardation*
    - 310 Borderline mental retardation—I.Q. 68-85
    - 311 Mild mental retardation—I.Q. 52-67
    - 312 Moderate mental retardation—I.Q. 36-51
    - 313 Severe mental retardation—I.Q. 20-35
    - 314 Profound mental retardation—I.Q. under 20
    - 315 Unspecified mental retardation
        (Patients whose intellectual functioning has not or cannot be evaluated precisely but which is recognized as clearly subnormal)
    - Clinical subcategories of mental retardation
        (Coded as fourth digit subdivisions following each of categories 310-315)

*Adapted from A Manual on Terminology and Classification in Mental Retardation, Willimantic, Conn., 1961, American Association on Mental Deficiency.

.0 Following infection and intoxication
Cytomegalic inclusion body disease, congenital
Rubella, congenital
Syphilis, congenital
Toxoplasmosis, congenital
Encephalopathy associated with other prenatal infections
Encephalopathy due to postnatal cerebral infection
Encephalopathy, congenital, associated with maternal toxemia of pregnancy
Encephalopathy, congenital, associated with other maternal intoxications
Bilirubin encephalopathy (kernicterus)
Postimmunization encephalopathy
Encephalopathy, other, due to intoxication
.1 Following trauma or physical agent
Encephalopathy due to prenatal injury
Encephalopathy due to mechanical injury at birth
Encephalopathy due to asphyxia at birth
Encephalopathy due to postnatal injury
.2 With disorders of metabolism, growth or nutrition
Cerebral lipoidosis, infantile (Tay-Sachs disease)
Cerebral lipoidosis, late infantile (Bielschowsky's disease)
Cerebral lipoidosis, juvenile (Spielmeyer-Vogt disease)
Cerebral lipoidosis, late juvenile (Kufs' disease)
Lipid histiocytosis of kerasin type (Gaucher's disease)
Lipid histiocytosis of phosphatide type (Niemann-Pick diesase)
Phenylketonuria
Hepatolenticular degeneration (Wilson's disease)
Porphyria
Galactosemia
Glucogenosis (von Gierke's disease)
Hypoglycemosis
.3 Associated with gross brain disease (postnatal)
Neurofibromatosis (neurofibroblastomatosis, von Recklinghausen's disease)
Trigeminal cerebral angiomatosis (Sturge-Weber-Dimitri disease)
Tuberous sclerosis (epiloia, Bourneville's disease)
Intracranial neoplasm, other
Encephalopathy associated with diffuse sclerosis of the brain:
 Acute infantile diffuse sclerosis (Krabbe's disease)
 Diffuse chronic infantile sclerosis (Merzbacher-Pelizaeus disease, aplasia axialis extracorticalis congenita)
 Infantile metachromatic leukodystrophy (Greenfield's disease)
 Juvenile metachromatic leukodystrophy (Scholz's disease)
Progressive subcortical encephalopathy (encephalitis periaxilis diffusa, Schilder's disease)
 Spinal sclerosis (Friedreich's ataxia)
Encephalopathy, other, due to unknown or uncertain cause with the structural reactions manifest

A Associated with diseases and conditions due to unknown prenatal influence
   Anencephaly (including hemianencephaly)
   Malformations of the gyri
   Porencephaly, congenital
   Multiple-congenital anomalies of the brain
   Other cerebral defects, congenital:
      Craniostenosis
      Hydrocephalus, congenital
      Hypertelorism (Greig's disease)
      Macrocephaly (megalencephaly)
      Microcephaly, primary
      Laurence-Moon-Biedl syndrome
.5 With chromosomal abnormality
   Autosomal trisomy of group G (trisomy 21, Langdon-Down disease, mongolism)
   Autosomal trisomy of group E
   Autosomal trisomy of group D
   Sex chromosome anomalies
   Abnormal number of chromosomes, other
   Short arm deletion of chromosome 5—group B (cri du chat)
   Short arm deletion of chromosome 18—group E
   Abnormal morphology of chromosomes, other
.6 Associated with prematurity
.7 Following major psychiatric disorder
.8 With psychosocial (environmental) deprivation
   Cultural-familial mental retardation
   Associated with environmental deprivation
.9 With other (and unspecified condition)

SUGGESTED READINGS

Birch, H. G.: Brain damage in children, Baltimore, 1964, The Williams & Wilkins Co.

Bowman, T. W., and Mautner, H., editors: Mental retardation, New York, 1966, Basic Books, Inc., Publishers.

Clarke, A. M., and Clark, A. D., editors: Mental deficiency. The changing outlook, ed. 2, New York, 1966, The Free Press.

Dittmann, L. L.: The mentally retarded child at home, a manual for parents, Washington, D. C., 1959, Department of Health, Education, and Welfare, Children's Bureau, publication no. 374.

Duhl, L. J.: Mental retardation, Amer. J. Ment. Defic. **62:**5, 1957.

Ellis, N. R., editor: Handbook of mental deficiency, New York, 1963, Mc-Graw-Hill Book Co.

Kanner, L. A.: A history of the care and study of the mentally retarded, Springfield, Ill., 1964, Charles C Thomas, Publisher.

Kramer, M., et al.: A method for determination of probabilities of stay, release, and death, for the mentally deficient, Amer. J. Ment. Defic. **62:**481, 1957.

Kugelmass, I. N.: The management of mental deficiency in children, New York, 1954, Grune & Stratton, Inc.

Lilienfeld, A. M.: Epidemiology of mongolism, Baltimore, 1969, The Johns Hopkins University Press.

Linn, L.: A handbook of hospital psychiatry, New York, 1955, International Universities Press, Inc., chap. 19.

Low, N. L., Bosma, J. F., and Armstrong, M. D.: Studies on phenylketonuria; V, EEG studies in phenylketonuria, Arch. Neurol. Psychiat. 77:359, 1957.

Luria, A. R.: The mentally retarded, New York, 1963, The Macmillan Co.

A manual on terminology and classification in mental retardation, Willimantic, Conn., 1961, American Association on Mental Deficiency.

Masland, R. L., Sarason, S. B., and Gladwyn, T.: Mental subnormality, New York, 1958, Basic Books, Inc., Publishers.

Menolascino, F. J., editor: Psychiatric approaches to mental retardation, New York, 1970, Basic Books, Inc., Publishers.

Noland, R. L.: Counseling parents of the mentally retarded: a sourcebook, Springfield, Ill., 1970, Charles C Thomas, Publisher.

Pasamanick, B., and Lilienfeld, A. M.: The association of maternal and fetal factors with the development of mental deficiency, J.A.M.A. 159:155, 1955.

Penrose, L. S.: The biology of mental defect, ed. 2, New York, 1963, Grune & Stratton, Inc.

Perry, S. E.: Some theoretic problems of mental deficiency and their action implications, Psychiatry 17:45, 1954.

Phillips, T., editor: Prevention and treatment of mental retardation, New York, 1960, Basic Books, Inc., Publishers.

Piaget, J.: The origins of intelligence in the child, London, 1953, Routledge & Kegan Paul, Ltd.

Robinson, H. B., and Robinson, N. M.: The mentally retarded child, New York, 1964, McGraw-Hill Book Co.

Tarjan, G.: Research and clinical advances in mental retardation, J.A.M.A. 182:617, 1962.

Tredgold, R. F., and Soddy, K.: A textbook of mental deficiency, ed. 10. Baltimore, 1964, The Williams & Wilkins Co.

3

THERAPEUTIC MEASURES

21
The psychiatric treatment team

As the multidimensional nature of many illnesses has become clearer, the focus of medical concern has begun to move from treating the illness to treating interacting dysfunctions of related systems which either exist within the patient (biological or physiological) or impinge upon the patient from without (environmental or social). To employ this complex concept of disease often requires a harmoniously effective team of specialists. This is particularly true in psychiatry, where disabling disorders may, in a sense, reside as much within the disturbed relationships surrounding the patient as within the patient himself. Here, therefore, the therapeutic task may involve working in a coordinated manner with several "patients"—for example, with the patient and his family or with the patient and his employer.

Depending upon the setting for treatment, whether state hospital, general hospital, clinic, school, or juvenile court, the professional identity of members of the treatment team varies considerably. Thus in a hospital, under supervision of the occupational therapist, a person trained primarily as a musician, artist, or teacher may perform a variety of socializing and ego supportive functions. Within the juvenile court, the probation officer or lawyer may be called upon to perform functions the aims of which do not differ, substantially, from the goals of supportive psychiatric treatment. In medical settings, the primary members of the team may commonly include the psychiatrist, internist, surgeon, pediatrician, social worker, psychologist, and nurse. For special problems the resources available from a mental health-oriented clergyman, dietitian, vocational guidance specialist, marriage counselor, physical therapist, library assistant, or volunteer aide should be kept in mind.

THE PSYCHIATRIST

Because of the complex nature of psychiatric disorders, the psychiatrist, more than most physicians, tends to become involved in administrative, educative, and professional leadership functions. His approach both to patients and to colleagues must be in some respects more collaborative and less authoritative than the approach of his brother physicians.

For example, when psychiatrist and social worker collaborate in the psychotherapy of a disturbed parent-child pair, the emotional relationship and communication pattern worked out between the two therapists is a dynamic factor powerfully affecting the new balance to be achieved within the family of the two patients. Energies spent in improving the individual self-awareness and group effectiveness of psychiatric team members will directly benefit patients. Traits of competitiveness, dominance over others, excessive need for approval, or indecisiveness in the team director should be scrutinized courageously by himself.

THE COLLABORATING PHYSICIAN

Commonly an internist, surgeon, pediatrician, or general practitioner may be involved at the time of referral, of disposition after the treatment, or when physical diseases accompany psychiatric disorders. The art of referring to a psychiatrist a patient who may be attached to "his" doctor and who believes his illness to be primarily somatic is indeed a difficult one. Later success in relating positively to the psychotherapist is much more likely if the outside physician consults with the psychiatrist before planning the timing and the rationale for the referral. For it is true that if the patient arrives on the psychiatrist's doorstep feeling rejected or insulted, or perhaps confused by a rather hurried explanation from his physician, the initial stages of forming constructive rapport are made more difficult than usual, if not impossible. In instances where the patient in psychotherapy is being attended regularly by another physician, it may occur that the latter's attitudes affect the patient's involvement in, and benefit from, psychotherapy. Some type of regular consultation is desirable between the two physicians to clarify the changing problems in the relationship each maintains with the patient.

THE SOCIAL WORKER

The psychiatric case worker is trained to undertake care of a great variety of social or emotional problems which are not so threatening to the organism as to require a physician's guidance. In addition, under supervision, experienced social workers may, on occasion, carry psychotherapeutic tasks. From her training, the social worker contributes to the team an alert awareness for family and cultural pressures which may be aggravating on the patient's symptoms. She is prepared to go into the patient's house or to meet the patient's employer at the latter's office in order to evaluate at first hand and report back upon the realities which face the patient. In the patient's efforts to make concrete changes in job or living arrangements, the social worker may function actively to encourage or to support the patient in defined directions.

In recent years a new type of social worker—the group worker—has been trained to function as an active participant with patients in group situations. These persons work to produce changes through sensitive environmental planning, group leadership, and intuitive on-the-spot guidance. In institutions and community organizations they have played vital roles in creating a therapeutic milieu.

THE PSYCHOLOGIST

Nurtured by an academic tradition rooted partly in philosophy and partly in the laboratory, the clinical psychologist is best prepared to represent behavioral science. Although psychological test instruments are still fairly crude and accurate predictions of important variables still difficult, it is the psychologist who is ready to aid the team in evaluating treatment results and in using the therapeutic setting for research purposes. Besides diagnostic and research functions, the clinical psychologist is also trained in psychotherapy (under medical supervision). In clinic practice it often happens that psychologist, social worker, and psychiatrist may among themselves carry three members of a family in treatment and then meet weekly in order collaboratively to evaluate progress.

THE NURSE

The nurse on the psychiatric ward combines a bewildering variety of functions. These include being responsible for the patient's immediate physical needs, mediating patients' requests for attention or special privileges, using her own intimacy with patients as a medium for behavior modification, supervising and training students and volunteers, participating with the occupational therapist or group worker in planning activities for patients, and assisting the doctor in physical modes of treatment. When intensive psychotherapy is being done within the hospital, a regular meeting between therapist and nursing staff is usually valuable both to the nurse, in providing her with insight into disturbed behavior, and to the psychotherapist, in understanding transference reactions and other disturbed behaviors both in and outside the interview. In some therapeutic wards an administrative separation is made between the personnel who are responsible for the patient (aide, nurse, and clinical director) and the psychotherapist; with responsibility taken off the psychotherapist for any decisions about the patient, it is hoped that the patient will feel free to trust the therapist, to express hostile or anxiety-laden impulses, and to work them through. Like the attendant or the activity therapist, the nurse becomes deeply involved in a patient's disturbed attitudes and actions and in some ways is in a unique position to observe and record for the physician subtleties of improvement or relapse.

ADJUNCTIVE THERAPISTS

Occupational therapy came to be regarded as a new profession, particularly from its important role in the rehabilitation of physically ill patients during World War I. Various forms of art (painting, sculpture), handicraft (wood, metal, leather, ceramics), dancing, music, and certain recreational therapies require specially trained personnel. Attempts to fit the activity to the patients' needs have taken the form of "occupational therapy prescriptions." Some hospitals prefer to give the patients a free choice in an unstructured workshop setting.

Industrial therapy is a most meaningful step toward returning the patient to community living. Such experience can lead to discharge for patients who need training in some marketable skill or vocation. Often mentally retarded patients who would otherwise spend an institutionalized lifetime can, through industrial training, graduate to a sheltered community workshop and special living arrangements apart from an institution. Hospitals may contract with local industries for piece work that can be performed in a hospital workshop and for which patients can earn wages even while still hospitalized.

Pastoral counseling attempts to meet the spiritual needs of patients through religious services for patients of several religious persuasions while they are hospitalized; the pastoral counselor also serves as an important link to the community and arranges for patients during the process of rehabilitation to attend community churches of their own choice. Very often the engagement in social activities with community religious groups can serve as an important step toward recovery. Increasingly, the clergy of community churches are seeking to gain psychiatric knowledge and counseling skills in order to better recognize incipent mental disorders and to learn proper management and referral techniques. In the mental hospital the pastoral counselor with special training participates in group therapy, counseling with special groups such as alcoholics, and learns to listen with a psychological as well as ecumenical religious ear to the problems of each client.

SUGGESTED READINGS

Barker, R. L.: Trends in the utilization of social work personnel, New York, 1966, National Association of Social Workers, Inc.

Caplan, G.: The theory and practice of mental health consultation, New York, 1970, Basic Books, Inc., Publishers.

Clark, D. H.: Principles of administrative therapy, Amer. J. Psychiat. **117:**506, 1960.

DePaul, A. V.: The nurse as a central figure in a mental health center, Perspect. Psychiat. Care **6:**17, 1968.

Deschin, C. S.: Future direction of social work. I. From concern with problems to emphasis on prevention, Amer. J. Orthopsychiat. **38:**9, 1968.

Fairweather, G.: Social psychology in treating mental illness, New York, 1964, John Wiley & Sons, Inc.

Peplau, H. E.: Principles of psychiatric nursing. In Arieti, S., editor: American handbook of psychiatry, New York, 1952, Basic Books, Inc., Publishers, vol. 2.

Schwartz, M. S., and Shockley E. L.: The nurse and the mental patient, New York, 1956, Russell Sage Foundation.

Stanton, A., and Schwartz, M.: The mental hospital, New York, 1954, Basic Books, Inc., Publishers.

Tudbury, M. A.: The psychiatric nurse in the general hospital, Springfield, Ill., 1958, Charles C Thomas, Publisher.

Weiss, J. M. A., editor: Nurses, patients and social systems, Columbia, Mo., 1968, University of Missouri Press.

West, W. L.: Changing concepts and practices in psychiatric occupational therapy, New York, 1959, American Occupational Therapy Association.

Zaslove, M. O., Ungerleider, J. T., and Fuller, M.: The importance of the psychiatric nurse: views of physicians, patients, and nurses, Amer. J. Psychiat. 125:482, 1968.

22
Individual psychotherapy

Of the many qualities of different psychotherapeutic relationships, we will present only those common aspects which seem to lend themselves to brief verbal description. The variety of experiences—whether from the physician's point of view or from the patient's—depends upon a multitude of factors, including differences in the participants' capacities for a continuing, intimate, creative relatedness, differences in their ideas concerning the goals of psychotherapy, and differences in their beliefs about the process of psychotherapy. Differences between settings for psychotherapy are relevant also although it cannot always be predicted how a given patient will be affected by whether he is seen in his hospital bed on the ward, sits in a bare, somewhat noisy clinic cubicle, lies down in a well-appointed private office, or receives psychotherapy in a soundproofed room with a listening tape recorder.

At the outset it is well to recognize that the interview as a form of communication need not be therapeutic. Many interviews are conducted for other purposes: social research, childhood education, moral suasion, authoritarian intimidation, selling merchandise, and so on. Whether an interview, or a series of interviews, has a therapeutic influence depends upon the motivations and psychological capacities of the participants, the structuring of communication, the subjective experiences fostered by the interviews, and the resulting encouragement or inner permission for the patient to experiment with new patterns of action. When the interview is therapeutic in intent and is successful, such an experience leads to increased mastery by the patient of his everyday social interactions and is accompanied by relief from symptoms.

The interview room should be quiet, comfortable, and conducive to inner contemplation without disturbance by telephone or street noises. Complete privacy of communication should be assured. Brief notes may be taken if they do not interfere with the therapist's attention. No furniture should intervene between the patient and physician (the stage should not be set for authoritative looks across a desk). A slight divergence of chairs in the face-to-face interview allows both doctor and patient a natural and easy avoidance of direct embarrassed stare.

Physician-patient contacts of whatever length, including the initial, history-taking interview, can be psychotherapeutic. It is recommended, however, that therapeutic interviews be scheduled regularly and that each last a definite period of time. Thirty-five to fifty minutes has been found, by experience, to be sufficiently long to permit the divulgence of worthwhile material, and yet not be too emotionally tiring for the patient. Shorter interviews may be indicated when the longer time produces too much anxiety. On the other hand, at the time of an acute emotional crisis, it may occasionally be valuable to stay with a patient for a prolonged period, until the storm has somewhat subsided. For intensive analysis of personality problems, interviews are held daily, 4 to 6 days a week. Less intensive psychotherapy is commonly carried on with interviews one to two times a week and, for supportive psychotherapy, as often as financial and geographical difficulties conveniently permit. When treatment is being terminated, even longer spacing of interviews may be used. Both therapist and patient should be punctual, as tardiness may indicate resistance to treatment. It is helpful for the therapist to take 10 minutes between patients to allow for relaxation and for organization of his notes.

The doctor is more than just a listener; he is an active participant whose attentive attitude, encouraging mood, and occasional words are calculated to help the patient uncover and clarify his feelings and behavior. Early, a question-and-answer technique may be necessary—particularly with passive, dependent patients. Gradually, however, the patient is encouraged to take more initiative and to discuss whatever topic comes into his mind. Initially, a brief explanation of therapy may be helpful and the patient can be given the following types of explanation:

"We seek to find an explanation for, and means to alter, repetitive ways of behavior in meeting conflict situations that make you uncomfortable and produce your symptoms."

"It will be necessary to review your life in considerable detail, emphasizing not only what you have done but also how you feel and have felt about what you have done and about important persons in your life."

"It is best for you to talk about whatever comes to your mind. As time goes on, you will be able to discuss matters that at first seem too personal or too emotionally painful to mention. It is very important that you learn to do this, because such areas of thought are usually the most important to study to help you get well. Our basic rule will be to say whatever pops into your mind, even if it does not always seem to make good sense at the time."

When the patient blocks, a period of silence may occur as the result of a thought that is important and so the therapist may, after a few moments of silence, inquire, "What is on your mind now?" or "What thought caused you to stop talking?" Yet, in helping the patient achieve greater spontaneity and insight, at times—for fear of mobilizing too much anxiety—care must be exercised not to press the patient into revealing too much too soon. The therapeutic sessions will never run short of material, for we are reviewing the patient's whole life; therapy could therefore occupy years. Practically, however, the subjects covered include all areas of life which are meaningful in terms of currently disturbed interpersonal relationships.

The therapist may obtain insight into facets of the patient's behavior of which he (the patient) is totally unaware. It is not so helpful to point this out to the patient directly as it is to lead him by means of carefully worded questions and directed associations to discover meaningful relationships for himself. Occasionally interpretations are given by the therapist in the form of "Could it perhaps be that this feeling toward your employer is like what you felt toward somebody else, your father, for example?" A "yes" answer from the patient, however, does not always imply emotional acceptance of the idea. Consequently his total (verbal and nonverbal) reaction to such interpretations should serve as clues to direct further exploration. At other times the patient may be confronted with some characteristic interview behavior or speech pattern that he is using to avoid emotional pain or to avoid serious contemplation of a central life issue.

The golden rule of therapy states, "It is more rewarding to listen than to speak." It is the patient who is being helped by verbalizing, confessing, and analysis—not the physician. Insofar as possible, considering the practical realities of living, it is well that patients not make major decisions while they are in treatment. One important goal of therapy is to help them mature so that they can make such decisions on their own. Even though it is obvious to the therapist what path should be followed, the patient is *not* the therapist; he has different goals, wishes, plans, etc.; hence, what would be a good solution for the therapist could well lead to further unhappiness for the patient. In this regard, remember that therapy is intended to preserve the individuality of the patient and is not a process of fashioning personalities in the likeness of the therapist. It follows from this that moral, religious, or ethical judgments are not implied by the therapist.

The content includes all mental productions of the patient and especially such topics as the following:

1. Subjective and somatic symptomatology
2. Family constellation and the complex emotional forces sensed within relationships to members of the family, in both the present and the past
3. Affects of fear, dread, loneliness, helplessness, confusion, anger, bitterness, depression, guilt, lust, hope, joy, and humor
4. Fantasy, dream material, and free association—with attention to recurrent or dramatic themes
5. Habitual interpersonal attitudes of clinging, isolation, defiance, accusation, complaint, domination, submission, provocation, rejection, inquiry, cooperation, helpfulness, or hero worship—as expressed to the psychotherapist or in other relationships
6. Recurrent patterns of action at work or at play, whether constructive or self-defeating

All psychotherapy is an elaboration and continuation of the original history-taking session. As time goes on, similar insights into similar problems begin to repeat themselves. This process, which follows the initial correction of distorted perceptions and which consists of numerous trial-and-error attempts at healthier solutions, is called *working through*. It may extend for weeks, months, or years. Indeed, after termination of psychotherapy this process can continue to operate. Psychotherapeutic alleviation of symptoms can occur soon after the first few interviews, during the middle of the working-through process, or not until close to termination.

THE DOCTOR-PATIENT RELATIONSHIP

The relationship between psychotherapist and patient occurs within certain broad psychosocial *structures* and utilizes a variety of interpersonal and intrapsychic *processes*. The societal position of the physician, a role defined through the ages as the healer, is a structure which fosters attitudes of dependence, trust, passivity, and suggestibility in all patients—without regard to personality or disease. As has been demonstrated in studies of the placebo effect, the popularity and public acceptance of any therapeutic agent contribute powerfully to its valuation by patients and staff and thereby to its objective influence. Another structural element in any doctor-patient relationship is the basic fit of their personalities. Does the physician have enough basic communality of personal experience with the patient to be able to establish a sensitive and genuine rapport? The beliefs and values held by the physician about matters of interpersonal influence, too, are important structural elements in the relationship, since they contribute to the goals and limits of the process. The nature of the patient's central conflicts, whether primitive and highly disorganizing to effective communication or less primitive and less disorganizing, contributes to the relationship. Similarly, the psychiatrist's own areas of continued immaturity, selective inattention, or latent anxiety will determine in a regular fashion those aspects of the patient's communication to which he can respond usefully.

Within the structure of a given doctor-patient relationship, many processes may be openly recognized and consciously utilized or, on the other hand, remain implicit or even relatively unimportant. The element of *hope,* the opportunity for the patient's hidden potentials for change and growth to be realized, remains implicit in many therapies and is utilized with greatest explicitness by the existential therapists. In nearly all psychotherapies, the therapist fosters some degree of *ambiguity* in the patient's knowledge of the therapeutic process and of him as a person. In the organismic approach of K. Goldstein, this is thought to be analogous to social isolation and sensory deprivation experiments which permit awareness of experiences bound to the less peripheral brain structures. Psychoanalytically oriented therapists also foster ambiguity as a way of *clarifying transference manifestations* and of *maximizing regression in the service of the ego*. On the other hand, in the client-centered approach of Carl Rogers, as well as in the psychobiological approach, the accent is more upon *acceptance of the patient as he is* and *clarification* of the patient's self-defeating, symptom-connected interpersonal operations. Most psychotherapists utilize *abreaction* or *catharsis,* the relief from tension obtained by simple impulse expression in a permissive setting. In all psychotherapies the therapist reinforces through his repeated, nonverbal patterns of response in the interview certain behaviors and tends to extinguish others. Learning-theory therapists tend to utilize the *operant conditioning processes* explicitly as a means of influence. The *educative* or psychopedagogical aspects of psychotherapy, in which the therapist acts as a parent or teacher in protecting or leading the patient, are recognized by all schools of therapy.

The psychobiologists particularly stress the value of *systematic rational review* of the patient's life history and symptom development. The *psychobiological point of view* is particularly adapted to psychotherapy within the traditional medical context and readily can be combined with physical examinations, drugs, or other physical therapies. It is based upon the principle of *negotiation*. The patient is encouraged to spell out his view of the nature of his symptom pattern and the physician then presents his view. Certain empirical attempts at trying this or that remedial behavior or attitude may serve to convince the patient or physician of the correct formulation or may bring to light new information. No rigid limits or requirements are placed upon the patient and any or all of the principles and processes described in this section may come into play at one time or another in this approach.

When patients displace upon the therapist irrational or infantile attitudes, originally developed in relation to early familial figures, the behavior is referred to as parataxic or prototaxic (by the Sullivanian therapists) or as a *transference manifestation*. Such inappropriate expressions often evoke emotional feelings or behaviors in the therapist. When consciously sensed and controlled, these *countertransference manifestations* are among the most informative psychotherapeutic phenomena. They may be further classified as to whether they are the outcome of a momentary *complementary identification* with the patient (in which the therapist's feeling of anger, for example, would complement the patient's provocativeness) or the outcome of a momentary *concordant identification* (in which the therapist's feeling of helplessness, say, agreed with the patient's experience). In the psychoanalytic frame of reference, constructive changes in patients are considered due to *transference cures* or to the *release of conflicted portions of the ego* to grow and make fresh identifications. The process of *identification,* unlike conditioning or rational learning, refers to the total shift in inner psychological forces rather than to changes in specific behaviors or feelings. While no therapist encourages his patients to emulate him, it is nevertheless true that patients can sense more useful ways of thinking, feeling, or reacting by relying on the therapist's understanding as a kind of borrowed ego. In instances in which the usual *nonjudgmental* and *nondirective* attitudes have been tried without effect over a long period of time or in which the patient seems on the verge of foolish, precipitous action the therapist can become quite active, giving *advice* or even exhorting. Such a direct approach, to be effective and scientifically based, must be eschewed on most occasions.

SUPERVISION AND CONSULTATION

Whether the psychiatrist is a beginner or an expert in psychotherapy, there will be cases in which regular sharing of his experiences and problems with a skilled outside therapist will serve to remove areas of selective inattention by the therapist and to clarify further the patient's problems. A collaborative atmosphere should be fostered in which the supervisor or consultant seeks to sense vicariously how the patient presents himself and his difficulties. Reporting by the psychotherapist may be by playing a tape recording, by reading from detailed notes, or by depending on memory of the patient's communications to summarize and formulate the latter's behavior. By presenting the interplay between patient and psychiatrist and focusing equally upon the experiences of both persons in the relationship, or by emphasizing heavily the psychotherapist's own subjective fantasies, feelings, and behavior while in the patient's presence, the consultant can clarify otherwise obscure facets of the treatment interaction. Each of these aspects may shed a somewhat different light upon the case. Perhaps in most successful supervision a mixture of all these processes takes place. The beginning psychotherapist would do well to avoid either too great a dependence upon or too great a competitiveness with his mentor.

TERMINATION OF PSYCHOTHERAPY

The question of when to end the relationship depends upon the needs and capacities of the patient and the goals set at the beginning. Symptomatic relief with some modifications in behavior can—in some patients—apparently be achieved in a very few interviews. With most patients, however, regardless of the frequency of interviews, it is well to plan on a period of several months to several years before closing the door. Even then it is well to leave with the patient the knowledge of a continued interest and of his freedom to return if necessary for further work. The neophyte psychotherapist would do well to regard any unexpected sudden desire, either on the patient's part or on his own, to end the relationship as a possible manifestation of transference or countertransference anxiety. Decision to terminate may take into consideration such factors as the current severity of symptoms, the current directions of change in the patient, the degree of stress or support in the patient's environment, the patient's latent potentiality for further constructive changes, and his motivation to undertake further psychotherapy.

SUGGESTED READINGS

Ellis, A.: New approaches to psychotherapy techniques, J. Clin. Psychol. 11:208, 1955.

Fenichel, O.: Problems of psychoanalytic technique, Albany, N. Y., 1941, The Psychoanalytic Quarterly, Inc.

Frank, J. D.: Persuasion and healing, Baltimore, 1961, The Johns Hopkins Press.

Frank, J. D.: Recent American research in psychotherapy, Brit. J. Med. Psychol. 41:5, March, 1968.

Friedman, M., and Simon, W. B.: How many public mental hospital inmates can benefit from psychotherapy? Psychotherapy: Theory, Research and Practice 5: Fall, 1968.

Imber, S. D., Nash, E. H., Hoehn-Saric, R., Stoen, A. R., and Frank, J. D.: A ten-year followup study of treated psychiatric outpatients. In Lesse, S., editor: An evaluation of the results of the psychotherapies, Springfield, Ill., 1968, Charles C Thomas, Publisher, chap. 5.

Kahn, R. L., and Cannell, C. F.: The dynamics of interviewing, New York, 1957, John Wiley & Sons, Inc.

Levine, M.: Psychotherapy in medical practice, New York, 1945, The Macmillan Co.

Lorr, M., McNair, D. M., and Weinstein, G. J.: Early effects of chlordiazepoxide (Librium) used with psycohtherapy, J. Psychiat. Res., 1:257, 1963.

Luff, M. C., and Garrod, M.: The after-results of psychotherapy in 500 adult cases, Brit. Med. J. 2:54, 1935.

Meyer, A.: The "complaint" as the center of genetic-dynamic and nosological teaching in psychiatry. In Winters, E. E., editor: Collected works of Adolph Meyer, Baltimore, 1951, The Johns Hopkins Press, vol. 3.

Rogers, C.: Client-centered therapy, Boston, 1951, Houghton Mifflin Co.

Uhlenhuth, E. H., and Duncan, D. B.: Subjective change with medical student therapists. II. Some determinants of change in psychoneurotic outpatients, Arch. Gen. Psychiat. 18:532, 1968.

VARIETIES OF PSYCHOTHERAPEUTIC APPROACHES
Psychoanalysis

The most elaborated conceptual frame of reference for psychotherapy is that developed by Sigmund Freud. Classical pyschoanalysis rests upon five points of view, each of them tied to rather extensive theoretical speculations and observations about human experience. While most psychotherapies draw upon various of Freud's discoveries, only psychoanalysis utilizes all five points of view. The *topographical* approach assumes that the mind contains three regions, the unconscious, the preconscious, and the conscious. The *genetic principle* states that present patterns of functioning shall be understood in terms of past experience and that neurotic phenomena are essentially manifestations of fixation at or regression to earlier developmental levels. Here lies the importance to the theory of the three stages of pregenital development: it provides a basis for classifying psychopathology according to whether the conflicts and defenses seem more to be oral, anal, or phallic. According to the *dynamic point of view* overt behavior and conscious experience are seen as outcomes of a struggle between the *instinctual impulses* to find expression and the counter forces *(countercathexes)* which operate to maintain self-control and self-esteem. The *economic viewpoint* states that the question of whether a patient is sick or well or whether he permits expression of impulses is a question of distribution of energies between the portions of the mind. If too large a proportion of energies is locked in unconscious conflict, fatigue and decreasing capacity for dealing with external stimuli *(reality)* result. The *structural point of view* is a working formulation which refers to the inner reservoir of basic aggressive and sexual energies (all unconscious) as the *id;* to the apparatus of control and mediation between action, sensation, and inner need as the *ego;* and to the internalized parental and guiding social models as the *super-ego* and *ego-ideal.* The psychic processes of the id are dominated by the *pleasure principle* and are referred to as *primary processes* (association by contiguity, displacement, condensation, and similarity). The functions of the ego are *perception, logical thought, memory, judgment, synthesis of experience,* and *control of motility* and are characterized as the *secondary processes* (association by logical, temporospatial, and causal relations).

The goal of psychoanalysis is to produce structural changes in the patient's ego by re-creating and resolving the *infantile neurosis.* The re-creation of the early pathogenic situation within the therapeutic relationship is called the *transference neurosis.* It is permitted to emerge by the use of the couch, with analyst sitting behind or out of the patient's line of vision, by meeting three to six times a week, and by encouraging the patient to follow the *basic rule of free association.* The patient is instructed to say everything which occurs to him, without censorship. As he listens the analyst adopts an *attitude of freefloating attention* in which he vacillates between vicarious emotional participation and objective evaluation and review. Classically the transference neurosis is resolved only through insight; that is, the analyst's *interpretations* are the instrument of cure. Early in the analysis interpretations are directed only at *resistances* to progress; later, basic conflicts are interpreted, as well. Following a prolonged period of *working through* in which the patient attempts to shift to new ways of handling life experience, and following resolution of the transference and countertransference distortions, the analysis is terminated.

SUGGESTED READINGS

Alexander, F., and French, T.: Psychoanalytic therapy, New York, 1946, The Ronald Press Co.

Brill, A. A.: Lectures on psychoanalytic psychiatry, New York, 1946, Alfred A. Knopf, Inc.

Fenichel, O.: Problems of psychonanalytic technique, Albany, N. Y., 1941, The Psychoanalytic Quarterly, Inc.

Freud, S.: The dynamics of the transference. In Collected papers, New York, 1959, Hogarth Press, Ltd., vol. 2.

Fromm-Reichmann, F.: Principles of intensive psychotherapy, Chicago, 1951, University of Chicago Press.

Glover, E.: The technique of psychoanalysis, New York, 1955, International Universities Press, Inc.

Greenson, R. R.: Variations in classical psychoanalytic technique: an introduction, Int. J. Psychoanal. 39:200, 1958.

Hendrick, I.: Facts and theories of psychoanalysis, ed. 2, New York, 1950, Alfred A. Knopf, Inc.

Kepecs, J. G.: Psychoanalysis today: rather lonely island, Arch. Gen. Psychiat. 18:161, 1968.

Knight, R. P.: Evaluation of the results of psychoanalytic therapy, Amer. J. Psychiat. 98:434, 1941.

Jungian psychotherapy

Carl Jung early split off from Sigmund Freud in his theory of personality. A basic difference arose between them as to the sources of psychic energy. While Freud viewed the libido as arising from some chemical substrate in the brain, Jung felt that the nature of psychic energy derived from evolutionary and primitive social myths and archetypes. He found evidence that in all peoples there are common symbols such as the mandala, the symbol of wholeness or the symbol of the whole self. He also pointed out the universality of phallic and other sexual symbols and the common content of fairy tales and religious rituals across different cultures. Jung's theory states that there are these universal unconscious sources of energy. Jung also differentiates within the unconscious specific personality tendencies referred to as "the shadow" and "animus" and "anima." The latter two refer to innate male and female character tendencies which are somewhat universal for all humanity but have a unique form in each individual.

Within this frame of reference the goal of Jungian psychotherapy is self-discovery and rebirth. By this, Jung means that psychotherapy should attempt to identify latent psychological tendencies arising from inner fantasies and feelings. The Jungian therapist tries to assist the individual to find means of expression for these repressed potentials leading to a revision of roles and functions in life. Thus the end result of Jungian psychotherapy is a new life style and a process referred to as individuation.

Underlying the Jungian psychotherapy process is a philosophy of time, space, and matter which differs from the prevalent empirical position of most scientists today. Jung believes that there are certain forces in people and in the universe which are not recognized by modern science but which find expression in extrasensory perception and in the expression of human purposes. He believes in a "synchronistic" or interactive relationship of psychological experience with the brain. Most psychologists today believe that psychological experience is based on neuronal events and on the functioning of the central nervous system. Jung, on the other hand, believes that there are independent psychological energies which interact with the brain within the person but are not dependent upon the nervous system.

In practice there are many competent Jungian therapists whose concern with individuation does not differ substantially from interests of other schools of psychotherapy except with regard to a greater concern for positive potentials arising from the unconscious.

SUGGESTED READINGS

Jacobi, J., and Hull, R. F. C., editors: C. G. Jung's psychological reflections: a new anthology of his writings 1905-1961, Princeton, 1970, Princeton University Press.

Jung, C. G.: Collected works, New York, 1953, Pantheon Books, Inc.

Jung, C. G.: Man and his symbols, Garden City, N. Y., 1964, Doubleday & Co., Inc.

The psychology of Alfred Adler

Alfred Adler, an early disciple of Freud, diverged to found his own school of individual psychology. Its approach differs from that of Freud in stressing goal-directed behavior and social adaptation.

Although emphasizing that persons differ in physical stature, predisposition to illness, etc., he believed it was less the actual inferiority itself than the *feelings of inferiority* in reaction to stresses, frustrations, and failures that shaped the *life style*. He felt that the human was neither a passive recipient of events from without nor of forces from within but rather that he had *innate capabilities* and a *creative power* to fashion his own life course.

Adler's psychology was not that of the individual alone. Innately friendly and cooperative, humans develop a trend to neurotic behavior if parents and teachers are overindulgent or overprotective or if they show the child hatred and rejection. He stressed the importance of birth order: the oldest being displaced by later siblings, the second having to cope with a stronger sibling, the youngest often being petted and indulged, and the only child suffering from lack of social interaction. Females, he felt, developed a *masculine protest* by reason of a world that puts greater premium on male status.

Adler felt that deep inferiority feelings were universal and normal, that they resulted from self-evaluation and led to a striving for superiority. Whereas the world initially appears chaotic to the child, he soon stabilizes it by the building of apperceptual schema (ideas about the world).

Each person develops a *life style* (self, ego, general methods of problem solving, total attitude) which is fixed by the time he is 5 years old. It affects the manner in which he strives to fulfill his goals and wishes in life's constant struggle to become superior. The very effort of striving makes a person seem more adequate. As much of it develops before the child can speak, it is unconscious; i.e., it cannot be verbalized.

Disturbed behavior is due to a maladaptive life style, with feelings of inadequacy and faulty compensatory responses. The same underlying principle exists for all failures or abnormalities, psychotic, neurotic, or whatever psychopathological entities.

The neurotic lives in fear that his exaggerated self-evaluation of superiority will be exposed, and he therefore develops self-guarding tendencies—"neurotic safeguards"—which include both aggressive acts and the seeking of distance by escape and avoidance (suicide, phobia, refusal to act, indecision, etc.); he further guards himself through limiting the sphere of action to that which he can control. Symptoms are formed at the point and time of crisis; hence, the onset of neurosis is seen as failure with life's major tasks (marriage, career, etc.).

To Adler, psychotherapy was essentially a social relationship applicable to all disorders in which the patient directed toward the therapist his habitual modes of reaction to significant persons in his life. By means of this relationship, the therapist could bring about a reduction in the feelings of inferiority and increase the patient's ability to meaningfully interact with others.

The therapist learns about the subjective responses of his patient by empathy and intuitive guessing, by eliciting reports from the patient, and by observing the interrelationships among situational events and the responses that occur in the presence of the therapist. The goals of treatment are (a) to reduce feelings of inferiority, (b) to correct erroneous perceptions and thinking, (c) to develop greater concern for the welfare of others with more affection and skills in interpersonal relations, (d) to reappraise goals, and (e) to increase initiative and courage to act in social situations.

Adler focused treatment on better understanding and felt that, when understanding was complete, improvement automatically followed. It was only necessary that the patient accept the need for change and for collaboration with a therapist whom he liked and trusted.

The therapist is required to remain attentive, sympathetic, and tactful and must maintain patience and tolerance in the face of hostility and resistance. The series of topics explored in therapy include childhood memories, childhood disorders, aggravating life conditions (including "organ inferiority"), family pressures, pampering, rivalry, neurotic patterns within the family, events that precipitate an aggravation of symptoms, birth order, dreams and fantasy, and expressive movements. He anticipated some initial partial improvement within 3 months.

Unfortunately, Adler's writings were poorly systematized; and although much of what he said presaged current interest in ego psychology and has been widely accepted in clinical practice, even in everyday language, yet as a system it has many deficiencies and has now been considerably outdated.

SUGGESTED READINGS

Adler, A.: What life should mean to you, New York, 1958, G. P. Putnam's Sons.

Adler, A.: Problems of neurosis, New York, 1964, Harper & Row, Publishers.

Ansbacher, A. L., and Ansbacher, R. R.: The individual psychology of Alfred Adler, New York, 1956, Basic Books, Inc., Publishers.

Otto Rank's psychotherapeutic approach

Otto Rank, onetime personal secretary to Freud, developed his own separate psychological system. Although his clinical experience was limited mainly to patients with compulsive neurosis and hysteria, he displayed considerable insight into human behavior and his writings have been widely read. Although his theories were loose and poorly organized, he became known for his concepts of *will, counter-will, life-fear, death-fear, birth trauma,* and *end-setting*. He believed that, although situational events played an important role in behavior, man had control over his own destiny. Rank postulated that, although individuals from birth had basic impulses (hunger, sex, thirst), the kinds of responses each showed were individualized and varied with learning. He postulated an original "trauma of birth," which represented a basic conflict and struggle, experienced by all men, between complete dependency and autonomous action. The individual, through exercise of his will, achieves a typical mode of adjustment so that he may live with his conflict in reasonable comfort. In this way Rank's approach was a precursor of more recent interests in existentialism in psychotherapy.

Rank conceptionalized humans as purposive, self-determining individuals with power to control primary physiological responses (drives) and affects (fear, guilt) and to select constructive, creative responses. Rank believed that neurotic behavior developed when fear and guilt became chronic or strong and when self-directing patterns were inadequate to control. The nature of the behavior disorder is determined by the nature of the patient's fear—either assertive-independent (life-fear) or submissive-helpless (death-fear). In this philosophy neurotics are considered not to be persons of action; they are thought to substitute thinking instead, and their self-evaluations are negative. Rank believed that an individual could stop his affective thoughts, could suppress them, and thereby reduce his discomfort. He rejected Freud's "psychology of the unconscious" as only furthering the neurotic attempt to avoid assuming responsibility for his own behavior.

The goals of treatment are (a) to change the patient's thoughts about himself from being critical and rejecting to approving and accepting and (b) to change the affective responses from negative to positive. With fear and guilt thus reduced and with self-confidence thus established, overt behavior could become constructive rather than avoidant. Man needs some kind of belief to be happy, and Rank's therapeutic attempts were directed toward giving him that belief in the form of faith in himself.

Rank outlined few techniques of therapy but felt that the therapist, from his own personal knowledge and experience, would develop a new technique tailored for each patient. After reducing his fears to a controllable level, the patient is encouraged to take the initiative in the treatment process. The therapy period focuses on discussing the here-and-now as an experience in living rather than as a mere discussion. Little attention is paid to content, but the therapist gets the patient to experience the full range of emotional expressions in the treatment situation and to learn to control and accept his emotional reactions toward others. The therapist makes no moral evaluation; he does not punish the patient through criticism, evaluation, or derogatory remarks. Past history is explored only if it leads to a clearer understanding of the current situation. The patient is encouraged to express openly all behaviors and connected emotions (fear, pride, shame, etc.). Dreams are discussed only in a symbolic way by discussing responses which were already conscious in another form. Free association is not used, as it would weaken the patient's control of directing his thoughts.

The patient is encouraged to react to the therapist emotionally as to human beings in general. The therapist guards against too strong a dependent emotional attachment through early establishment of a date the treatment process will terminate *(end-setting)* and manipulating the length of time of the therapy session as a reality factor. This planned ending of psychotherapy is believed to assist the patient to reexperience with greater mastery earlier separation and birth traumas.

SUGGESTED READINGS

Rank, O.: Will therapy and truth and reality, New York, 1950, Alfred A. Knopf, Inc.
Rank, O.: Otto Rank, New York, 1958, Julian Press, Inc.
Taft, J.: The trauma of birth, New York, 1952, Robert Brunner.

Psychotherapy in the mode of Karen Horney

Dr. Horney was one of the first of the early psychoanalytic group to join with Harry Stack Sullivan and to emphasize the importance of the social environment and the cultural stresses in accounting for neurotic phenomena. She fully accepts the basic concepts of psychoanalysis such as repression, the unconscious, and the use of defense mechanisms but emphasizes much more in her dealing with patients a careful analysis of actual, present-day life stress. Thus, Horney has contributed to a reorientation of psychiatry toward current conflicts (marital, job, and cross-cultural) as now expressed in the recent A.P.A. classification under the heading of "Social Maladjustment."

Horney, like Jung, has felt that the task of psychotherapy lies in the direction of clarification of the individual's identity and preferred social mode of functioning. Unlike Jung and Freud, however, she places less emphasis on working to understand innate or inner conflicting tendencies, such as conflicts between the drives, and places greater emphasis on the psychological tasks of resolving pressures from current and past social relationships. For example, in relation to understanding dream content she would be somewhat more likely to interpret dream material as expressions of actual life choices and alternatives rather than simply as expressions of primitive biologically based conflicts.

Horney's view of anxiety again has depended somewhat less on the structural theory of the personality and more upon unresolved social conflicts.

SUGGESTED READINGS

Horney, K.: The neurotic personality of our time, New York, 1937, W. W. Norton & Co., Inc.

Horney, K.: Self-analysis, New York, 1942, W. W. Norton & Co., Inc.

Horney, K.: Neurosis and human growth, New York, 1950, W. W. Norton & Co., Inc.

Client-centered psychotherapy

Client-centered psychotherapy was developed by Rogers and his school in the period from 1938 to 1950. The use of the word *client* was intended to underscore a focus on the internal phenomenological world of the client, indicating that the individual seeking help was perceived as a self-responsible person rather than as an object (patient) for treatment. The distinctive characteristics of this therapy include (a) the hypothesis that certain attitudes in the therapist constitute the necessary and sufficient conditions for treatment, (b) the concept that the therapist is immediately accessible to the client in the experiencing of the treatment relationship, (c) a continuing focus on the phenomenological world of the client, (d) the theory that therapeutic process is marked by a change in the client's manner of experiencing, along with an increased ability to live more fully, (e) a continuing emphasis on the self-actualizing quality of a human organism as the motivational force in therapy, (f) a focus on the process of personality change rather than upon the structure of the personality, (g) an emphasis on the need for continued research upon the method of psychotherapy, (h) the belief that the same principles of psychotherapy apply to psychotic, neurotic, and normal individuals, and (i) the opinion that psychotherapy is but one specialized example of all constructive interpersonal relationships.

In client-centered psychotherapy it is stressed that success in treatment is not so much dependent upon the technical training or skills of the therapist as it is upon the presence of certain attitudes in the therapist. Therapeutic progress and personality change depend upon the communication of these attitudes and their perception by the client. These important attitudes include (a) the therapist's genuineness or congruence, (b) his complete acceptance and unconditional positive regard for his client, and (c) a sensitive empathic understanding of the client. Throughout the treatment process the therapist openly reflects the feelings and attitudes which he is experiencing via his own self-awareness. His genuine positive regard for the client is communicated in a warm acceptance of the client's expressions regardless of their nature. It is important not to imply disapproval of painful, hostile, defensive, or abnormal feelings but to accept them in the same manner as good, positive, and mature feelings without the necessity of making judgment. Thus the therapist creates a "safe" environment in which the client is motivated to explore his own deepest thoughts and feelings and to share them with another human being. The therapist develops an empathy in which he is completely at home in the client's world. He senses and understands the client's inner world of personal private meanings as if it were his own world.

It is important for therapeutic success that the client reciprocate the therapist's attitudes, that, in an atmosphere of complete acceptance, he express his thoughts and feelings little by little, and that he become increasingly able to listen to communications from within himself. He realizes best at a time when he is angry, frightened, or experiencing feelings of love that he can reveal these hidden and "awful" aspects of himself without changing the therapist's regard for him, and slowly he moves toward adopting this same attitude toward himself, i.e., accepting himself as he is. Finally, he is free to change and grow in the directions which are natural to the maturing organism. From a position of remoteness he moves toward an immediacy of experiencing to discover its current meaning. There is no time limit on the therapy, and, indeed, it is felt that even in a relatively limited number of hours significant changes in personality attitudes and behavior can be produced.

SUGGESTED READINGS

Rogers, C. R.: Client-centered therapy, Boston, 1951, Houghton Mifflin Co.

Rogers, C. R.: On becoming a person, Boston, 1961, Houghton Mifflin Co.

Rogers, C. R., Gendlin, E. T., Kelser, D. J., and Truax, C. B.: The therapeutic relationship and its impact: a study of psychotherapy with schizophrenics, Madison, 1967, University of Wisconsin Press.

The learning theory approach to psychotherapy

The learning theory approach to psychotherapy leans heavily on the assumption that individual behavior is shaped by patterns of response from the social environment. As with behavior in animals, human behavior is considered to be learned in an automatic fashion; man's freedom to direct his own behavior is more apparent than real. In the course of growth and development, each person is taught by others ways of handling and reducing the intensity of such drives as hunger, thirst, curiosity, and sex. External events connected with these satisfactions acquire for him an individual and motivating significance. Fear is a normal response which initiates protective behavior. It may, however, become intense, inappropriate, and too generalized; such a fearful person must learn to reduce the intensity of the fear so that other functionally important behavior is not disrupted. The richness of behavior in man, as compared with animals, is made possible by thoughts which can stand in the place of action.

The kinds of habit patterns, both of action and of thought, learned in dealing with drives and emotions, are characteristic for each individual. The acquisition of disordered behavior follows these same principles of learning as does normal behavior. Neurosis is thus seen as the result of faulty child-rearing practices and the pressures of unhealthy social customs. Thus the environment may have taught the child a conflict between the sex drive and the need to reduce fear. Besides conflict based upon incompatible drives, there can be conflict stemming from incompatible rewards and punishments presented simultaneously from the environment.

The learning theorists speak of *avoidance conflicts* (of which fear is the most important) and *approach conflicts* (in which incompatible goals exist). The gradient concept relates to increase of intensity with either a spatial or temporal proximity to the conflict. Conflict may be solved temporarily by running away for a time, by the suspension of all activity, by suppression, or by repression. Repression places a conflict beyond conscious awareness and thus renders neurosis inaccessible to ready verbal examination, as is also true of conflicts formed in the child before speech patterns were developed.

Factors predisposing to a neurosis include poor childhood training and inconsistent behavior on the part of teachers and parents, particularly when children are small and helpless and easily influenced due to a limited choice of behavioral action. Society often provides a matrix with built-in conflicts, relating especially to patterns associated with eating, elimination, sexual responses, and aggressive behavior. In some cases a chance exposure to some emotion-provoking event triggers the neurosis.

The symptoms that develop from fear and anxiety are both physiological—cardiac, gastrointestinal, etc.—and learned —phobias, compulsions, etc. Thus the patient appears both miserable and, due to his maladaptive behavior, somewhat stupid.

The learning theorists believe that removal of symptoms is not a sufficient goal of treatment but rather that the underlying conflict must be searched out and relieved. Therapeutic goals are designed to help the patient acquire a conscious control over his thoughts, to help him unlearn the consequences of inhibition and inadequate responses, and to help him learn to consciously delay responses and substitute more adequate and discriminative responses by the use of higher mental process.

The therapist seeks to discover the kinds of events that elicit anxiety and the kinds of responses involved. The patient is taught through free association to reveal his full train of thoughts and emotional sensations. The therapist demonstrates his art through an ability to observe carefully and to accurately identify crucial behavior sequences. He judges which events he can manipulate to achieve intended behavior modification by helping the patient *extinguish* (get rid of) old, inadequate responses and *learn* new, adaptive ones. In the interview situation he must give the appearance of a nice kind of person with whom the patient can identify, yet he must be sufficiently neutral so that the patient can generalize, in his interaction with the therapist, patterns and responses he uses with others. It is not enough that new behavior patterns are discussed; they must also be tried out in real life; and if failure occurs, they can be discarded or tried differently anew.

The therapist must remain free from emotional involvement and unaffected by the acts and emotions of his patient. He must show restraint and must have sufficient sensitivity to the feelings of others to empathize with the patient, to maintain a positive attitude, and to instill sufficient motivation to continue treatment.

The actual work in the treatment hour consists of maintaining a verbal productivity, keeping the patient focused on productive themes, and overcoming hesitance and blocking by explanations or interpretations of any resistance to speak and to explore. The therapist points out responses that are occurring but should not occur, and he initiates responses that are not occurring but should occur. He unmasks the true meaning of acts and thoughts that are but repetitive or symbolic. He points out ways to modify the fear response. He helps the patient identify and appropriately label attitudes and emotions, and he leads the patient toward satisfying episodes of behavior. He uses the therapeutic interaction as a real life model; movies, video tape, or specially designed group experiences may be presented regularly so that, in graded fashion, the appropriate responses may be seen in others and learned by imitation of these others in action.

SUGGESTED READINGS

Dollard, J., and Miller, N. E.: Personality and psychotherapy: an analysis in terms of learning, thinking and culture, New York, 1952, McGraw-Hill Book Co.

Hilgard, E. R.: Theories of learning, New York, 1956, Appleton-Century-Crofts.

Mowrer, O. H.: Learning theory and the symbolic process, New York, 1960, John Wiley & Sons, Inc.

Hypnotherapy

The history of hypnosis has been characterized by periods of great interest and of rejection. Beginning with Franz Mesmer (1734-1815), its proponents have included James Esdaile

(1808-1859), a Scottish surgeon; James Braid (1795-1860), a Manchester physician; A. A. Liebeault (1823-1904), a French country physician in Nancy; Hippolyte Bernheim (1837-1919), a professor of medicine who worked with Liebeault; Jean Charcot (1825-1893), of the Salpêtrière in Paris; Joseph Breuer (1841-1925), a Viennese physician; Sigmund Freud (1856-1939); Morton Prince (1854-1929), founder of the Harvard Psychological Clinic; Clark Hull, Professor of Psychology at Yale; and, more recently, Grinker, Spiegel, Brenman, Gill, Erickson, Wolberg, Hilgard, Barber, Orne, and others. Recent experimental work has suggested a physiological predictor (EEG) of hypnotizability and has shown that changes in brain electrical activity with hypnosis differ from the EEG patterns of moderate or deep sleep and rather suggest a state of increased vigilance.

Hypnosis has been widely used in obstetrics, dentistry, and surgery and has found many applications in medicine, including psychiatry, where its appropriate use in selected cases can expedite and shorten the process of psychotherapy. The concept of the "hypnotist" is to be rejected. Rather hypnosis should be considered a useful tool, an extension of the doctor-patient relationship which can affect the ease and speed of communication. Hypnotizability is the ability to accept uncritically and to act upon a verbal or nonverbal suggestion, given either directly or indirectly, either deliberately or inadvertently. It is an intrinsic characteristic of the human mind, present in all individuals to a variable degree, and operative more or less all of the time. It is our experience that the great majority of patients can achieve a degree of hypnosis that is helpful to treatment.

There is probably in all of medicine no technique in which the doctor plays so active, directive, and authoritative a role and in which, on occasion, his ministrations can gain such prompt and dramatic results as with hypnosis. It should be remembered, however, that behavior and mood alteration or even symptom removal during the trance state is no substitute for an understanding of the dynamics, nor is an abreaction alone so valuable as the integration of acquired insights into conscious awareness.

A good doctor-patient relationship, rapport, and positive

suggestion blend imperceptibly into hypnosis. Patients vary greatly in the extent to which they show signs of deep hypnosis (amnesia, somnambulism, and posthypnotic suggestion). About 20% of all persons can achieve a deep hypnotic trance on the first attempt, and practically all can be helped by light hypnoidal states or simply positive suggestion.

Hypnosis is readily accomplished. Many elaborate induction methods and rituals are described in readily available texts. Most of these however simply involve principles of restricting the perceptual field (visual fixation), monotonous suggestion ("sle-e-e-e-p, relax, sle-e-e-e-p, relax," etc.), visualization ("TV screens"), and confusing verbalization ("When you are sure you can't open your eyes, try to open them to make sure you can't."). A simple method is to have the subject gaze upward at a pencil until the eyes feel tired and close. "You feel so relaxed and sleepy—relax, relax, let yourself go—away-y-y in-n-n." "When you are sure your eyes won't open, try to open them." "Let your head fall." Words are repeated in a low voice and monotonous manner. Successful suggestions tested by successful challenges deepen the trance. (Suggest and test for anesthesia, suggest arm levitation, etc.)

The skillful hypnotist tailors his technique to the needs of his patient (i.e., uses visual techniques with those who visualize well, arm levitation with tense, poor visualizers, etc.). The trance should be structured so that something useful can be accomplished. The ultimate purpose should be a more traditional psychiatric approach in which hypnosis is merely one tool. In exploring the patient's past life, it may be important to relive earlier life periods. This can be helped by *age regression* accomplished by hypnosis. The patient may play-act events of earlier years. Other useful techniques include *hypnotic dream induction, automatic writing, visualization under hypnosis, role playing of hypnotically induced conflicts,* and *abreaction.* The therapeutic process can continue after the treatment hour by means of *posthypnotic suggestions.* Here by the setting of a predicted, neutral, and nonembarrassing time for their appearance, significant memories may be brought to consciousness.

In summary: (1) People are suggestible and may be helped by positive suggestion, given deliberately or under hypnosis.

(2) Formal hypnotic techniques may be used as a part of, but not as a substitute for, the psychotherapeutic approach. (3) Properly used, hypnosis is a useful adjunct to psychotherapeutic methods and may greatly shorten the time needed to reach the desired therapeutic goal.

SUGGESTED READINGS

Barber, T. X.: Hypnotizability, suggestibility and personality; part V, a critical review of research findings, Psychol. Rep. **14**:229, 1964.

Brenman, H., and Gill, M.: Hypnotherapy, New York, 1947, International Universities Press, Inc.

Kline, M. V.: Clinical correlations of experimental hypnosis, Springfield, Ill., 1963, Charles C Thomas, Publisher.

Meares, A.: A system of medical hypnosis, Philadelphia, 1960, W. B. Saunders Co.

Orne, M. T: Hypnosis, motivation and compliance, Amer. J. Psychiat. **122**:721, 1966.

Ulett, G. A., Akpinar, S., and Itil, T. M.: Hypnosis—physiological, pharmacological reality, Amer. J. Psychiat. **128**:7, 1971.

Ulett, G. A., and Peterson, D. B.: Applied hypnosis and positive suggestion, St. Louis, 1965, The C. V. Mosby Co.

Winn, R. B.: Dictionary of hypnosis, New York, 1965, Philosophical Library, Inc.

Wolberg, L. R.: Medical hypnosis, New York, 1948, Grune & Stratton, Inc., vols. 1 and 2.

Psychotherapy through reciprocal inhibition

The *reciprocal inhibition* approach to psychotherapy represents a serious alternative to the repression theory approach. It is based upon the assumption that neurotic habits are learned and can best be eliminated through unlearning. It is only necessary that the therapist arrange for the proper sequence of events.

The therapeutic model is based upon the *drive reduction* conditioning theories of Clark Hull.

Habits result as a recurring response to a given stimulus. Such a response may be generalized to other situations which are similar or contain an element in common even though inappropriate. Habits become stronger when rewarded and tend to become inhibited when reward is lacking. Other stimuli occurring simultaneously interfere with a habit's reoccurrence on future occasions.

A special case of conditioned inhibition occurs when a response antagonistic to the response to be extinguished is associated with it, as both responses cannot occur simultaneously. Thus, through proper association, one can be strengthened and the other extinguished. Wolpe, with whose name this approach is commonly associated, states that neuroses are learned behavior patterns, basically unadaptive, conditioned anxiety reactions. The resultant anxiety disrupts major aspects of an individual's life or restricts or limits his behavior. Predisposing conditions are physiological differences in reactivity to anxiety-provoking situations. Some persons, through previous learning, have already acquired many inappropriate anxiety responses. Other predisposing factors are fatigue, drugs, hormones, etc.

Precipitating events produce severe anxiety. Fear may be associated with any of a number of events that were present at the time of the major fear stimulus. Previously conditioned childhood emotions may serve as a focus of restriction of the number of responses in a person's repertoire and may result in inadequate responses as may also a misinterpretation of the situation. Not only events but also thoughts can become anxiety elicitors. Associated events that have occurred at the same time as anxiety is produced may also elicit anxiety—shadows, odors, noises, etc.; it only demands that they make an impression on the central nervous system. Associated with the anxiety may be physiological changes, such as increased pulse rate or respiration, and these in turn may also become elicitors. Once anxiety becomes a habitual occurrence, it may impair other aspects of a person's behavior. Muscle tension may produce headaches, thinking may be disrupted, and psychosomatic symptoms, stomach reactions, etc., may occur. These symptoms produce more anxiety, and a vicious circle results.

The patient himself may learn to control anxiety by (a) physical avoidance, (b) displacing his attention, (c) the use of drugs, alcohol, etc., (d) the development of excessive and compulsive behavior which exerts control, or (e) amnesia—forgetting the content of the emotional response.

The goals of therapy are (a) to alter or extinguish the symptoms and (b) to help the patient unlearn the anxiety response to inappropriate events.

In order to effect behavioral change, anxiety-eliciting situations must be presented to the patient under circumstances in which responses other than anxiety will occur. The first step is to identify the troublesome anxiety sequences and to select the appropriate treatment procedures. The patient is presented with events, situations or responses, or symbolic representations of such events which inappropriately elicit anxiety and symptoms, and these learned conditions are then weakened. A sufficient number of repetitions must occur so that the troublesome connections will be abolished and more adaptive behavior will take place.

Among techniques used by the therapist are (a) assertive responses, including anger or friendly responses, (b) sexual responses, (c) muscular relaxation, (d) respiratory responses using CO_2, (e) competitively conditioned motor responses, (f) anxiety relief responses, (g) pleasant responses in life situations, e.g., with drug enhancement, and (h) interview-induced emotional responses and abreactions.

The therapist collects data on which to judge events: the patient's behavior, present life situation, etc.; he determines what stimuli do or can evoke symptoms at the present time; and he collects data on developmental history with emphasis on habitual emotional responses in each setting. Such tests as the Bernreuter Self Sufficiency questionnaire and the Willoughby Personality Schedule (a kind of systematic interview) are employed.

The goals of therapy include symptom improvement, increased productiveness, increased adjustment to and pleasure in sex, improved interpersonal relationships, and improved ability to handle and to change psychological conflicts and reality stresses. Improvement is judged by the patient's report, the reports of others, clinical assessments, and changes in the Willoughby scale. The first step to changing neurotic behavior is by acting, not by thinking.

Therapy relationship as a general procedure is a human interaction which provokes emotions, friendly sympathetic experiences. Assertive responses are used in life situations—aggressive, relaxing, affectionate, sexual—only when anxieties are provoked by interpersonal situations. The therapist sells the patient on the idea of trying it in a real life situation and then discusses and corrects the patient's performance. Behavior is shaped by consequences—systematic desensitization occurs during interviews. The therapist establishes a list of circumstances eliciting anxiety, from the strongest to the weakest. He trains the patient to muscle relaxation with hypnosis, he forces the patient's attention on anxiety-provoking circumstances, and he then helps him relax. Progress is made from the simplest to the more difficult visualized scenes. CO_2 respiratory responses may be used for freefloating anxiety. CO_2 produces muscle relaxation and is antagonistic to anxiety. Competitive motor responses are produced in the presence of conflict situations—through the patient's imagery in the treatment situation. Mild shocks may elicit other motor responses than those usually associated with anxieties. Real life behavior is the most effective therapeutic tool, and the patient is urged to experience success in the community.

Proponents of this theory believe that the majority of candidates for psychotherapy can be significantly helped, with a relatively small number of sessions.

SUGGESTED READINGS

Bugenthal, J. F. T.: Search for authenticity, New York, 1965, Holt, Rinehart & Winston, Inc.

Eysenck, H. J.: Behavior therapy and the neurosis, New York, 1960, Pergamon Press, Inc.

Eysenck, H. J., and Rachman, S.: The causes and cures of neurosis, San Diego, Calif., 1965, R. R. Knapp.

Franks, C. M., editor: Conditioning techniques in clinical practice and research, New York, 1964, Springer Publishing Co., Inc.

Parker, B.: My language is me, New York, 1962, Basic Books, Inc., Publishers.

Strupp, H. H.: Psychotherapists in action, New York, 1960, Grune & Stratton, Inc.

Ulman, L. P., and Krasner, L., editors: Case studies in behavior modification, New York, 1965, Holt, Rinehart & Winston, Inc.

Wolpe, J.: Psychotherapy by reciprocal inhibition, Stanford, Calif., 1958, Stanford University Press.

Wolpe, J.: The experimental foundations of some new psychotherapeutic methods. In Bachrach, A. J., editor: Experimental frontiers of clinical psychology, New York, 1962, Basic Books, Inc., Publishers.

Brief therapy

Most commonly patients come for relief of symptoms of less than 6 months' duration or symptoms referable to a recent life situation which has led to intensification of a chronic set of difficulties. In many such cases it is possible to set rather limited goals and yet provide the patient with substantial symptomatic relief as well as some opportunity for psychological growth. The initial *ventilation of feelings* and *uncovering of major current sources of anxiety* can most effectively be done in the first or second interview while the patient is suffering and highly motivated to receive help. Such an initial contact may extend for 2 hours in order to obtain a full account and demonstrate the physician's concern. The work of psychotherapy in such situations tries the observational and intuitive capacities of the therapist. He needs to thresh out the wheat of the precipitating life crisis from the chaff of accumulated but generally manageable dissatisfactions. This can sometimes be done through a focus on the situation surrounding the development of the most recent or acute symptom. Once the nidus of current stress has been defined, a confrontation of the patient with the nature of the situation may give considerable relief through insight, provided the patient's personality is sufficiently resilient. In patients who exhibit diffuse symptomatology, panic, confusion, social withdrawal, or bizarre attitudes, an underlying severe personality defect may be suspected, and a more gentle *supportive approach* be employed. Here the therapist may utilize his own understanding as a basis for *giving advice* or *clarifying certain assets* in the patient which the latter may be overlooking. At any rate, in brief therapy one must take special pains to present material to the patient in ways consistent with the later's self-esteem, since time has not permitted much testing out of the therapist or development of a deep rapport.

SUGGESTED READING

Small, L.: The briefer psychotherapies, New York, 1971, Brunner/Mazel, Inc.

23
Group therapy

Since ancient times many leaders of men, particularly state or religious leaders, have recognized the power of a unified group in producing certain psychological changes within individual members of the group. Wherever individuals form such a stable group for the purpose of relieving symptoms or of strengthening certain personality functions, group therapy may be said to exist. Although some of the qualities of a group and part of the direction in which it proceeds depend upon the personality of the group leader, it is important to recognize that any group has the latent power of self-direction; it may, in one way or another, resist a leader who tries to produce changes which are too divergent from the standards, beliefs, or defenses of the members. The effects a group has upon participants' personality or social adjustments seem to be influenced by the tolerance developed within the group for emotional expression, for self-scrutiny without loss of self-esteem, for attempting corrective emotional experiences, and for identifying or empathizing with each other.

In the United States, group therapy was originated by Pratt in 1905 when groups of patients suffering from tuberculosis were brought together to discuss their reality problems, to help each other solve these problems through discussion, and to receive emotional support. In Vienna, Moreno used this technique in 1910 with a group of prostitutes and later in dealing with children's emotional problems. In 1929 Wender began experimenting with group therapy with psychoneurotics and became convinced that for certain patients it was a more powerful tool than individual therapy. Since then, with

Marsch's report in 1931 of group therapy with psychotics, with Schilder's and Slavson's use of psychoanalytic concepts in group therapy during the 1930's, and with Moreno's development of psychodrama during the same period, group techniques have had increasing application. Group therapy permits treatment of more patients by a single therapist and therefore has economic advantages. Partly because the military psychiatrist needed to treat many patients at once and partly because of the communality of soldiers' problems, the use of group therapy was greatly increased during World War II.

Very recently there has been a movement toward group experience as the "in thing," a popular way to help people learn by experience how to relate more easily and happily to other people. Such "sensitivity groups" are also known as T-groups, intensive group encounters, personal growth groups, and marathons. That such groups can have a beneficial effect upon a person's day-to-day relationships is attested to by the wide use of this technique by industry in management training. The best of such groups are run by trained professional leaders. Without trained leadership, danger exists that unstable personalities will be overstimulated and stressed to the point of acute emotional disturbances.

No matter what the type of group therapy, special problems arise which make the experience quite different from individual psychotherapy. At the outset it is desirable to plan to group patients together who are sufficiently similar so that sharing of attitudes and experiences will not be made too difficult without, however, having patients so similar that they will rigidly reinforce each other's perceptual distortions or anxieties. In fitting patients together the leader may consider how aggressive or inhibited a candidate seems compared to other members, how anxious he will be made by anticipated behaviors of others, and whether his cultural background and value system have enough in common with the others. If both sexes are included in the group, special problems arise which make a rough balance in numbers of men and women desirable. In a group of rather conforming or inhibited patients it is valuable to consider adding one or two individuals who have greater capacity for open expression of primitive impulses. While the usual size of a psychotherapeutic group is a workable 5 to 8 members, in dealing with psychotics a larger group of 12 to 15 members has been found to have advantages. It is usually important that those in the group not have outside obligations to one another. Some experiences indicate that after the first dozen or so sessions of a coherent group it becomes increasingly difficult to add new members.

Like individual psychotherapy with children or psychotics, group psychotherapy tends to put the therapist much more "on the spot" and to bring into operation his own neurotic tendencies. Since patients have tended to attack the leader quite freely at times and may not spare the leader's own sources of anxiety, it is well for the therapist to have some type of supervision. Members of the group will react sensitively to whether the therapist genuinely is able to accept their hostility and anxiety without being too disturbed.

It is possible to describe roughly a number of phases of this process. Particularly with passive leadership, initial anxious silences are common. Soon thereafter one or two members may impulsively "confess" a great deal; this may frighten the more isolated, inhibited patients, particularly if pressure is put on them to do likewise. Before long, rivalries appear and the formation of shifting subgroup allegiances. At times a member may attempt to usurp leadership through incessant talking. Throughout the experience the therapist works to help the group clarify the meaning of individual behavior and to establish reality.

At the present stage of our knowledge, group therapy cannot be said to have any specific indications. Recent experiences suggest that the following disorders may sometimes be handled better in groups than by individual psychotherapy: alcoholism, severe psychosomatic disorders, ambulatory psychoses, transient situational neuroses, student counseling, vocational guidance problems, and adjustment problems such as new patients' adapting to a hospital ward situation. In addition, group therapy has been found of value as a preparation for individual therapy in persons who are not sure of their own motivation for individual therapy and as an adjunctive therapy providing social contacts and emotional support for severely disturbed immature characters, chronic psychotics, or psychopaths.

To the extent that human beings change their behavior through corrective action and identification with others rather than through detailed personal insight, group therapy may be potentially more effective than individual therapy. There is less time for each individual member to discuss his problems; on the other hand, inappropriate reactions, when expressed in the group, may be more visibly pathological than in individual therapy. Thus, if a patient on various occasions expresses a neurotic attitude, in relation to first one and then another member of the group, it soon becomes evident to all that this is a problem of the patient rather than of the other members. Group therapy may be arbitrarily divided into several types, each determined by the goals of the group and the leader's behavior.

PSYCHOANALYTIC GROUP PSYCHOTHERAPY

In the psychoanalytic group type of therapy the group aims at considerable insight and personality modification and the leader assumes a rather passive role. This form mobilizes the most anxiety and the most acting-out behavior within the group. Concepts of transference and countertransference are utilized in analyzing members' perceptual distortions and in understanding the outbursts of affect.

SOCIAL GROUP WORK

At the opposite pole from the first type named is social group work, a way of modifying individual and group behavior through skillfully designed patterns of group action. The goal here is to employ unused personal assets and to encourage their further growth. Analysis of symptomatic behavior is usually attempted only as required to remove obstacles to growth. The curative effects of settlement houses, clubs, political organizations, activity groups, religious orders, and schools may be said to fall within this general category. The active community group leader utilizes the energies of persons so that they receive emotional satisfaction from the action and the emotional interplay and so that healthy behavior patterns become stabilized.

The *life-space interview* or *marginal interview* is a psychotherapeutic approach appropriate in the group activity setting. It provides a well-timed opportunity to bypass defenses against discussion of interpersonal conflicts in a more formal interview. Disturbed behavior has been demonstrated before the eyes of the participant therapist and is thus more accessible to exploration.

PSYCHODRAMA

An elaborate theory and set of techniques for psychodrama have been worked out over the years since 1914 by J. L. Moreno. Many of the basic psychodynamic postulates are similar to those underlying psychoanalysis, but benefit is sought through action expression, reliving on the therapeutic stage, and working through in action. Moreno refers to *resistance* and employs special techniques (*warming up* the group, having the patient's role taken by a *double,* assisting dramatic expression of conflict through *auxiliary egos*) to overcome resistance. The patient is referred to as the *protagonist* and may portray on the stage either his own inner problems or a central problem of concern to the therapeutic group.

FLEXIBLE GROUP PSYCHOTHERAPY

The term "flexible group psychotherapy" designates a variety of forms of therapy which aim at sufficient insight and personality change to achieve relief of symptoms or improved social adaptation. Patients are encouraged to express their problems in a permissive family atmosphere. Behavior patterns are discussed in historical terms but interpretation of transference feelings may be avoided. The patient learns new ways of meeting specific life situations through discussion, redefining his conflicts, and corrective emotional experiences. The leader may vary his behavior considerably from time to time and, where desirable, may introduce psychodrama, role-playing, or play therapy techniques to assist the group's progress.

SUGGESTED READINGS

Boszormenyi-Nagy, I., and Framo, J. L., editors: Intensive family therapy, New York, 1965, Hoeber Medical Division, Harper & Row, Publishers.
Frank, J. D.: Group therapy in the mental hospital, monograph series no. 1, Washington, D. C., Dec., 1955, American Psychiatric Association.
Friedman, A. S., et al.: Psychotherapy for the whole family, New York, 1965, Springer Publishing Co., Inc.

Gans, R.: Group co-therapists in the therapeutic situation, Int. J. Group Psychother. **12**:82, 1962.

Goodrich, D. W., Mazer, J., and Cline, B.: Fostering the involvement of the psychiatric patient in group activities, Psychiatry **21**:259, 1958.

Hinckley, R. G., and Hermann, L.: Group treatment in psychotherapy, Minneapolis, 1952, University of Minnesota Press.

Howells, J. G.: Theory and practice of family psychiatry, New York, 1963, Brunner/Mazel, Inc.

Jones, M.: Beyond the therapeutic community: social learning and social psychiatry, New Haven, Conn., 1968, Yale University Press.

Laqueur, H. P., Wells, C. F., and Agresti, M.: Multiple family therapy in a state hospital, Hosp. Community Psychiat. **20**:13, 1969.

MacLennan, B. W.: Group approaches to problems of socially deprived youth: the classical psychotherapeutic model, Int. J. Group Psychother. **18**:481, 1968.

Moreno, J. L.: Psychodrama. In Arieti, S., editor: American handbook of psychiatry, New York, 1959, Basic Books, Inc., Publishers, vol. 2.

Mullan, H., and Sanguiliano, I.: The therapists' contribution, Springfield, Ill., 1964, Charles C Thomas, Publisher.

Powdermaker, F., and Frank, J.: Group psychotherapy, Cambridge, Mass., 1953, Harvard University Press.

Rogers, C.: On encounter groups, New York, 1970, Brunner/Mazel, Inc.

Slavson, S.: Analytic group psychotherapy with children, adolescents and adults, New York, 1950, Columbia University Press.

Thelen, H.: Dynamics of groups at work, Chicago, 1954, University of Chicago Press.

Yalom, I.: The theory and practice of group psychotherapy, New York, 1969, Basic Books, Inc., Publishers.

24
The physical therapies (EST, insulin, sleep, etc.)

ELECTROCONVULSIVE THERAPY

The production of convulsive seizures by pharmacological means was introduced by von Meduna as a treatment for schizophrenia. Later (1937) Cerletti and Bini introduced the simpler method of electroshock or electroconvulsive therapy (EST, ECT). The manner in which treatments of this type produce remission from emotional disorder is not understood, but their ability to relieve the symptoms of psychotic depression is universally accepted. Their effectiveness in other psychiatric disorders, however, is still open to question. Although early observations suggested that the use of antidepressant drugs might ultimately replace ECT, it is now apparent that ECT still remains the treatment of choice for severe suicidal depressions that require hospitalization. Because of the slow onset of action of these drugs, there exists a delay of 3 to 21 days in treatment results, during which period suicide may occur. To cope with this problem the antidepressant drug can be given concurrently and following the administration of ECT, with the goal of earlier termination of the course of electroshock and a reduction in the number of ECT treatments that are required.

Indications. The best results with electroshock therapy have been obtained in patients with involutional psychotic reaction (depressed type) or manic-depressive reaction (depressed type). The duration of the depression is shortened and the incidence of suicide is decreased, resulting in a higher recovery rate.

There is no evidence that a course of electroshock therapy prevents subsequent attacks or alters the frequency of recurrences. In manic-depressive reaction, manic type, the manic attacks may be shortened, but treatments may have to be given intensively (once daily or oftener). In schizophrenia, those patients in whom prognosis is judged to be good regardless of treatment (young patients with short duration of illness, with acute onset, and with pronounced affective component) seem to have remission within 2 to 6 weeks when electroshock treatments are used. There is much debate regarding the use of electroshock therapy for patients with psychoneurosis and other disorders. In such cases where the depressive element is marked, ECT may be of some help in a combined therapeutic approach. Maintenance ECT given every 4 weeks is used prophylactically in patients with recurrent psychotic depressions.

Technique. Prior to electroshock treatment, the patient should be given a thorough physical examination with special attention to cardiac and pulmonary status. Chest x-ray films, an electrocardiogram, and a signed permit from relatives should be obtained. Lateral x-ray views of the spine and an electroencephalogram are advisable.

Preparation of patient. Before the patient receives an electroconvulsive treatment, the following steps should be taken.

1. Allow only clear fluid after midnight and give no breakfast.

2. It is important to prepare the patient psychologically for the treatment, with understanding reassurance. Apprehensive patients may receive a sedative the night before or intravenously prior to treatment. This also tends to lessen the postshock excitement, and its effect on raising the convulsive threshold is usually not sufficient to interfere with the treatment.

3. Nauseated patients and those who have a tendency to vagal crises may be given 1/200 grain atropine. This is a routine precaution in many hospitals. Larger doses, 1 to 2 mg., are given I.V. 3 to 5 minutes prior to the treatment as a preventive for cardiac complications.

4. Instruct patient to void bladder and bowels just before treatment.

5. Remove dentures and hairpins. Search for chewing gum or other loose bodies in the mouth.

6. Loosen tight clothing.

7. Succinylcholine chloride (SCC) may be used to soften the convulsion in patients with orthopedic or cardiac complications, but it must be used with great caution and with full realization that the muscles of respiration may be completely paralyzed and that artificial respiration is often necessary. Such muscle relaxants are used routinely by many psychiatrists, with a variety of techniques for administration. Combination with Pentothal sodium is used to suppress the apprehension that may occur. When adequate relaxing doses of such drugs are given, positive-pressure oxygen is often necessary. The objection to the use of muscle relaxants is that, although decreasing the rate of fracture complication, they unquestionably increase the chance of fatal accident. Some hospitals require the presence of a trained anesthetist during this procedure.

Position of patient. Hyperextend the back with a pillow.

Treat on a hard stretcher or with a bedboard under the mattress and use a mouth gag.

Hold lightly to prevent extreme motions and immediately after shock watch the patient, during the confusional period that may follow treatment, to avoid his rolling from the stretcher or bed.

Electrode placement. Usually electrodes are placed approximately over the lower motor area (bitemporal). It has been proposed that posterior placement (i.e., hypothalamic, so-called) is better for the relief of anxiety whereas anterior placement is better for treating depression. A midvertex lead is sometimes substituted for one of the lateral leads, thus permitting stimulation of one hemisphere only. Other special techniques have been described for use primarily with unidirectional currents: One uses multiple leads; another is the so-called monopolar stimulation, in which a large indifferent lead is placed on the right arm and the stimulating lead is moved over the scalp to the approximate region of the brain to be stimulated. Placement of a small electrode in the nasopharynx and a large electrode on the scalp is said to concentrate stimulation upon basal brain structures. The advantages of these several methods of electrode placement over the conventional bitemporal application are still matters of individual opinion.

Number of treatments. Usually treatments are given three times a week. For psychotic depressions, 12 to 14 in a series are often used although, with concurrent administration of antidepressant drugs, this number can be reduced to as few as 3 or 4 treatments; 15 to 25 are usually considered necessary for schizophrenics. Patients have been given hundreds of treatments administered over many months without clinically obvious psychological or neurological deficit. The administration of several treatments per day over a period of several days produces the picture of a severe organic psychosis with confusion and loss of control over body functions. This so-called regressive shock therapy (REST, RECT) has found but little acceptance.

Complications. Potential complications in the use of ECT are suggested briefly below.

Death rate. The overall death rate is usually given as about 0.08%. This varies from as much as 0.5% in patients over 60 years of age to as little as 0.02% in patients under 30 years of age.

Fractures and dislocations. These are estimated to occur in 25% of cases. The number reported varies considerably from series to series and with the care in which x-ray films of the spine are taken and read. Fractures are detected much less frequently if one relies only upon the patient's complaints and clinical findings than if the dorsal vertebrae are studied carefully with x-ray films before and after treatment.

Respiratory arrest. In case of such arrest, give artificial respiration. A rebreathing bag and oxygen tank should be available for emergency use.

Cardiovascular difficulty. Cardiac arrest can occur. One may give atropine prophylactically.

Psychiatric complications. Blurring of memory is the most common complication. In many patients the dramatic symptoms of a Korsakov type psychosis may develop. It is important to recognize this organic syndrome so as not to give more shock, because it will clear spontaneously and symptoms are only prolonged by more electroshock. It is believed by some that in older persons with confusion, niacin, 400 mg. per day, should be given a trial prior to shock, as ECT may aggravate the organic picture.

EEG changes. Changes in EEG occur almost universally.

Slowing is seen in all leads, progressing maximally by 10 or 12 treatments and disappearing in most cases within a few weeks. Such induced cerebral dysfunction has been reported to be a necessary but not sufficient cause for the induced behavioral alterations, in that it may provide the means for a change in adaptation of the subject to his environment.

Mode of action. Although many theories exist as to the mechanism by which improvement occurs with ECT, we still lack a definitive answer to this problem. There is evidence that repeated convulsions are necessary to obtain therapeutic results and that the method by which the seizure is produced is of little importance. Confusion and memory loss are apparently not necessary for therapeutic success. Fink has presented his conclusions in a neurophysiological-adaptive hypothesis which states that the changes in brain function that follow repeated convulsions produce a necessary substrate which facilitates mechanisms for behavioral change and improvement. The induced biochemical changes, which may be reflected in EEG or spinal fluid studies, permit changes in thinking, mood, and affect, which in turn depend upon the subject's personality for their expression and duration. This theoretical view thus combines both the physiological and psychological data of electroshock research.

Contraindications. There are few absolute contraindications to the use of ECT, inasmuch as it in itself is frequently a treatment of emergency nature or desperation. All ages have been treated, from 3 to 80 years, and patients in all stages of pregnancy. In patients with tuberculosis electroshock can activate a lesion. Insulin (IST), however, is more dangerous in this regard. Patients with bone and joint disease are treated after medication with succinylcholine. Patients with aortic aneurysm, once thought to be an absolute contraindication to ECT, have now been successfully treated with SCG-Pentothal—modified convulsive therapy. Coronary disease makes one reluctant to give shock. With disease of the myocardium one would sedate and otherwise avoid exhausting the patient. A contraindication to ECT is the presence of brain tumor. In patients with hypertension, ECT may lower the blood pressure. Serious and even fatal complications have been reported from giving electroconvulsive therapy to patients receiving reserpine.

However, combined chlorpromazine-ECT has been reported as a safe procedure and of help in those patients who fail to respond to either treatment alone. The daily dose of chlorpromazine should be kept under 750 mg. and probably should not be administered in the period just preceding treatment.

Equipment. In principle, no complex apparatus is required to induce a therapeutic convulsion electrically. Any electrical stimulus capable of irritating the cerebrum sufficiently to produce excitation of the motor cortex can induce a seizure. A patient of ours once treated himself by tearing a lamp cord apart and holding the frayed ends to his temples.

The shock machines in current use have controls to permit the administration of measured amounts of current for controlled periods of time, as most psychiatrists seek to produce the seizure with a minimal stimulus. In most equipment the voltage is held constant and the milliamperage of current delivered is varied, although in some equipment the voltage can also be altered. The electrical stimulus usually employed is the commercially available alternating current at 60 cycles per second.

Attempts to produce a gentler onset of the seizure resulted in the glissando control which permits an initial build-up or rise of current during a second or more, rather than the instantaneous application of the full stimulus. Unfortunately, if the rise is slow enough to effectively alter the severity of seizure onset, the patient is uncomfortably aware of the treatment, and intravenous barbiturates must be administered before a course of such treatments.

Other attempts to improve upon conventional ECT resulted in the so-called unidirectional current stimulators (Reiter, Liberson-Offner B.S.T., etc.) which use forms of rectified current interrupted and modulated variously by different manufacturers. These modifications have not satisfactorily eliminated the complications of ECT, although they in general seem to induce milder seizures with less confusion and less alteration of the brain wave pattern than seen with conventional ECT. Unfortunately, however, it is often necessary to give a greater number of these milder treatments to achieve the desired therapeutic result.

OTHER TECHNIQUES

In an attempt to broaden the usefulness of ECT a number of cerebrostimulation procedures have been developed. Much careful work utilizing matched control groups must be done before the effectiveness of such methods can be known.

Subconvulsive and stimulative electrocerebral therapy

Subconvulsive (ESnc) and high-frequency stimulative electrocerebral therapy (Sedac) are produced, using unidirectional stimulating equipment. In these techniques only sufficient current is used to induce clonic movements and autonomic effects. Since the patient remains conscious and has an unpleasant memory of this procedure, it is usually given only after the prior intravenous administration of sodium Amytal or Pentothal sodium. Following this, the stimulation is given until the anesthetic wears off. Recent work seems to indicate that at least part of the effect of this treatment comes about through stimulation of the peripheral sensory nerves of the head; therefore, similar effect may be achieved by a method of peripheral stimulation in which the electrodes are applied against the legs and the small of the back, with the treatment otherwise given similarly.

Recent controlled studies of subconvulsive treatment using both electrical and photoshock methods seem to indicate that this method is without significant effect either in patients with psychotic depressions or in patients with anxiety states. Nonconvulsive electrostimulation immediately following a grand mal seizure (countershock) has been shown to have no value in alleviating the amnesia that may follow ECT.

Electrosleep

For many years Russian scientists have been investigating the properties of electrosleep as a therapeutic tool. More recently, considerable interest has been shown by American investigators. The term "electrosleep" has been considered inappropriate due to the fact that sleep is not induced in all subjects. It has been suggested that the term be replaced by "transcerebral electrotherapy."

To date there is no convincing evidence to suggest that electrosleep apparatus is significantly effective, either in inducing sleep or in treating minor forms of mental illness. An element of suggestibility is definitely present and is considered an important factor in the results obtained. Considerable research is necessary in this field.

In electrosleep therapy negative electrodes are applied over the eyes, and positive electrodes are placed over the mastoid processes. A weak, pulsed current (up to 1.5 mA and up to 50 V) for a total period of one hour per treatment session is used. Treatments may be given daily.

Pharmacological treatments

Generalized seizures can be produced pharmacologically by a variety of substances. Therapeutic convulsions induced by Metrazol were early abandoned for a number of reasons, which included undependability of seizure production, severity of seizures, unwanted multiple seizures, and production of marked apprehension in the patient during the period of induction. Other convulsant drugs for intravenous administration are now available which seem to obviate at least some of the above drawbacks.

Some workers have reported using currents of high voltage—but of brief duration—in conjunction with analeptics and anticonvulsants in an attempt to produce maximal stimulation of deeper structures in the brain.

Indoklon, hexafluorodiethyl ether, a convulsant ether, has been utilized for the production of generalized seizures. It is inhaled by the patient during a procedure of administration that is similar to that utilized with any gas anesthetic. Indoklon may also be given intravenously.

Photoshock

Photoshock is a treatment in which the intravenous injection of an analeptic such as hexazole (4-cyclohexyl-3-ethyl-1,2,4-triazole) is given in conjunction with intermittent photic stimulation of a stroboscope set to give 15 flashes per second. The resulting treatment is at least as effective as electroshock and appears to be gentler and produces less confusion in the patient.

Insulin therapy

The use of insulin (IST) to induce severe hypoglycemic states for the treatment of psychoses was reported by Manfred

Sakel of Vienna in 1933. This treatment has shown a marked decline since World War II. The term "insulin shock" refers to the state of vasomotor collapse induced by this method.

Indications. Schizophrenia of recent onset.

Contraindications. This treatment is time-consuming and not without danger. It requires careful attention to technique. Specific contraindications are cardiovascular disease, especially coronary disease or pulmonary tuberculosis, febrile illness, diabetes, acute or chronic diseases of liver, kidney, pancreas, thyroid, or adrenals.

Preparation. Complete physical examination, posteroanterior x-ray films of chest, and an electrocardiogram. Give preliminary test for insulin sensitivity (use 5 to 10 units regular insulin subcutaneously, examine in 6 hours for wheal, and watch for hypoglycemia the first hour).

Technique. Insulin therapy may be used for either subcoma or coma.

Subcoma. Regular insulin (not crystalline or PZI) is given subcutaneously at 6:00 A.M. to patients fasting and in bed. An initial dose of 15 U. is increased by 10 U. until desired effect is achieved. From time to time it may be necessary to decrease or increase the dose by 5 to 10 U. to hold the patient at the required level.

GOAL. The goal is to produce hypoglycemic reactions of drowsiness or sleep for $\frac{1}{2}$ to 1 hour.

TERMINATION. Oral administration or gavage of 400 ml. orange juice with glucose, 2 Gm. per unit of insulin, or 10 to 50 ml. 50% glucose intravenously.

COURSE. Depending upon the clinical course of the patient, 20 to 100 treatments.

Coma. Give regular insulin, 15 U., subcutaneously; increase by 10 U. each day until brief periods of coma occur (usually around 100 U.); then proceed with greater caution until goal of 1 hour's coma is reached. Alter to maintain; usually can decrease by 5 U. per day. If no coma occurs with 400 U., increase by 25 to 50 U. At 500 U., try zigzag reduction (350, 150, 300, 75, etc.).

Alternatively, use a multiple-injection technique, with increasing daily dosages to 20-20-20 or 30-20-20 U. of insulin given 15 minutes apart.

GOAL. Comatose reactions of 60 minutes' duration. Watch for a dangerous stage in which contracted pupils fail to respond to light, corneal reflexes are absent, pulse rate runs between 50 and 60, and respiratory difficulties and muscular hypotonia occur. This deep coma is reputedly therapeutic but should not be maintained for over 20 minutes. Immediate termination is indicated if systolic blood pressure drops below 100 mm. Hg and pulse below 55.

TERMINATION. Give 50 ml. 50% glucose intravenously (or 500 ml. by stomach tube) followed by oral orange juice with 2 to 400 Gm. glucose (i.e., 2 Gm. per insulin unit given) or glucagon injected intramuscularly in 1 to 5 mg. doses. Patient is then encouraged to eat breakfast and all meals during the day. Sugar-fortified orange juice in midafternoon is a precaution against delayed insulin reactions, which are not uncommon.

COURSE. Coma is produced 6 days a week for 2 weeks to 3 months if necessary.

Combined IST and ECT. Both electroconvulsive therapy (ECT) and Metrazol convulsions have been used in combination with and to terminate insulin coma treatments in cases refractory to insulin alone. The increased possibility of lasting organic brain alteration makes this combination a treatment of desperation.

Complications. Prolonged irreversible coma, respiratory and circulatory complications, intracranial hemorrhage, and death sometimes follow insulin therapy.

Prompt recognition of prolonged coma is essential. If comatose patient does not begin to revive in 10 to 15 minutes following normal gavage, administer 30 to 50 ml. 50% glucose intravenously. If no signs of arousal appear in 5 minutes, suspect prolonged coma.

Treatment of prolonged stupor is by use of intravenous glucose and dehydrating agents such as 50 ml. 50% sorbitol solution intravenously. Fifty milliliters 50% concentrated lyophilized human serum solution may also be given. Adrenocortical hormones should be used and are said by some, if given prophylactically, to prevent prolonged coma. Thiamine and blood plasma may be repeated every 2 or 3 hours until recovery. If the stupor continues for longer than 12 hours, adequate provision must be made for parenteral fluids, proteins, and carbohydrates to maintain an optimal state of nutrition. The therapist must be prepared for a long wait. It should be kept in mind that episodes of prolonged stupor often serve to sensitize the patient to the effects of insulin, so that if treatment is continued the dose of insulin may be decreased as much as nine tenths of the previous amount and irreversible stupors still can result.

Convulsions may be avoided by the administration of phenobarbital or Dilantin at the time insulin is given. If subcoma is employed in patients over 45 years old and those with cardiovascular complications, special care must be taken to avoid coma.

Results. Results obtained with insulin therapy depend upon the factors included in case selection. Studies of patients followed for 5 to 10 years after treatment reveal remission rates from 13% to 84%. As in all treatment of schizophrenia, good prognosis is augured by youth, short duration of disease, precipitation of attack by external events, pyknic or athletic habitus, and good premorbid personality adjustment. A weight gain of 30 pounds or more during treatment is a favorable sign.

Insulin hypoglycemia produces marked slowing in the EEG, and there remains the question of permanent localized damage. Although insulin coma treatment has been largely replaced by psychopharmacology and ECT, there are some who believe it still has a role in the therapy of treatment-resistant patients.

Other coma-inducing techniques that have been used include acetylcholine (Fiamberti, 1937) and atropine (Forrer, 1951).

Carbon dioxide therapy

Carbon dioxide therapy was introduced by Meduna in 1945 as a treatment for psychoneurosis. A mixture of 30% CO_2 and 70% O_2 is used with an ordinary anesthesia mask, rubber bag, and reducing valve arrangement, with the patient in a supine position. Usually from 15 to 50 inspirations are needed to induce narcosis. The patient may abreact or report dreams.

Continuous sleep therapy

One of the oldest treatment methods in psychiatry is prolonged sleep therapy. This received considerable attention during World War II and is widely used in Russia today but is little used in civilian psychiatry in the United States. The once popular Cloetta's mixture (paraldehyde, 0.4864 Gm.; amylene hydrate, 0.1593 Gm.; chloral hydrate 0.1157 Gm.; alcohol, 92%, 0.1747 Gm.; isopropyl-allyl-barbituric acid, 0.0409 Gm.; Digalen, 0.0330 mg.; and ephedrine hydrochloride, 2.4600 mg.) rectally administered has more recently been replaced by mixtures of tranquilizers and barbiturates given orally. One such mixture that has been used consists of Seconal (short-acting), 100 mg.; Nembutal (moderate-acting), 100 mg.; sodium Amytal (long-acting), 150 mg.; and chlorpromazine, 50 mg.

In this treatment the nursing care and the adjustment of drug schedule and periods of awakening for elimination and food intake are critical. Pneumonia is a complication requiring cessation of sleep treatment and administration of antibiotic medication. The course of continuous sleep may be from 2 weeks to 2 months. Some excellent results reported from combat fatigue cases in wartime have not been duplicated in civilian medicine. Patients treated by this method range from those with psychoneurosis to those with chronic psychotic illness.

Hydrotherapy

The remedial use of water for mental ills had its origin in the baths of ancient times, and today swimming pools (group hydrotherapy) still play a role in the activities therapy programs of a number of mental hospitals. Individual hydrotherapy, however, is today rarely used in the hospital management of psychiatric patients. Prior to the advent of psychotropic drugs, it was widely applied in the form of continuous tub baths, showers, sprays, douches, and wet sheet packs.

SUGGESTED READINGS

Alexander, L.: Treatment of mental disorder, Philadelphia, 1953, W. B. Saunders Co.

Azima, H.: Prolonged sleep treatment in mental disorder, J. Ment. Sci. **101**:593, 1955.

Esquibel, A., Kurland, A., and Mendelsohn, D.: The use of glucagon in terminating insulin coma, Dis. Nerv. Syst. **19**:485, 1958.

Fink, M.: The mode of action of convulsive therapy: the neurophysiologic-adaptive view, J. Neuropsychiat. 3:231, 1962.

Fink, M., Kahn, R. L., Karp, E., Pollack, M., Green, M. A., Alan, B., and Lefkowitz, H. J.: Inhalant-induced convulsions: significance for the theory of the convulsive therapy process, Arch. Gen. Psychiat. 4:259, 1961.

Forrer, G., and Miller, J.: Atropine coma: a somatic therapy in psychiatry, Amer. J. Psychiat. 115:455, 1958.

Geller, M. R.: The treatment of psychiatric disorders with insulin, 1936-1960, a selected annotated bibliography, Washington, D. C., 1962, U. S. Department of Health, Education, and Welfare, Public Health Service.

Goldman, D.: Brief stimulus electric shock therapy, J. Nerv. Ment. Dis. 110:36, 1949.

Gordon, H.: Fifty shock therapy theories, Milit. Surg. 103:397, 1948.

Itil, T. M., Gannon, P., Akpinar, S., and Hsu, W.: Quantitative EEG analysis of electro-sleep using frequency analyzer and digital computer methods, Dis. Nerv. Syst., 1972.

Janis, I. L.: Psychologic effects of electric convulsive treatments, J. Nerv. Ment. Dis. 111:359, 1950.

Johnson, L. C., Ulett, G. A., Johnson, M., Smith, K., and Sines, J. O.: Electroconvulsive therapy (with and without atropine), Arch. Gen. Psychiat. 2:324, 1960.

Jones, C. H., Blachly, P. H., and Brookhart, J. M.: The analeptic action of peripheral electrical stimulation in hypoglycemic coma, Arch. Neurol. Psychiat. 73:560, 1955.

Jones, C., Shanklin, J. G., Dixon, H. H., Brookhart, J. M., and Blachly, P. H.: Peripheral electrical stimulation, a new form of psychiatric treatment (preliminary report), Dis. Nerv. Syst. 16:323, 1955.

Kalinowsky, L. B., and Hoch, P. H.: Somatic treatments in psychiatry; pharmaco-therapy; convulsive, insulin, surgical and other methods, New York, 1969, Grune & Stratton, Inc.

Laquer, H., and La Burt, H.: Coma therapy with multiple insulin doses, J. Neuropsychiat. 1:135, 1960.

Lewis, W., Richardson, D., and Gahagan, L.: Cardiovascular disturbances and their management in modified electrotherapy for psychiatric illness, New Eng. J. Med. 252:1016, 1955.

Meduna, L. J., editor: Carbon dioxide therapy, ed. 2, Springfield, Ill., 1958, Charles C Thomas, Publisher.

Nussbaum, K., and Kurland, A.: Bis (2,2, 2-trifluorethyl) ether (Indoklon) modified with succinylcholine (Anectine) as a convulsant in psychiatric treatment, J. Neuropsychiat. 5:143, 1963.

Ottoson, J.: Experimental studies of the mode of action of electroconvulsive therapy, Acta Psychiat. Scand. 35(supp. 145):5, 1960.

Polonio, P., and Slater, E.: A prognostic study of insulin treatment of schizophrenia, J. Ment. Sci. 100:442, 1954.

Reynolds, D. V., and Sjoberg, A. E.: Neuroelectric research: electroneuroprosthesis, electroanesthesia and nonconvulsive electrotherapy, Springfield, Ill., 1971 Charles C Thomas, Publisher.

Rinkel, M., and Himwich, H.: Insulin treatment in psychiatry, New York, 1959, Philosophical Library, Inc.

Sargant, W. W., and Slater, E. T.: An introduction to physical methods of treatment in psychiatry, ed. 4, Baltimore, 1963, The Williams & Wilkins Co.

Tokizane, T., and Sawyer, C. H.: Sites of origin of hypoglycemic seizures in the rabbit, Arch. Neurol. Psychiat. 77:259, 1957.

Ulett, G. A., Gleser, G., Caldwell, B., and Smith, K.: The use of matched groups in the evaluation of convulsive and subconvulsive photoshock, Bull. Menninger Clin. 13:138, 1954.

Ulett, G. A., Smith, K., and Biddy, R.: Shock treatment. In Spiegel, E., editor: Progress in neurology and psychiatry, vol. 17, New York, 1962, Grune & Stratton, Inc.

Ulett, G. A., Smith, K., and Gleser, G.: Evaluation of convulsive and subconvulsive shock therapies utilizing a control group, Amer. J. Psychiat. 112:795, 1956.

Wayne, G. J.: Use of succinylcholine chloride in electroconvulsive therapy, Dis. Nerv. Syst. 21:149, 1960.

Wageneder, F. M., and Schuy, S.: Electrotherapeutic sleep and electroanaesthesia, International Congress Series No. 136, New York. 1967. Excerpta Medica Foundation.

West, F., Bond, E., Shurley, J., and Meyers, C.: Insulin coma therapy in schizophrenia; a fourteeen-year follow-up study, Amer. J. Psychiat. 111:583, 1955.

Wright, R.: Hydrotherapy in psychiatric hospitals, Boston, 1940, The Tudor Press.

25
Psychosurgery

Techniques of operating upon the human brain for the relief of psychiatric disorder originated from pioneer work of the Swiss psychiatrist Burkhardt (1888), that of Moniz and Lima of Portugal (1936), and subsequent popularization of the procedure in the United States by Freeman and Watts. Despite thousands of operations, however, the subject of lobotomy remains controversial. In part this stems from the tendency to reserve this brain-mutilating procedure for patients who have failed with all other measures of treatment. Naturally the number of cures in such material will not be great. As with other modes of therapy the best results are obtained if grossly deteriorated patients are avoided and operation is reserved for patients who preserve some evidence of vigorous emotional life. Whether such techniques have value in present-day psychiatry has yet to be answered by carefully controlled studies comparing psychosurgery with other modern treatment modalities and in the light of findings from more recent refined methods using implanted wire electrodes for EEG recording, focal stimulation, and the production of small discrete brain lesions.

Indications. Psychosurgery was most commonly used for schizophrenics who had been chronic institutional problems, for severe chronic obsessive-compulsive neuroses, chronic anxiety neuroses, and severe chronic depressive states. With the widespread use of tranquilizing medications, psychosurgery is now rarely used. The most common indication today is for the relief of intractable pain, as in the case of terminal malignancy or severe hypochondriasis. Depth electrode stimulation methods have shown promising results for patients with chronic anxiety states and compulsive and phobic neuroses.

Techniques. The various operations for prefrontal lobotomy have been designed to sever the connections to or remove tissue from, primarily, areas 9, 10, 11, 12, 13, 14, 44, 45, 46, and the anterior cingulate area (area 24). It is felt that cutting the projection pathways from the anterior and dorsomedial thalamic nuclei (i.e., the fiber tracts passing in the lower quadrants of the frontal lobe) is of greatest importance. Areas 13, 14, and 24 also have hypothalamic connections; lesions here produce alterations in autonomic functioning. Startle and rage effects can be lessened if area 13 is protected during surgery.

Lobotomy. Literally, lobotomy is a cutting into the lobe, whereas *leukotomy* is a severance of white matter. There are several techniques used in lobotomy.

OPEN. Open lobotomy is performed under direct vision through large superior trephine openings.

CLOSED. Lateral small burr holes are used. Operation is blind, but with careful measurement from external landmarks the surgeon can limit section to superior or, more usually, inferior quadrants. A variation of this technique has been described by Grantham and consists of electrocoagulation of the lower and upper medial quadrants of the frontal lobe through medially placed burr holes. Putnam has described a technique in which a preliminary test for effects of lobotomy is made by initially injecting iodized procaine in oil transorbitally.

TRANSORBITAL. This so-called "ice-pick" operation was sometimes done using ECT as the anesthetic agent. A leukotome is plunged through the conjunctival sac and orbital plate into the orbital surface of the frontal lobe, where an arc swing of the instrument cuts the inferior quadrant of the lobe.

ULTRASONIC. A technique of some promise is the destruction of the deep white matter with ultrasonic vibrations.

Lobectomy. Radical removal of all frontal areas as well as orbital surface is involved in lobectomy.

Gyrectomy. This open operative removal of cortical tissue (gyri) was termed "topectomy" by the Columbia-Greystone Project Group who removed areas 9, 10, and 46 by subpial dissection.

Cingulectomy. Cingulectomy is the removal of the cingulate gyrus.

Thalamotomy (Spiegel and Wycis). Thalamotomy uses a stereotaxic apparatus to produce lesions deep in the thalamus.

The choice of psychosurgical procedure, in particular the decision of whether a minimal or a radical destruction of tissue is indicated, is governed by the age of the patient (minimal operation in the aged), the duration of the disease (more radical surgery in more chronic illnesses), and the personality organization (more radical procedures being indicated in the more severely disturbed patients). Unilateral procedures appear to be less reliable than bilateral procedures.

Complications. Estimated morbidity is about 1%. Neurological complications are 10% to 20%, including operative hemorrhages, parasurgical cysts and necrosis, epileptic seizures (rates vary with the type of operative procedure), and a persistent urinary incontinence. Little mention is made in the literature of patients who are made clinically worse by the operation, possibly because of the nature of the patients chosen for the procedure. However, alterations in personality can occur that are most distressing and embarrassing to relatives who are typically quoted in the literature as saying, "For him the operation did miracles; if only we did not have to live with him." Postoperatively, there may be apathy, a lack of creative drive, little foresight, and in general an attitude of not caring. Impulsive, aggressive behavior can at times result.

Results. By conservative estimate, over one third of chronic, hospitalized psychiatric patients treated by lobotomy are returned to the community; another third remain unchanged. Some optimistic studies boost the number recovered to well over 50% and compare this to control groups (in which permission for the operation was refused by the relatives) where over 90% remained unchanged. Obviously such figures are not too meaningful without careful description of the types of cases selected and without a matched control series given an equal amount of hospital attention. Studies of 1000 patients of all types followed for 1 to 16 years after lobotomy (Freeman) reveal satisfactory adjustment out of the hospital. Results are better in those cases in which the duration of the illness is short, and results become progressively worse with increasing chronicity. Results in obsessive neurotics and in patients with involutional psychosis are, on the whole, better than in those with schizophrenia.

Psychological studies reveal no significant change in I. Q. Self-reference, self-consciousness, and concern over poor performance are alleviated—with a frequent shift from tension to apathy. Impairment of abstract thinking, concept formation, and planning is seen, along with perseveration and stereotypy.

Sociological studies of postlobotomy patients have indicated a trend toward improved work and family adjustment, but in neither of these areas were pre-illness achievements attained. The degree of acceptance by members of the family of the postoperative patient and lapses of judgment and of modesty have been observed to be important factors in determining whether the patient can make a community adjustment.

SUGGESTED READINGS

Freeman, W., and Watts, J. W.: Psychosurgery, ed. 2, Springfield, Ill., 1950, Charles C Thomas, Publisher.

Fulton, J. F.: Frontal lobotomy and affective behavior, New York, 1951, W. W. Norton & Co., Inc.

Grantham, E. C.: Prefrontal lobotomy for relief of pain, J. Neurosurg. 8:405, 1951.

Greenblatt, M., and Solomon, H. C.: Studies of lobotomy, Res. Pub. Ass. Res. Nerv. Ment. Dis. 35:15, 1958.

Lindstrom, P.: Prefrontal ultrasonic irradiation—a substitute for lobotomy, Arch. Neurol. Psychiat. 72:399, 1954.

Mettler, F. A.: Selective partial ablation of the frontal cortex, New York, 1949, Paul B. Hoeber, Inc.

Moniz, E.: Tentatives opératoires dans le traitement de certaines psychoses, Paris, 1936, Masson et Cie.

Oltman, J. E., and Friedman, S.: Long-term results of frontal lobotomy in schizophrenic patients, Amer. J. Psychiat. 118:70, 1961.

Putnam, T. J.: Procaine base in iodized oil introduced transorbitally as a test for the effects of lobotomy, Trans. Amer. Neurol. Ass. 75:125, 1950.

Rylander, G.: Personality analysis before and after frontal lobotomy, Proc. Ass. Res. Nerv. Ment. Dis. 27:691, 1948.

Sem-Jacobsen, C. W.: Depth-electrographic stimulation of the human brain and behavior: from fourteen years of studies and treatment of Parkinson's disease and mental disorders with implanted electrodes, Springfield, Ill., 1968, Charles C Thomas, Publisher.

Shobe, F. O., and Gildea, M.: Long-term follow-up of selected lobotomized private patients, J.A.M.A. 206:327, 1968.

Sykes, M. K., and Tredgold, R. F.: Restricted orbital undercutting: a study of effects on 350 patients over the 10 years 1951-1960, Brit. J. Psychiat. 110:609, 1964.

Wittenborn, J R., and Mettler, F. A.: Some psychological changes following psychosurgery, J. Abnorm. Soc. Psychol. 14:548, 1952.

Wood, M. W., and Rowland, J. P.: Bilateral anterior thalamotomy for the hyperactive child, Southern Med. J. 61:36, 1968.

26
Chemotherapy in mental illness

The treatment of the mentally ill by means of drugs is not new, but certainly it has been the focus of a renewed interest in the past few years. Unlike the antibiotics, whose action is against known etiological agents, drugs in psychiatry are, for the most part, used to alleviate undesirable symptoms. Initially, therefore, states of mania, delirium, and anxiety were treated with morphine, with chloral hydrate, and with paraldehyde. Such drugs often had the desired quieting effect on motor behavior but produced in addition an undesirable somnolence and lethargy which prohibited the patient's participation in other therapeutic activities. The newer ataractics produce tranquilization of behavior without lethargy and recently introduced antidepressants relieve the mood disturbances with fewer side effects than the earlier stimulating drugs.

BARBITURATES

The barbiturates, a most important group of drugs widely used in the treatment of mentally ill persons, were introduced in 1903. These may be divided into two chemical groups, those containing a phenyl radical and possessing anticonvulsant and sedative properties (e.g., phenobarbital) and those containing only aliphatic substituent groups and possessing little or no anticonvulsant action. Barbiturates have varying degrees of hypnotic power and differ as to rapidity of action and duration of effect. Suitable for prolonged narcosis is barbital. If an effect lasting several hours with gradual onset is desired, sodium Amytal or pentobarbital is more appropriate.

Pentothal sodium is commonly employed for a rapid hypnotic result of brief duration but it has greater tendency to depress respiration and vascular tone.

In the administering of intravenous barbiturates a 2.5%, freshly prepared solution should be employed. Periods of apnea or laryngospasm may be avoided by slow induction but experience is required before the correct dosage and rate of administration of the quick-acting barbiturates will be clear to the physician. Very anxious or overactive patients will require a rapidity of administration of Pentothal which might lead to serious complications in normal or retarded individuals. Special caution should be used in elderly patients (smaller dose), in those with nephritis (avoidance of long-acting barbiturates), and in those with cardiovascular or respiratory disorders. Caution should be observed when administering barbiturates in the presence of liver disease.

As an adjunct to certain phases of psychotherapy, a sufficient intravenous dose of Amytal, Pentothal, or other fairly rapidly acting hypnotic to produce mild drowsiness and release of inhibitions* has a number of uses during an interview. Instead of hypnosis, or as an adjunct thereto, it may be used with suggestion to remove hysterical conversion symptoms; greatest success appears with conversion symptoms of recent onset. In the treatment of acute combat anxiety or hysterical reactions, these drugs (often with hypnosis) enable patients to abreact hidden terrors and to face and accept the traumatic situation by repeatedly reliving it during narcoanalysis. In any such situation where strong catharsis of feeling results, the therapist must play the role of a powerful, understanding being who actively points out reality and suggests alternate ways of handling these matters. In addition this method of producing relaxation and release of inhibitions has been used to help patients recover forgotten but disturbing memories and commonly as a diagnostic adjunct where the differential diagnosis of such conditions as hysteria, early psychosis, malingering, or epileptic seizures is in question.

---

*Methamphetamine hydrochloride (Methedrine, Pervitin, Desoxyn, Desoxyephedrine) has also been used to release inhibitions through exciting the central nervous system.

TRANQUILIZERS

The tranquilizers have produced a considerable change in the management of disturbed psychotic patients. Like the barbiturates, these drugs have a quieting or calming effect; but, unlike the older hypnotic agents, these new ataractics accomplish the desired result without producing marked drowsiness. The tranquilizers have become one of the most frequently used drugs in medicine. The literature in this field is vast and confusing. These agents are probably neither specific nor "curative"; yet when they are properly selected for the individual patient and administered in high dosage over a sufficiently long time, social restitution has occurred in cases where the prognosis otherwise seemed extremely poor. Their use is apparently for symptoms, and although some patients appear to respond better to one agent than another, claims of superiority must be carefully weighed against comparability of dose given with each agent and the frequency of side effects at effective dose levels. As with other new drugs, tranquilizers are often poorly selected, used when not needed, or used unwisely. In serious psychosis, large doses of the drugs may be necessary, and patients may be continued on maintenance doses for many months or years. (Be alert for drug habituation.) **Some studies** hint that the price of psychotic symptom control may, for some, be in the form of lasting neurological symptoms ("tardive dyskinesia").

In general the *major tranquilizers* are useful for the following conditions: (1) schizophrenia—aggressive outbursts, noisiness, and destructive behavior, particularly; (2) affective disorders—hypomanic and manic states, paranoid disturbance, and agitated states in involutional psychoses; (3) acute brain syndrome— states of intoxication, delirium, and hallucinations; and (4) chronic brain syndrome—restlessness, violent outbursts, and destructive behavior. The *minor tranquilizers* are used for anxiety, irritability, and muscle tension. In neurotics an impairment of motor function, slowing of intellectual functioning, and feelings of depersonalization may be produced by the major tranquilizers, which are less well tolerated by the neurotic than by the psychotic patient.

ANTIDEPRESSANTS

Another important group of psychotropic drugs is the antidepressants. This group includes *imipramine type drugs* (thymoleptics) (iminodibenzyl derivatives, tricyclic antidepressants, dibenzepines); *monoamine oxidase* (MAO) *inhibitors* (thymerethics) (hydrazine); and *psychomotor stimulants*. Studies have shown the best of these drugs to be about as effective as ECT. However, the slower onset of symptom relief with drugs may be a factor of treatment selection in the severely depressed and suicidal patient. The combined use of drugs and electroconvulsive therapy reduces the number of ECT treatments necessary. Of those few patients who do not respond to drugs, approximately 50% will respond to ECT.

Patients vary in their response to the antidepressant agents. Thus one drug may be ineffective in a patient but another type of drug produce a dramatic effect. Amitryptaline and other imipramine type drugs appear to be most effective for serious endogenous depressions and are slightly safer than the MAO inhibitors. Side effects from the MAO inhibitors— especially hypertensive crises with intracranial bleeding, headache, stiff neck, and vomiting—may follow the ingestion of food high in tyramine content, especially highly ripened cheeses (Camembert, Liederkranz, Edam, and cheddar) and such foods as yogurt, fava beans, Bovril, cream, alcohol, beer, and wine. Symptoms can also occur when an MAO inhibitor is given in combination with an imipramine type drug, or when the latter is used to replace an MAO inhibitor, without allowing a sufficient (7 to 10 days) interval of time.

The above drugs seem to be truly and specifically antidepressants, with little or no effect on normal persons. The psychomotor stimulants, by contrast, are euphoriants and stimulants of psychomotor activity, especially where there is fatigue. The use of such stimulants in depression seems open to question, from the results of recent placebo control studies. In contrast, the use of amphetamine to reduce and control hyperkinetic behavior in children is well documented. Recently, there has been increasing interest in the use of lithium salts for the treatment and prevention of the manic state in manic-depressive psychosis.

HALLUCINOGENS

LSD$_{25}$ (lysergic acid), mescaline, mushroom derivatives, and related compounds have recently drawn attention, both for research production of "model psychosis" and as an aid to psychotherapy. Beginning with 25 μg. of LSD orally and increasing by 50 μg. daily, toxic reactions are achieved usually by 75 to 150 μg. The effects last for several hours and include hallucinations, abreactions, intense states of belief and religious experiences. Such states are certainly influenced by suggestion, and the clinical usefulness of these agents is in need of critical evaluation. If it has any value, this type of treatment appears to be the most promising with alcoholics and in some personality disorders.

• • •

The field of psychopharmacology is exciting and active, with an ever-increasing number of new agents being made available to the psychiatrist. The final chapter has not yet been written on the mechanism of action of these agents, but research in this field may well offer important insights into the etiology of psychiatric illness. The following list and tables itemize various drugs and doses which the psychiatrist may wish to use in the treatment of patients:

Central nervous system depressants

Sodium bromide	(Oral) 1 Gm.
Chloral hydrate	(Oral) 0.5-2 Gm.; can be administered rectally in olive oil; not to be given to patients with liver or kidney damage
Paraldehyde	(Oral) 3-15 ml.; given best in orange juice or rectally with 2 parts olive oil

Barbiturates:

Pentothal (ultrashort action)	(I.V.) 0.5 Gm. in 20 ml. at rate of 1 ml./min. until asleep
Seconal (short action)	0.1-0.2 Gm.
Amytal (moderate action)	0.05-0.2 Gm.
Pentobarbital (moderate action)	0.05-0.1 Gm.
Barbital (long action)	0.3-0.5 Gm.
Phenobarbital (long action)	0.1-0.2 Gm.

Anticonvulsants
See Table 4, p. 126, "Anticonvulsant drugs"

Central nervous system stimulants

Picrotoxin — (I.V.) 3 mg. dose repeated with caution at 3-minute intervals until signs of reflex activity appear; dangerous and rarely used

Pentylenetetrazol (Metrazol)
- (Oral) 0.1 Gm. t.i.d.
- (I.V.) 0.3-1.0 Gm. to produce a convulsion; rarely used and with caution

Nikethamide (Covamine) — (I.V.) 5-10 ml. followed by 5 ml. q. 5-30 min.

Methylphenidate HCl (Ritalin) — (I.M. or Sub. Q.) 10 mg. 1-3 times daily; mild cortical stimulant; also useful in narcolepsy

Caffeine sodium benzoate — (I.M.) 0.5 Gm.

Antihistaminics

Pyribenzamine — (Oral) 50 mg.

Benadryl (diphenhydramine) — (Oral) 25-50 mg.

*Muscle relaxants**

d-Tubocurarine chloride — (I.V.) 3 mg./40 lb. body weight, given slowly over 1-2 min.

Succinylcholine chloride (Anectine) — 20 mg. recommended for male patients of athletic habitus, although doses of 50-70 mg. not uncommonly used; dose adjusted as necessary for individual patient and given in single injection; loses potency on standing a few minutes, if mixed with Pentothal

Analgesics

Morphine sulfate — (Hypo) 8-20 mg.

Codeine sulfate — (Hypo) 15-60 mg.

Methadone (Dolophine, Amidone) — (Oral) 5-10 mg.

Meperidine hydrochloride (Demerol) — (Oral or hypo) 50-150 mg.

Acetylsalicylic acid — (Oral) 0.3-1 Gm.

---

*Use these drugs only when someone skilled in the administration of supplemental and controlled respiration and the facilities for such procedures are present.

Vitamins

Thiamine hydrochloride	(I.M.) 10 mg. b.i.d.
	(Oral) 10 mg. t.i.d.
Riboflavin	(I.M.) 10 mg.
	(Oral) 5-10 mg. daily
Nicotinic acid (niacin)	(Oral) 100 mg. 5 times per day
	(I.V.) 25 mg. 2-4 times per day
Ascorbic acid	(Oral) 0.5-1 Gm. daily in divided doses

Drugs stimulating structures innervated by adrenergic nerves

Epinephrine (Adrenalin)	(Hypo) 0.1-0.5 ml. of 1:1000 solution
Ephedrine hydrochloride or sulfate	(Oral) 15-50 mg.
Amphetamine sulfate (Benzedrine)	(Oral) 5-10 mg.
d-Amphetamine sulfate (Dexedrine)	(Oral) 5 mg.

Drugs inhibiting structures innervated by adrenergic nerves

Dibenamine hydrochloride	(Oral) 10 mg., 2-20 tablets per day
	(I.V.) 0.5-2 mg./kg. in 500 ml. isotonic salt solution, over 60 min.
Tetraethylammonium chloride	(I.V.) 200-500 mg. 10% solution administered over 2 min.
Priscoline	(Oral) 25 mg.

Drugs stimulating structures innervated by cholinergic nerves

Acetyl-β-methylcholine chloride (Mecholyl)	(Hypo) 15-50 mg.; test with small dose first
	(Oral) 50-500 mg. t.i.d
Carbamylcholine chloride (Doryl)	(Hypo) 0.25 mg.

Drugs inhibiting structures innervated by postganglionic cholinergic nerves

Atropine sulfate	(Hypo) 0.5-1.0 mg.
Belladonna tincture	(Oral) 0.6 ml.
Extract of belladonna	(Oral) 0.015 Gm.
Scopolamine hydrobromide	(Oral or hypo) 0.5 mg.

Synthetic anticholinergic agents

These agents are used to control drug-induced parkinsonism and spasticity. They reduce akinesia, rigidity and tremor, masklike facies, inertia, and propulsive gait, also control excessive flow of saliva and oily skin, and lessen frequency and intensity of oculogyric crises.

Side effects include dry mouth, blurred vision, mild tranisent hypotension, nausea, and constipation. There is rarely a transient decrease in urinary flow and occasionally short periods of euphoria or disorientation.

Doses must be individually and gradually adjusted. Observe caution in patients with glaucoma.

Biperiden (Akineton)	Tablet: 2 mg. Ampule: 5 mg./1 ml.	2 mg. 1-3 times daily 2 mg. I.M.; repeat p.r.n. up to 4 doses in 24 hr. period
Trihexyphenidyl HCl(Artane)	Tablets: 2 and 5 mg. Sequels (sustained release): 5 mg. Elixir: 2 mg./5 ml.	1-15 mg. daily
Methanesulfonate (Cogentin)	Tablets: 2 mg. Ampules: 1 mg./2ml.	1-4 mg. 1-2 times daily 2 ml. I.M.
Procyclidine HCl (Kemadrin)	Tablets: 5 mg. (scored)	2.5-5 mg. t.i.d.; maximum to 30 mg. daily
Caramiphen HCl (Panparnit)	Coated tablets: 12.5 and 50 mg.	12.5-50 mg. 5 times daily

(Tables 6 to 8 and Figures 4 and 5 follow.)

Table 6. Neuroleptics (major tranquilizers, antipsychotics)

Drug	Manufac- turer	Form	Dosage	
			Minimum	*Maximum*
		Phenothiazine derivatives		
		Dimethylamine phenothiazine derivatives (aromatic)		
Chlorpromazine (Thorazine)	Smith, Kline & French	Coated tablets: 10, 25, 50, 100, and 200 mg. Injectable: 25 mg./ml. Spansule capsules: 30, 75, 150, 200, and 300 mg. Concentrate: 30 mg./ml. Syrup: 10 mg./5 ml. Suppositories: 25 and 100 mg.	10–25 mg. t.i.d. Children: ¼ mg./lb.	1500–200 mg. dai To 100 r daily
Promazine (Sparine)	Wyeth	Tablets: 10, 25, 50, 100, and 200 mg. Syrup: 10 mg./5 ml. Concentrate: 30 mg. and 100 mg./ml. Injectable: 25 mg./ml. (I.V. use), 50 mg./ml. (I.M. use)	25–200 mg. t.i.d. Children: Over 12 yr. 10–25 mg. t.i.d.	1000 mg daily
Triflupromazine (Vesprin)	Squibb	Tablets: 10, 25, and 50 mg. Injectable: 10 and 20 mg./ml. Suspension: 10 mg./ml.	25 mg. b.i.d. Children: 30–150 mg. daily	400 mg. daily
		Piperazinyl phenothiazine derivatives		
Acetophenazine (Tindal)	Schering	Coated tablets: 20 mg.	20 mg. b.i.d.	80 mg. daily
Carphenazine (Proketazine)	Wyeth	Tablets: 12.5, 25, and 50 mg. Oral concentrate: 50 mg./ml.	25–50 mg. t.i.d.	400 mg. daily
Fluphenazine (Prolixin)	Squibb	Coated tablets: 1, 2.5, and 5 mg. Elixir: 5 mg./ml. Injectable: 2.5 mg./ml. (Enanthate): Vials of 5 ml. 25 mg./ml.	1–5 mg. daily (Enanthate): 25 mg. (1 ml.) q. 2nd week	20 mg. daily
(Permitil)	Schering	Coated tablets: 0.25, 1, 2.5, 5, and 10 mg. Chronotabs (slow action): 1 mg. Oral concentrate: 5 mg./ml.	0.5 mg. daily	2 mg. dail

Use	*Side effects and precautions*	*Foreign equivalents*
itation, hyperac- ity, and anxiety psychoses (schizo- renia, manic-de- essive states, and ganic psychoses)	Incidence of various side effects varies widely (from 0% to 50 %), depending upon drug used, size of dose, and individual sensitivity of patient Physician to be on alert for following: jaundice, liver damage, leukopenia, agranulocytosis, urticaria, contact dermatitis, photosensitivity, gastrointestinal syndrome, parkinsonism, blurry vision, convulsive seizures, hypotension, depression, constipation, urinary difficulty, vomiting, drowsiness, fatigue, cataleptic seizures, dyskinetic syndrome, akathisia, and galactorrhea	Aminasin, Aminazin, Ampliactil, Ampliactyl, Amplictil, Chlorbromasin, Chlorderazia, Chloropromazin, Chloropromazina, Contomin, Fenactil, Hibanil, Hibernal, Hibernol, Klopromex, Klorpromazine, Klorpromex, Largactil, Largactyl, Largaktil, Largaktyl, Megaphen, Neuropromazin, Novomazina, Opromazin, Phenathyl, Plegomazin, Prazil, Promactil, Promazil, Propaphenin, Prozil, Thorazene, Torazina, Wintermin
	These drugs also potentiate C.N.S. depressants (alcohol, barbiturates, etc.) Hypotension, convulsive seizures, and blood dyscrasias (leukopenia and agranulocytosis) more common with dimethylamine phenothiazines	Alofen, Ampazine, Apacergil, Centractil, Centractyl, Eliranol, Esparin, Lemazina, Lete, Liranol, Neo-Hibernex, Neuroplegil, Piarine, Prazine, Proma, Promacina, Promantine, Promanyl, Promazinon, Promilene, Promwill, Propazine, Protactil, Protactyl,Pro-Tan, Pro-Tran, Prozine, Sediston, Statazine, Talofen, Tomil, Verophen
ychoneurosis, be- .vior disorders, d alcoholism allucinations, delu- ⟩ns, and insomnia		Adazin, Esprivex, Fluomazina, Flumazin, Fluorofen, Flupromazine, Nivoman, Psyquil, Siquil, Vespral, Vetame
		Phenothoxate
	Dystonic reactions (parkinsonism, cataleptic seizures, and akathisia) seen more commonly with piperazinyl phenothiazines	
		Antasol, Anatensil, Anatensol, Flumazine, Flufenazine, Flumezin, Lyogen, Moditen, Omca, Pacinol, Sevinal, Sevinol, Siqualine, Siquoline, Tensofin, Trancin, Vespazin
⎧Relief of anxiety ⎨ and tension on ⎩outpatient basis	⎧Side effects infrequent ⎨at daily dosage of 2 mg. ⎩or less	

Continued.

Table 6. Neuroleptics (major tranquilizers, antipsychotics)—cont'd

Drug	Manufac-turer	Form	Dosage	
			Minimum	*Maximum*
Perphenazine (Trilafon)	Schering	Tablets: 2, 4, 8, and 16 mg.; 8 mg. Repetabs (delayed release) Suppositories: 2, 4, and 8 mg. Concentrate: 16 mg./5 ml. Syrup: 2 mg./5 ml. Injectable: 5 mg./ml. (1 ml. ampules and 10 ml. vials)	2 mg. t.i.d.	64 mg. daily
Piperacetazine (Quide)	Dow	Tablets: 10 and 25 mg.	10 mg. b.i.d.—q.i.d.	160 mg. daily
Prochlorperazine (Compazine)	Smith, Kline & French	Tablets: 5, 10, and 25 mg. Injectable: 5 mg./ml. Spansule capsules: 10, 15, 30, and 75 mg. Concentrate: 10 mg./ml. Syrup: 5 mg./5 ml. Suppositories: 2.5, 5, and 25 mg.	15–20 mg. daily Children: 5–25 mg. daily	75–150 mg. daily
Trifluoperazine (Stelazine)	Smith, Kline & French	Coated tablets: 1, 2, 5, and 10 mg. Injectable: 2 mg./ml. Concentrate: 10 mg./ml.	2 mg. t.i.d.	80 mg. daily
Piperidine phenothiazine derivatives				
Butaperazine (Repoise)	A. H. Robins	Tablets: 5, 10, and 25 mg.	5–10 mg., 3 times daily	100 mg. daily
Mepazine (Pacatal)	Warner-Chilcott	Tablets: 25, 50, and 100 mg. Injectable: 25 mg./ml.	25 mg. t.i.d. Children: 25 mg. b.i.d.	300 mg. daily
Thioridazine hydrochloride (Mellaril)	Sandoz	Coated tablets: 10, 25, 50, 100, 150, and 200 mg. Concentrate: 30 mg./ml.	10 mg. t.i.d. Children: 10 mg. t.i.d.	800 mg. daily
Thioxanthene derivatives				
Chlorprothixene (Taractan)	Roche	Tablets: 10, 25, 50, and 100 mg. 12.5 mg./ml. in 2 ml. ampules Concentrate: 100 mg./5 ml.	30 mg. oral daily 12.5 mg. I.M. (vomiting) 75 mg. I.M. (agitation)	600 mg. oral daily 25 mg. I.M. (vomiting) 200 mg. I.M. (agitation)
Thiothixene (Navane)	Roerig	Capsules: 1, 2, 5, and 10 mg.	2 mg. t.i.d.	60 mg. daily
Butyrophenone derivatives				
Haloperidol (Haldol)	McNeil	Tablets: 0.5, 1, and 2 mg. Concentrate: 2 mg./ml.	1–2 mg., 2–3 times daily	2–5 mg., 2–3 times daily Mainte-nance: 1 mg., 3–times daily

Use	Side effects and precautions	Foreign equivalents
		Chlorpiprazin, Chlorpiprozin, Decantan, Etaperazine, Etapirazin, Ethaperazine, Fentazin, Grenolon, Perfanazin, Perfenazin, Perfenazina, Perphenan, Perfenazine, PZC, Trilifan
		Capazine, Chlormeprazine, Dicopal, Meterazine, Nipodal, Nipprodal, Novamin
		Eskazine, Eskazinyl, Jatroneural, Terfluzin, Terfluzine, Tranquis
		Randolectil, Megalectil
		Lacumin, Mepasin, Mepazine, MPMP, Nothiazine, Pacatol, Pactal, Papital, Paxital
		Mallerol, Malloryl, Meleril, Melleretten, Melleril
	Mild dermatitis, occasional vertigo, tremor	Chlorprotixen, Chlorprotixin, Quinlan, Tactaran, Taractaran, Tarasan, Tarassan, Truxal
		Orbinamon
	Not in children under 12 years	Aldol, Haloperidol, Serenace, Serenase, Serenelfi

Continued.

Table 6. Neuroleptics (major tranquilizers, antipsychotics)—cont'd

Drug	Manufac-turer	Form	Dosage
		Rauwolfia **alkaloids**	
Serpasil	Ciba	Tablets: 0.1, 0.25, 1, and 2 mg.	0.25 mg. b.i.d. starting dose Maintenance: 0.25 mg. daily hypertension and mild e tional disturbance

Table 7. Antianxiety drugs (minor tranquilizers)

			Dosage	
Drug	Manufac-turer	Form	Adults	Children
		Glycol and glycerol derivatives		
Meprobamate (Equanil)	Wyeth	Tablets: 200 and 400 mg. Suspension: 200 mg./5 ml. Continuous release capsules: 400 mg.	400 mg. b.i.d.-q.i.d.	100 mg. t.i.d. 200 mg. 3 yr. and over
(Miltown)	Wallace	Tablets: 400 mg. Meprospan capsules (sus-tained release): 200 and 400 mg. Injectable (ampules): 400 mg./5 ml.	400 mg. I.M. q. 4 h.	Infants: 125 mg. I. q. 6 h.
Oxanamide (Quiactin)	Merrell	Coated tablets: 400 mg.	400 mg. q.i.d.	
Ethchlorvynol (Placidyl)	Abbott	Capsules: 100, 200 and 500 mg.	500 mg. h.s., 100 mg. b.i.d., 200 mg. t.i.d. daytime dose	
Ethinamate (Valmid)	Lilly	Diskets: 500 mg.	1-2 tablets before retiring	
Glutethimide (Doriden)	Ciba	Tablets: 125, 250, and 500 mg. Capsules: 500 mg.	500 mg. h.s., 250 mg. t.i.d.	125 mg.
Methyprylon (Noludar)	Roche	Tablets: 50 and 200 mg. Capsules: 300 mg.	200-400 mg. bedtime 50-100 mg. 3-4 times daily	Adjust to age and weight

Use	Side effects	Precautions	Foreign equivalents
pression, anxiety, ten- , psychosomatic disor- s, alcohol intoxication; d in combination with nothiazines for psychoses, ital deficiency, schizo- enia, etc.; used with ECT increase effectiveness; intain after discontinuing T; adjunct to psycho- rapy	Dry mouth, blurred vision, insomnia, dizziness, head- ache, nausea, skin rash, tremor; transient eosinophi- lia, jaundice, or agranulocy- tosis are rare; occasionally drowsiness, constipation, or G.I. disturbances	Do not give with a mono- amine oxadase inhibitor: use with care in patients with convulsive disorder; use with caution in patients with glaucoma or a propen- sity to urinary retention	Deprinol, Imizin, Irmin, Melipramin, Promiben, Sur- plix
			Adepril, Horizon, Laroxyl, Saroten, Sarotex, Triptanol, Tryptanol, Tryptisol, Tryp- tizol, Uxen
			Acetexa, Allegran, Aventyl, Noritren, Noritilen, Sansi- val, Vividyl
pression of all types, in- ding both psychotic and choneurotic; also depres- ı with chronic illness	Hypertensive crises (hyper- tensive reaction with head- ache, nausea and vomiting, palpitations, and rarely in- tracranial bleeding), pre- sumably a result of sym- pathomimetic actions of phe- nelzine and tranylcypro- mine, have been reported immediately following ad- ministration of ampheta- mine or ingestion of certain foods which contain tyra- mine, such as well-ripened cheeses and fava beans, yo- gurt, beer, wine, alcohol, and creams Constipation and delayed micturition, edema, blurred vision, dry mouth, sweating, occasional weakness, leth- argy, headaches, occasional skin rash, and occasional nausea Large doses may produce overstimulation, with anx- iety, restlessness, and in- somnia	Observe for effects of over- stimulation Suicide always a danger dur- ing recovery from depres- sions Contraindicated in patients with cerebrovascular and cardiovascular disorders Do not give in combination with other monoamine oxi- dase inhibitors or sympatho- mimetics, or in combination with Tofranil or Elavil	Maraplan, Marplan
			Epsril, Nuredal
			Alacine, Feneizina, Kalgan, Monofen, Monophen, Nar- delzine, Phenalzine, Stiner- val

Continued.

Table 8. Antidepressants—cont'd

Drug	Manufac-turer	Form	Dosage Start	Dosage Treatment
			Psychomotor stimulants	
Dextro amphetamine (Dexedrine)	Smith, Kline & French	Tablets: 5 mg. Spansule capsules: 5, 10, and 15 mg. Elixir: 5 mg./5 ml.	Up to 30 mg./day Spansule capsule gives 10–12 hr. therapeutic effect Children: 2.5–10 mg. daily in divided doses before 4 P.M.	
Methamphetamine (Desoxyn)	Abbott	Tablets: 2.5 and 5 mg. Long-release tablets (Gradumet): 5, 10, and 15 mg. Elixir: 3.3 mg./5 ml.	2.5 mg., b.i.d. or t.i.d., before breakfast and at noon Long-release tablets given once daily in morning	
Methylphenidate (Ritalin)	Ciba	Tablets: 5, 10, and 20 mg. Injectable: 100 mg. multiple-dose (10 mg./ml.)	Oral: 10–20 mg. t.i.d. Injectable (I.V., I.M., or subcutaneously): 10–50 mg. q. ½ h. or as indicated	

Use	Side effects and precautions		Foreign equivalents
d depression and leth- y; hyperactive children, avior disorders	Sympathomimetic effects May potentiate epinephrine	Check blood pressure with repeated doses	Afatin, Afettine, Amsustain, Dephadren, Dexamed, Dexedrina, Dextroanfetamina, Lentanet, Maxiton, Obesedrin, Phenpromin, Phetadex, Proptan, Proptane, Tempodex
d stimulant and antidessant; stimulates freer oalization			
rotic and psychotic desion			Amedrine, Desfedran, Desoxyephedrin, Desoxyephedrine, Dexosyn, Eufodrin, Eufodrinal, Isophen, Metanfetamina, Methedrinal, Methedrine, Methylamphetamine, Pervitin, Philopon, Psykoton
ug - induced depressions 1 *Rauwolfia* or phenoth- 1e compounds			
			Phenidylate, Rilatin, Rilatine

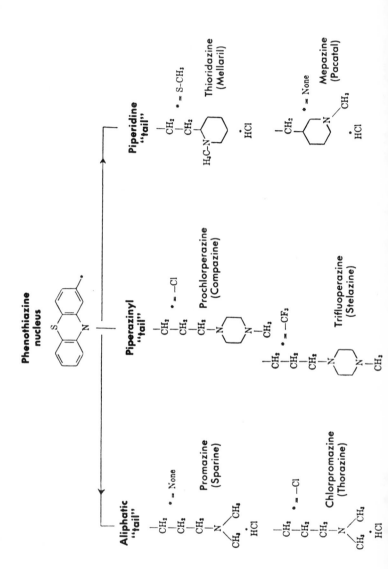

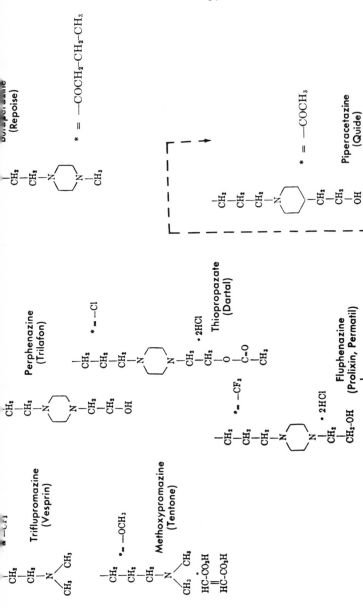

Figure 4. Psychotropic drugs derived from the phenothiazine nucleus.

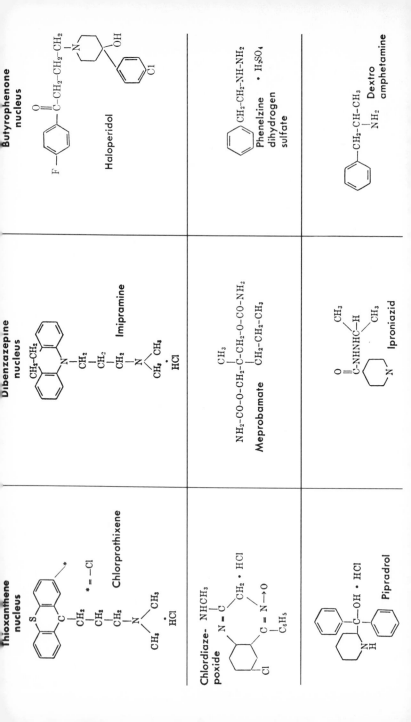

SUGGESTED READINGS

AMA drug evaluations, AMA Council on Drugs, Chicago, 1971, American Medical Association.

Ban, T. A.: Psychopharmacology, Baltimore, 1969, The Williams & Wilkins Co.

Beecher, H. K., and Rinkle, M.: A quantitative approach to psychopharmacology, New York, 1963, Philosophical Library, Inc.

Benson, W. M., and Schiele, B. C.: Tranquilizing and antidepressive drugs, Springfield, Ill., 1962, Charles C Thomas, Publisher.

Black, P., editor: Drugs and the brain: papers on the action, use, and abuse of psychotropic agents, Baltimore, 1969, Johns Hopkins University Press.

Caldwell, A. E.: Psychopharmaca—a bibliography of psychopharmacology, 1952-1957, Washington, D. C., 1958, U. S. Government Printing Office.

Cohen, S., and Ditman, K. S.: Prolonged adverse reactions to lysergic acid diethylamide, Arch. Gen. Psychiat. 8:475, 1963.

Cole, J. O., and Gerald, R. W.: Psychopharmacology—problems in evaluation, Washington, D. C., 1959, National Academy of Science, National Research Council.

DiMascio, A.: Clinical handbook of psychopharmacology, New York, 1970, Science House, Inc.

Engelhardt, D. M., Rosen, B., Freedman, N., and Margolis, R.: Phenothiazines in prevention of psychiatric hospitalization. IV. Delay or prevention of hospitalization—a reevaluation, Arch. Gen. Psychiat. 16:98, 1967.

Galbrecht, C. R., and Klett, C. J.: Predicting response to phenothiazines: the right drug for the right patient, J. Nerv. Ment. Dis. 147:173, 1968.

Gittleman-Klein, R., and Klein, D. V.: Long-term effects of "antipsychotic" agents: a review. In Efron, D. H., editors: Psychopharmacology—a review of progress, 1957-1967, Public Health Service Pub. No. 1836, Washington, D. C., 1968, U. S. Government Printing Office.

Goldman, D., and Ulett, G. A.: Practical psychiatry for the internist, St. Louis, 1968, The C. V. Mosby Co.

Goodman, L., and Gilman, A.: The pharmacological basis of therapeutics, ed. 4, New York, 1970, The Macmillan Co.

Haase, H. J., and Janssen, P. A. J.: The action of neuroleptic drugs, Chicago, 1965, Year Book Medical Publishers, Inc.

Itil, T. M., Keskiner, A., and Fink, M.: Therapeutic studies in "therapy resistant" schizophrenic patients, Community Psychiatry 7:488, 1966.

Klein, D. V., and Davis, J. M.: Diagnosis and drug treatment of psychiatric disorders, Baltimore, 1969, The Williams & Wilkins Co.

Klerman, G. L.: Modes of action of antidepressant drugs. In Cole, J. O., and Wittenborn, J. R., editors: Pharmacotherapy of depression, Springfield Ill., 1966, Charles C Thomas, Publisher.

Levine, J., Schiele, B., and Bouthilet, L., editors: Principles and problems in establishing the efficacy of psychotropic agents, Public Health Service

Pub. No. 2138, Washington, D. C., Jan., 1971, U. S. Government Printing Office.

Lipman, R. S., Hammer, H. M., Bernardes, J. F., and Park, L. C.: Patient report of significant life situation events (methodological inplications of outpatient drug evaluation), Dis. Nerv. Syst. 26:586, 1965.

Marks, J., and Pare, C. M. B., editors: The scientific basis of drug therapy in psychiatry, New York, 1965, Pergamon Press, Inc.

Overall, J. E., Hollister, L. E., Kimbell, J., Jr., and Shelton, J.: Extrinsic factors influencing responses to psychotherapeutic drugs, Arch. Gen. Psychiat. 11:89, 1969.

Rinkel, M., editor: Specific and nonspecific factors in psychopharmacology, New York, 1963, Philosophical Library, Inc.

Schou, M., and Baastrup, C.: Lithium prophylaxis in recurrent affective disorders, Brit. J. Psychiat. 118:133, 1971.

Smith, W. L.: Drugs and cerebral function, Springfield, Ill., 1970, Charles C Thomas, Publisher.

The cheese reaction, editorial, Lancet 1:540, Mar. 7, 1964.

Uhr, L. M., and Miller, J. G., editors: Drugs and behavior, New York, 1960, John Wiley & Sons, Inc.

27
Management of suicidal patients

INCIDENCE

In the United States, suicides account for 20,000 deaths a year. This is the tenth leading cause of death. There are about 10 attempted suicides for each 1 that is successful. Suicide is not a product of modern civilization but is influenced by social factors. Anthropologists have found it to be completely absent in some cultures, very common in others. The suicide rate decreases in time of war and in prosperity. Ireland, Chile, New Zealand, and Norway are among countries with low suicide rates. Sweden, Denmark, and Japan, among the highest. Suicide depends, however, not only upon broad social factors but also upon immediate environmental pressures and differences in individual personality structure.

Recent studies show that suicide occurs almost exclusively in persons clinically ill and that two thirds of these suffer from either manic-depressive psychosis or alcoholism. Over 80% are older than 40 years and men outnumber women two to one. Seemingly more vulnerable are persons who live alone (single, divorced, or widowed) and those concerned over the death of a loved one or about personal ill health. Less serious attempts may occur after drinking and marital quarrels. The number of attempted suicides far exceeds the number of completed suicides.

Two thirds of successful suicides communicated their intent to someone prior to the act. A smaller number of unsuccessful ones communicated such intent. One fourth of all attempted suicides and over one half of successful suicides have made previous attempts. One in ten has a family history of successful or attempted suicide. Most successful suicides have received medical or psychiatric care prior to the act.

Attempts to explain the dynamics of suicide include Freud's suggestion that anger toward others is turned inward against the self; that suicide is only a further step for a patient already "emotionally dead"; that the patient feels he will be reunited with loved ones after death; that he gains a feeling of omnipotence by destroying a life, though it be his own; or that suicide is welcomed as a form of punishment for feelings of worthlessness. Much that has been written about a "death instinct" was neatly summarized by Zilboorg (1937): "To say the death instinct gains the upper hand over the life instinct is merely an elaborate way of saying that man does die or kill himself." Hendin says it is worthwhile to inquire of everyone who attempts suicide concerning his attitudes toward death, about presumed events after death, and about his thoughts regarding the suicidal act.

The most common methods of attempting suicide in the United States include drug ingestion, cutting, and gas inhalation. In other countries favorite methods vary. The most common methods used in *successful* suicides are hanging, shooting, drug ingestion, and asphyxiation by gas. Drowning, shooting, and hanging are more commonly seen in men and poisoning in women. Barbiturate ingestion accounted for 21% of all suicides in San Francisco in 1947. More subtle methods of suicide are the physiological such as, for example, the coronary patient who refuses to reduce his work schedule and the diabetic who suddenly is unable to balance his insulin and diet. Another form of chronic suicide is exhibited by alcoholics and addicts. Delirious patients, seen most often on medical and surgical wards, present a different type of suicidal risk in that they may take their lives in a state of anxious confusion in which, for example, they can mistake a window for a door.

It has been found that suicide is rare among neurotics who show predominately an anxiety reaction. The hysteric's attempts at environmental manipulation through suicidal gesture may, however, perhaps from misjudgment, have a fatal outcome. The whole problem of evaluating the suicidal danger in neurotics is complicated by the frequent mislabeling as neurotic of those persons suffering from mild degrees of manic-depressive disorder. Commonly, however, a psychoneurotic (with obsessive-compulsive reaction, hysteria, etc.) may experience symptoms of depression as an episode of his basic neurosis.

PREVENTION

In evaluating suicidal danger, one must remember that suicidal thoughts or ideas, considered in more than a passing manner, have been found in as many as 50% of normal persons by some investigators. Hysterical and psychopathic individuals use attempted suicide as a means of revenge or spite, or to achieve their own way. In the chronic psychoneurotic or other unstable personality, acute alcoholism may release inhibitions and arouse strong feelings of guilt, fear, or aggression—with consequent suicide. The psychoneurotic with whom suicide is an obsessive rumination or in whom the suicidal thought is in the form of a fear instead of a desire presents less danger. In the case of persons who act out their problems it must be remembered that what is begun as merely a suicidal gesture may result in a successful attempt.

Even here, however, there is awareness of the possibility that the attempt may be successful; this action, in fact, has the nature of a gamble with death. The depressed patient is a potential suicide, and no suicidal talk is to be considered lightly. The agitated depressive who admits no delusions is a likely candidate, as is the patient with delusions of worthlessness, guilt, and need for punishment. It should not be forgotten that suicide is an important cause of death among chronic alcoholics. Feelings of futility in adolescence and in old age should be heeded as warning signals. Marked insomnia should also place the physician on his guard; early morning hours are a favorite time for suicide. A history of previous attempts or of suicides in the family may be important, and suicidal desire may yet lurk behind the smiling countenance in a rapidly recovering patient with depression. Evidence of bodily tension such as hand wringing may be the only warning sign that remains. The Rorschach and other tests can sometimes reveal suicidal intentions.

Recently there are community efforts to organize suicide-prevention centers with 24-hour telephone coverage and available consultants. Although such centers appear very worthwhile in assisting persons with various types of emotional trouble, it would appear that persons calling in are not always those who have made suicidal attempts. A real focus of effort should be upon the high-risk patients who have been identified as making serious suicidal attempts.

Immediate hospitalization of the acutely depressed or suspected suicidal patient on a closed ward may be a lifesaving measure. But do not leave the patient alone while you step out to call the hospital! Adequate suicidal precautions can be observed only on a psychiatric division. A well-meaning companion is often little better than no preventive measure. In a general hospital setting, delirious patients should be evaluated when at their worst (during the evening hours) and should be kept on the ground floor and near the nurses' station. The use of antidepressant drugs is an effective tool to combat depression. As there is some delay in achieving an effective level with these drugs, electroconvulsive therapy is often necessary during the early stages of drug therapy.

Often the psychiatrist takes a calculated risk and follows the mild depressive as an outpatient. Here psychotherapy is not only of remedial benefit but also permits the psychotherapist to repeatedly evaluate the current suicidal risk. Adequate chemical sedation at night combined with Dexedrine in the morning has long been a useful routine. The antidepressants are extremely useful for cases of depression followed in the outpatient clinic. In selected cases ECT is also an outpatient procedure.

SUGGESTED READINGS

Bosselman, B. C.: Self-destruction, Springfield, Ill., 1958, Charles C Thomas, Publisher.

Dublin, L.: Suicide: a sociological and statistical study, New York, 1963, The Ronald Press Co.

Durkheim, E.: Suicide, a study in sociology (translated by J. Spaulding and G. Simpson), Glencoe, Ill., 1951, The Free Press.

Fisch, M.: The suicidal gesture, Amer. J. Psychiat. 111:33, 1954.

Freud, S.: Mourning and melancholia. In Collected papers, London, 1949, Hogarth Press, Ltd., vol. 4.

Hendin, H.: The psychodynamics of suicide, J. Nerv. Ment. Dis. 136:236, 1963.

Hendin, H.: Suicide and Scandinavia, New York, 1964, Grune & Stratton, Inc.

Menninger, K.: Man against himself, New York, 1938, Harcourt, Brace & World, Inc.

Robins, E., et al.: Some clinical considerations in the prevention of suicide based on a study of 134 successful suicides, Amer. J. Public Health 49:888, 1959.

Ulett, G. A., Martin, D. W., and McBride, J. R.: The Rorschach findings in a case of suicide, Amer. J. Orthopsychiat. 20:817, 1950.

Weiss, J. M. A.: Suicide: an epidemiologic analysis, Psychiat. Quart. 28:225, 1954.

Wolff, K.: Patterns of self-destruction: depression and suicide, Springfield, Ill., 1970, Charles C Thomas, Publisher.

28
Management of psychiatric problems in the military setting

The role of the psychiatrist in a military setting is strucured, defined, and limited by the needs and mission of the Armed Forces. Even more than in civilian practice, the needs of the social group are preeminent, whereas the expectations of the individual patient and the physician are secondary. The therapeutic aim, however, is the same, namely, to help the patient to function effectively and comfortably within the current situation.

The psychiatrist should strive for intelligent utilization of personnel. Most psychoneurotics make as good soldiers as anyone else. Evaluation of the military patient should include assessment not only of the diagnostic symptoms (their type and severity) but also of the premorbid personality, the degree of the precipitating stress, and on the basis of these a prognostic opinion of the patient's ability to function in the military situation and of the degree and type of stress he may be able to withstand. The psychiatrist must be cautious in evaluating the patient's own story, for he may too readily accent his past inadequacies and problems in the conscious or unconscious hope that he may be found unsuited for service.

In practice the military psychiatrist should furnish that kind of brief therapeutic program which will enable the patient better to adjust to military life and to return to duty as quickly as possible. Severe and chronic cases are transferred to military psychiatric centers not too far from the front lines for intensive physical and psychotherapeutic endeavors. From the initial contact with the patient, throughout all phases of treatment, the expectation is for him to return to duty; if any other outcome is even subtly fostered, secondary gain from illness will alone prevent rehabilitation. Ultimate transfer to Veterans Adminstration facilities or medical discharge to civilian life is possible. Patients with severe personality disorders may be discharged for the convenience of the government and for the best interests of both the Service and the individual concerned. Before decision for such discharge is reached, however, the psychiatrist should carefully consider the possibility of reassignment and trial at another type of duty.

In the zone of combat, patients with combat exhaustion may manifest varying degrees of personality disintegration, conversion symptoms, panic states, or even psychotic symptomatology. It should be noted, however, that apart from these transient reactions the incidence of major psychosis is no greater than in civilian life. Apart from the psychological elements involved, fatigue is a potent factor and the treatment should include food, rest, sleep (with or without sedation), as well as brief psychiatric interviewing. It has been found that the immediate management of these cases by an experienced psychiatrist, close to the area of battle, may permit a return to combat duty in 50% to 90% of such cases. The report of the physical examination should be discussed with the patient. If the facts warrant it, and in the light of our universal cultural belief that illness relieves a man of his responsibilities, an early positive statement should be made as to the absence of medical justification for the separation of the patient from military service. Psychotherapy is brief and involves techniques of ventilation, reassurance, persuasion, and firm suggestion that the patient will improve and rejoin his combat outfit. The discussion is directed at feelings of resentment, hostility, and self-pity, with focus on the current problem and avoidance of a discussion of symptoms and bodily complaints. The key to therapy is solution of the conflict between the *short-term gain* of evacuation to safety and the *long-term guilt* engendered by thoughts of leaving his buddies and by failure to perform with the degree of honor required by his superego, the family, and the community, as he sees it.

Throughout, the physician must be firm, decisive, fair, and moderate. He must not leave decisions conditional upon the patient's improvement. Newcomers to military psychiatry and those stationed in rear echelons tend to identify with the patient, have their anxiety stirred by his tales of combat, and may find it difficult to function without guilt feelings when returning men to a duty more dangerous and arduous than their own. On the other hand, the psychiatrist who is himself a part of the combat team becomes closely identified with the welfare of the group and can more readily accept the attitude that it is for the best interests of the individual to rejoin his outfit.

Intravenous Pentothal sodium to produce catharsis and abreaction has been used less frequently as other methods proved more successful. Its primary indication now seems to be either for use in severe or resistant cases in which the ultimate goal is recovery for noncombatant status or for relief of grossly incapacitating symptoms resulting from recent traumatic experiences.

In summary, and quoting Colonel D. B. Peterson from his experience in the Korean campaign, "The military psychiatrist should, while maintaining good liaison with both line and medical command, at all echelons appropriate to his location: treat as far forward as possible, avoid hospital atmosphere, expedite return to duty, and aid the patient to define the reality situation and his part in it."*

---

*From Peterson, D. B.: Amer. J. Psychiat. **112**:23, 1955.

SUGGESTED READINGS

Glass, A. J.: Psychotherapy in the combat zone, Amer. J. Psychiat. **110**:725, 1954.

Glass, A. J., Artiss, K. L., Gibbs, J. J., and Sweeney, V. C.: The current status of Army psychiatry, Amer. J. Psychiat. **117**:673, 1961.

Gonzalez, V. R.: Psychiatry and the army brat, Springfield, Ill., 1970, Charles C Thomas, Publisher.

Greenhill, M. H.: Clinical features of the psychoneuroses in World War II veterans, N. Carolina Med. J. **7**:585, 1946.

Grinker, R., and Spiegel, J.: Men under stress, New York, 1963, McGraw-Hill Book Co.

Menninger, W. C.: Psychiatry in a troubled world, New York, 1948, The Macmillan Co.

Peterson, D. B., and Chambers, R. E.: Restatement of combat psychiatry, Amer. J. Psychiat. **109**:249, 1952.

Solomon, H. C., and Yakovlev, P. I.: Manual of military neuropsychiatry, Philadelphia, 1944, W. B. Saunders Co.

Weiss, J. M. A.: The role of the psychotherapist in military training centers, Milit. Med. **118**:95, 1956.

29
Forensic psychiatry

The psychiatrist deals with persons whose chief symptom is deviation in behavior, and he frequently must testify in court. For this reason he should familarize himself with medicolegal procedures. In the courtroom, as a special witness, his sole job is to give scientific facts or psychiatric opinions, not to defend the psychotic or to bring a criminal to justice. On the witness stand he should use clear and concise language that a lay jury can understand. He should be prepared to undergo cross-examination, even endure cajolery or threat to his personal esteem, and behave always in a modest and unemotional manner. However, a psychiatrist with an adequate workup of the patient and convinced of his position will rarely be subjected to detailed cross-examination by an experienced trial attorney.

COURTROOM TESTIMONY

Although the psychiatrist is called into court as a scientist and expert, he may be asked to give opinions as well as facts. He would do well to prepare his testimony beforehand with the advice of the trial lawyer who has called upon him, in order to know the kind of question he may be asked. He can appear very foolish, and indeed be of little help to anyone if he cannot give the kind of information needed by the court. He should remember that the information needed from his mental status examination will be different from case to case. Most courts will not permit the psychiatrist to decide whether the patient knows right from wrong or is or is not competent. They merely want his *opinion* of how the patient is functioning mentally—his mental state at some designated time—and possibly a psychiatric diagnosis. A physician usually cannot quote history taken by himself or by someone else, as this is hearsay evidence and not admissible. Of most importance are the findings on examination of the patient, with careful note taking at the time of such examination. The court will be interested in the logic leading to the diagnosis. The court may require "yes" and "no" answers in order to arrive at its verdict; however, it is possible to ask the judge for permission to explain.

CRIMINAL RESPONSIBILITY

A psychiatrist is frequently called upon to testify in criminal cases. He may be asked to give opinions in accordance with rules laid down in 1843 in the famous *McNaughton case* where in Scotland in 1843 a paranoid patient, David Mc-Naughton, shot and killed the secretary to Prime Minister Robert Peel. The rule that was established then asks: "Was the accused laboring under such a defect of reasoning from a disease of his mind as not to know the nature and quality of the act he was doing, and if he did it, he did not know that what he was doing was wrong?" The majority of American psychiatrists today, as well as enlightened jurists, feel that this test is unsatisfactory, yet frequently some answer to it must be given. More recently there has been introduced the concept of *irresistible impulse* as a criminal defense. Although in itself not a good term, it implies psychiatrically acceptable doctrine that some individuals are less able to adhere to the right, by reason of abnormal urges which they have little power to control. This problem is closely allied to the question of the existence of *temporary insanity*, which, although almost nonexistent from the medical point of view, is a concept with which the forensic psychiatrist should be familiar. Ideally, the psychiatrist should give evidence to show: (1) whether the individual was suffering from a medically recognized disorder and (2) whether the disorder had distorted his social judgment and interfered with the exercise of customary social control. Proof of a mental disorder may serve to reduce the degree of crime (e.g., from murder to manslaughter).

The Durham decision in the District of Columbia provided

a most hopeful shift in the handling of psychiatric testimony. Under the *Durham Rule* the behavior of the accused is considered as to whether it is a product of mental disorder. If it is judged to be so, the individual is committed rather than sentenced. Whereas many legal minds have feared that this criterion would result in the community's being flooded with psychopathic characters, the fact is that a very small percentage of criminals have successfully proved their behavior to be the result of mental illness. The doctor's role is to give evidence relating to the presence of a mental illness, not to express an opinion that the accused should be restrained or imprisoned for his offense. His function is not to recommend punishment or even to express an opinion as to the defendant's potential for crime or that he "undoubtedly" would commit similar crimes in the future if unrestrained.

COMMITMENT PROCEDURES

The procedure for commitment of insane patients or mentally ill persons varies from state to state but in general three basic methods are used: (1) examination by one or usually two physicians appearing before a judge, with a jury hearing on demand of the patient or at the judge's discretion; (2) in a few states a hearing before a commission consisting of a judge and two physicians or a physician and a lawyer; and (3) commitment upon certification by a physician, with hearing only upon appeal by the person being certified.

The widespread use of court commitment procedure was instituted to protect the sane person from being railroaded into a mental hospital, in the days when institutionalization was considered a putting away, rather than a procedure for purposes of medical treatment. Such commitment procedures involving public hearings with the patient present are cumbersome, expensive, and heartless, and they place the patient under needless and possibly harmful stress. The procedure is analogous to that in conviction for a crime and with paranoid persons may dangerously involve those who give testimony. It is hoped that in a more enlightened future a court-appointed commission of physicians can commit directly by certification.

In many states *observation commitment* is permitted for a

brief, stated length of time, as an emergency procedure. This is accomplished by permission of the relatives and a statement by two qualified physicians. Most states today permit *voluntary commitment,* or informal procedures in which the patient may seek hospitalization for himself, if there is room and if the hospital admitting authority feels the patient will benefit from such hospitalization. In most cases he can obtain release a few days after written request unless by that time he has been formally committed. Patients who feel they are being restrained illegally may request a hearing through a *writ of habeas corpus.*

The commitment of mental defectives and alcoholics is, in some states, provided for under separate statutes. Voluntary admission of alcoholics has not been entirely satisfactory, because of their early demand for release when they become sober. Recent legislation that frowns upon repeated arrest and incarceration in jail for public drunkenness will surely bring greater hospital admission rates of persons whose main symptom is alcoholism.

PRIVILEGED COMMUNICATION

Communications between a patient and his physician are, in 32 of the states, held to be confidential and such information cannot be released without the written permission of the patient or unless the patient calls the physician to testify in court on his behalf. Although this rule applies only to information pertaining to litigation, yet there is the moral and professional ethical obligation against disclosure of such information to any person other than those concerned with the patient's immediate health care. Recently there has been concern over the accessibility of medical records stored in a computer. In actuality, it is more difficult to break into computer storage than into an ordinary medical record library; hence, if due precaution and some of the new user identification techniques are utilized, such fears are unwarranted.

SEXUAL OFFENSES

Because of emotion aroused in the public by the report of deviant sexual activities, legislation has been enacted from time to time dealing with such offenders. Although some states have laws dealing with exhibitionism, bestiality, homosexuality, adultery, and prostitution, those who commit such acts are often not dangerous to others.

The "sexual psychopath" clause is directed mainly toward pedophilia (sex relations with children) and rape (including statutory rape [sexual intercourse below the age of consent], incest, or forced rape). Ideally the purpose of such laws is to permit a truly indeterminate sentence of from 1 day to life imprisonment with the ultimate aim that the patient be incarcerated as long as is deemed necessary to protect the public but with the intention that he might be rehabilitated by psychiatric treatment and be released whenever it appeared that he was a good risk on parole. The wording of such laws varies from state to state, and thus difficulties have arisen in their administration.

Actually we know little of the practical dynamics of sexual psychopathy that would lead to an efficient treatment or cure of such conditions, and one defect in a law of this type is that it implies that we can predict who is likely to demonstrate socially dangerous sexual behavior. Some states permit hospitalization only after a criminal offense has been committed. Studies have shown that sex offenders have no single category of mental pathology and that men who are sex offenders often commit other types of crime and vice versa.

As Guttmacher points out, there is as much difference between the average exhibitionist and a rapist as between a shoplifter and a safecracker. Also there is no evidence that sexual criminals progress from minor offenses such as exhibitionism to major offenses like forced rape.

MENTAL INCOMPETENCY

The psychiatrist is frequently called upon to judge a patient's testamentary capacity or mental competency and to help the family with the institution of *guardianship* proceedings. In such cases, the significance of emotional disability is often overlooked by the court. In deciding competency, one should consider the background and experience of the person and also whether competency for only a specific act is to be judged (e.g., executing a will or some particular business transaction). It is important that the psychiatrist not consider competence generally but understand that the question is, instead, "competence for what particular purpose." Therefore, his mental status examination should be tailored to throw light upon the specific question.

Guardianship proceedings in most states are, in some ways, similar to commitment procedures. A petition is made to the court by friends or relatives and the patient is notified. The case may be tried by the judge alone in a probate or county court, although in a number of states a jury trial is still used and the patient has the right of counsel.

The adjudication that a person is mentally ill does not establish that such a person is incompetent. Thus mental illness may coexist with good mental capacity. A patient committed without a decision about his competency enjoys all of his civil rights, including the right to contract, to transfer property, to sue, and to be sued. In some states, however, statutes expressly declare that persons committed to state institutions are legally incompetent to contract.

In the case of *competence regarding the making of a will,* the fact that the patient had to be prompted to recall his property is not sufficient to prove unfitness to make a will. For testamentary purposes it is sufficient that the testator understand the condition of his estate, his obligation toward his relatives, and the importance and effect of the provisions of his will. Because senile persons may have increased suggestibility, the court may deem it important to ascertain whether undue influence was used when the will was made. Courts have sometimes ruled that it takes less mind to make a will than to make a contract.

It is of increasing importance that the physician have the consent of the patient before proceeding with any treatment procedure. This is especially true in connection with electroconvulsive therapies. A patient's mere signing of a routine release form is not sufficient. In recent suits for malpractice it has been important that evidence be presented to show that the possible side effects and complications of the procedure were fully explained. Where competence of the patient is in doubt, informed consent should be obtained from the next of kin. For emergency practices and for research procedures, a human rights committee can stand in judgment that the patient's rights were not abused. Research procedures should be of value for the patient himself and not merely for the good of humanity.

MARRIAGE AND DIVORCE

About half the states have laws intended to prevent insane persons from marrying; but in many the responsibility falls on the license clerk, who can hardly be expected to judge upon mental competency. Marriages of such persons are considered void or voidable and thus open to annulment, although children born of such void marriages are not considered legally illegitimate. Incurable insanity is a ground for divorce in more than half the states.

SUGGESTED READINGS

Allen, R. C., Ferster, E. A., and Rubin, J. G., editors: Readings in law and psychiatry Baltimore, 1968, The Johns Hopkins Press.

American Bar Foundation, Lindman, F. T., and McIntrye, D. M., editors: The mentally disabled and the law, Chicago, 1961, University of Chicago Press.

Bearcroft, J., and Donovan, M. D.: Psychiatric referrals from courts and prisons, Brit. Med. J. 2:1519, 1965.

Biggs, J., Jr.: The guilty mind: psychiatry and the law of homicide, Baltimore, 1967, The Johns Hopkins Press.

Freedman, L. Z.: Social and legal considerations of psychiatric therapy in a general hospital. In Kaufman, M. R., editor: The psychiatric unit in a general hospital, New York, 1965, International Universities Press, Inc.

Glueck, S.: Law and psychiatry, Baltimore, 1962, The Johns Hopkins Press.

Guttmacher, M. S.: Critique of views of Thomas Szasz on legal psychiatry, Arch. Gen. Psychiat. 10:238, 1964.

Guttmacher, M. S.: The role of psychiatry in law, Springfield, Ill., 1968, Charles C Thomas, Publisher.

Hollender, M. H.: Privileged communication and confidentiality, Dis. Nerv. Syst. 26:169, 1965.

Jeffery, C. R.: Criminal responsibility and mental disease, Springfield, Ill., 1967, Charles C Thomas, Publisher.

MacDonald, J. M.: Psychiatry and the criminal: a guide to psychiatric examinations for the criminal courts, Springfield, Ill., 1969, Charles C Thomas, Publisher.

Polier, J. W.: The rule of law and the role of psychiatry (Isaac Ray Lectures), Baltimore, 1968, The Johns Hopkins Press.

Rappeport, J. R., and Lassen, G.: Dangerousness—arrest rate comparisons of discharged patients and the general population, Amer. J. Psychiat. 121:776, 1965.

Robitscher, J. B.: Pursuit of agreement: psychiatry and the law, Philadelphia, 1966, J. B. Lippincott Co.

Shindell, S.: The law in medical practice, Pittsburgh, 1966, University of Pittsburgh Press.

Solvenko, R.: History of criminal progress as related to mental disorders, Psychoanal. Rev. 55:223, 1968.

Special Committee on Mental Illness: Due process and the criminal defendant, New York, 1968, Fordham University Press.

Whitlock, F. A.: Criminal responsibility and mental illness, London, 1963, Butterworth & Co. Ltd.

30
The psychiatrist and community mental health

THE PROBLEM

Mental illness is a serious public health problem. One half of all hospital beds in the United States are devoted to the care of the mentally ill. Estimates have been variously given that 1 in every 20 persons will spend some part of his life within a mental hospital and that many Americans (approximately 1 in 5) are afflicted with less serious emotional maladies requiring treatment. Suicide alone accounts for 20,000 deaths a year, and there are an estimated 5 to 6 million chronic alcoholics in the United States. Studies by Essen-Möller in Sweden, by Srole in midtown Manhattan, and by Leighton and Leighton in Stirling County, a Canadian rural area, indicate that from one third to two thirds of the population studied showed symptoms suggestive of psychiatric disorder. Such figures, large though they may be, give only a partial picture of the amount of mental and emotional disturbance—in terms of their cost as measured by man-hours lost to industry and tax dollars spent for treatment and custodial care and the indirect cost—such as the personal and community tragedies of delinquency, crime, personal isolation, boredom with work, purposelessness in day-to-day living, alcoholism, and drug addiction. The characteristics of clinic outpatients which were studied by Rosen, Bahn, and Kramer in 1961 clarify which disorders are now receiving diagnostic and some therapeutic attention in the United States. Approximately 200 per 100,000 population received clinic attention that year. The highest rates were for boys 10 to 14 years of age and girls 15 to 17 years of age. The lowest rates were for children under 5 years and adults over 65 years. Rates of first admission to state mental hospitals increase steadily with age and are higher for men than for women in every age group. Married adults are less likely to receive clinic care than are the unmarried adults. Rates for organic brain syndromes are relatively high during the first 10 years of life, low in adolescence and young adulthood, and high again toward the end of the life-span. Among adults, psychoneuroses account for more of the female rate, whereas personality disorders account for more of the male rate. There is also evidence that clinics tend to devote more of their resources to these disorders than to the mentally retarded or to the delinquent.

Introduction of psychotropic drugs in 1955 had a considerable impact on public psychiatry. Since then, and for the first time in the long history of public mental hospitals, there has been a decrease in the number of hospitalized patients, dropping from 558,922 in 1955 to 370,849 in 1970. President John F. Kennedy, speaking before Congress in 1963, predicted a 50% decline in state hospital patients in a 10- to 20-year period. It is notable that the present reduction has occurred in the face of a 7% yearly increase in admission rate.

PREVENTIVE PSYCHIATRY

The concept of preventive psychiatry includes programs for reducing the incidence of mental disorders (primary prevention), reducing the duration of disorders (secondary prevention), and reducing the impairment resulting from disorders (tertiary prevention). Inasmuch as the etiology of most psychiatric illness is not known, primary prevention today refers to educational programs and other methods of giving help to individuals at naturally occurring transition points in their lives and when coping with crises. Secondary prevention deals with early case finding, with population screening, and with making more effective treatment facilities available for larger numbers of persons. Tertiary prevention or rehabilitation refers to programs aimed at strengthening the links between the hospital and the community to help and supervise the discharged patient. Good aftercare programs prevent hospital readmissions. Perhaps one of the most heartening functions of the psychiatrist or of other mental health workers who move into the community is case finding. Partly because of primitive social taboos against mental disturbance and partly because of internal anxiety which may be mobilized by the effort of beginning to face one's fears, emotional disorders tend to be diagnosed correctly only after months or years of suffering. As with other chronic illnesses, however, treatment is increasingly effective and economical the earlier the diagnosis is made. At present there exist no proved tests for mass screening comparable to the chest x-ray program for tuberculosis.

THE PSYCHIATRIST IN THE COMMUNITY

It is evident that the public health psychiatrist does not confine his interest to the medical setting as such but is concerned with the total course of lives of individuals living in the community. This concern becomes focused on a diversity of biological, socioeconomic, and cultural conditions ranging from the poor hydration and nutrition of working class pregnant women in the south during the summer (which has been shown to be associated with prenatal brain damage), to the legal precedents for judging a criminal to be insane, to the value systems in our culture which define acceptable or unacceptable family behavior patterns. On national and community levels, the psychiatrist becomes involved in educational campaigns which seek to remove the stigma of mental disease, to educate the public about existing facilities, and to create a greater demand for adequate treatment for the mentally ill.

These activities are conducted frequently by service-minded volunteers working in collaboration with social agencies, social workers, educators, clergymen, courts, and others. The psychiatrist is frequently sought out by these persons for information about mental health and illness and he should be aware of the fact that whereas it is relatively easy to describe the warning signs of definite psychiatric disorders it is most hazardous to be dogmatic about mental health. Yet it is true that certain psychotherapeutic-like principles are involved in establishing an enlightened school system, an enlightened penal system, or an enlightened personnel system for a large organization. The psychiatrist is beginning to bring to these areas methods directed at uncovering the causes of individual or group malfunction, as well as problem-solving attitudes and techniques.

Even if he is sought out or welcomed by lay groups, the psychiatrist may encounter difficulties once he is out of a traditional medical setting. One of the first tasks here is to make a kind of diagnosis of the real purpose, sometimes hidden, for which psychiatric guidance is sought. Not infrequently community groups have hopes that the psychiatrist in some magical way can dispatch a vexing social problem. Here clearly the consultant's role is to aid the group in mastering its anxiety and to provide orientation about psychiatric aspects of the problem; but at the same time he should keep clear with all concerned where responsibility belongs. For example, if the psychiatrist is called upon in desperation after an outbreak of delinquent behavior in a high school, it is obviously dangerous for him to let the school believe that any single simple remedy is available for the complex problems of which such an outbreak may be symptomatic.

In these situations a useful tool is group discussion, led in a nonauthoritarian manner, which focuses upon a few specific questions which are of genuine concern to the group and with which they have had firsthand experience. Excellent movies or plays now available through mental health associations can present a wide range of vital questions concerning childhood (discipline, tantrums, sex information), adolescence (gangs, dating, struggle for independence), young adulthood (courtship, marriage, pregnancy), or later life (parenthood, job adjustment, retirement). The psychiatrist here encourages maximal group participation—through proper program planning, limiting the size of the group, arranging the chairs in a circle, setting up a cheerful and relaxed group atmosphere. He keeps the focus of discussion clarified and sets limits to group members who wish to dominate or wander too far off the topic. At the end he summarizes for the group lest they leave this somewhat unusual educational experience with an anxious feeling that they have "done all the work without getting any answers." After such emotionally involving, sensitively led group discussions, individuals can sometimes move in the direction of defining a psychological problem close to their own lives in a more constructive manner and, where necessary, seek therapeutic assistance.

MANAGEMENT OF CIVILIAN DISASTER

As part of his community responsibility a psychiatrist may be called upon to assist with sudden community catastrophes.

Exposure to unexpected personal danger, the witnessing of threatened or actual gruesome damage to loved ones, and experiencing separation from family and friends can tax the strongest personalities. Whether or not disaster produces an acute emotional disorder seems to depend upon a variety of factors. Degree and duration of physical stress, geographical closeness to the area of greatest danger, and previous susceptibility to anxiety apparently influence the likelihood of breakdown.

Disaster can produce many of the acute syndromes usually observed in psychiatric practice. Most individuals will show some signs of stress and are best treated by a word of encouragement and assignment to a constructive relief job. *Individual panic (blind flight)*, while infrequent, is dangerous in a crowd because of its contagion. A few individuals who lose control completely can precipitate a mad mass flight and therefore should be quickly segregated with gentle firmness by two or more attendants and remain attended until self-control is regained. Punitiveness (using cold water, slapping the face) should be avoided. *Obtunded reactions* occur in some persons who suddenly seem devoid of emotional reaction and act dazed or as though there were no danger. *Manic-like reactions* with inappropriate joking, rapid speech, and overactivity may occur.

Chronic psychiatric disorders may develop after a disaster, and where supportive measures fail, removal to a psychiatric hospital is indicated.

During the days and weeks following a disaster, the psychiatrist may be helpful in various ways through supportive group meetings with teachers, parents, other relatives of patients, and community leaders by demonstrating that it is safe to admit emotional disturbance following trauma and that realistic appraisal of unpleasant adjustments is more constructive than is denial of upsetting feelings.

THE COMMUNITY PSYCHIATRY MOVEMENT

Concern over mental health problems resulted in passage of Public Law 182 by Congress in 1956. This law established the Joint Commission on Mental Illness and Health, whose final report, *Action for Mental Health,* 1961,* pointed out major problems that exist in psychiatry in the United States today. Cited were the great professional manpower shortage, an overemphasis upon treatment techniques inappropriate to the economic and social aspects of the problem, and a low level of service in state public psychiatry that results in custodial care in large crowded facilities. The report stressed the need for early and adequate treatment in smaller units and for a strengthening of community resources in the mental health field.

In 1963 President Kennedy recommended, and Congress passed, Public Law 88-164, which enabled local communities to obtain matching federal funds to construct local community mental health centers. These centers combine a variety of services, both inpatient and outpatient, for children and adults, partial (day/night) hospital services, 24-hour emergency care, consultation, education, and research. Each center is designed to service a population area of 75,000 to 200,000 persons. In 1965 Congress passed P.L. 89-105 appropriating funds to assist in the staffing costs for these units. Although specifically suited to the needs of more populous areas and those more plentifully supplied with mental health professionals, some aspects of this plan have been imaginatively implemented in most states. In some less populous areas the program has included a few beds of a local county hospital, in other areas psychiatric consultation needs have been met via closed circuit television, and in others an administrative sectioning of large state hospitals into smaller units has served

---

*In Canada, a committee of psychiatrists appointed by the Canadian Mental Health Association made a similar study. Their report, entitled *More for the Mind,* 1963, gives a summary of similar problems that exist in that country together with practical suggestions for their solution.

to focus upon and better meet the needs of given regional geographic units of the community.

Such a nationwide effort to upgrade public psychiatric care was indeed impressive but like many public programs has recently failed to receive adequate continuing financial support. However, no such program can achieve great success without the training of additional psychiatrists who are willing to accept careers in public service. Another major concern is the lack of continuity in the conduct of public health programs as a result of high turnover of top administrative personnel. The ultimate solution to the costly and vexing problems of mental illness must, however, await the development of more effective treatment methods.

Major improvements in the delivery of mental health care are being accomplished through the application of modern electronic data-processing techniques to both the administrative and the clinical areas of psychiatry. This gives promise of great assistance with problems about patient records, personnel, statistics, and communication. Such methods will permit an actuarial approach to diagnosis and the prescription of more effective treatments. Computerized patient data files foster research upon sufficiently large case samples to give more meaningful answers to questions that have long troubled psychiatrists. Through these methods, widely separated psychiatric centers can agree upon and participate in a standard system of psychiatry, and with the ever increasing substitution of facts for theory a major revolution within psychiatry will surely occur worldwide.

SUGGESTED READINGS

Action for mental health, final report of the Joint Commission on Mental Illness and Health, New York, 1961, Basic Books, Inc., Publishers.

Albee, G. W.: Emerging concept of mental illness and models of treatment: the psychologic point of view, Amer. J. Pyschiat. 125:870, 1969.

Bandler, B.: American Psychoanalytic Association and community psychiatry, Amer. J. Psychiat. 124:1037, 1968.

Bellak, L., editor: Handbook of community psychiatry and community mental health, New York, 1964, Grune & Stratton, Inc.

Caplan, G.: Principles of preventive psychiatry, New York, 1964, Basic Books, Inc., Publishers.

Cranshaw, R.: Reactions to disaster, Arch. Gen. Psychiat. 9:157, 1963.

Duhl, L.: Psychiatry and the community, Int. J. Soc. Psychiat. 1:42, 1955.

Epps, R. L., Barnes, R. H., and McPartland, T. S.: A community concern, Springfield, Ill., 1965, Charles C Thomas, Publisher.

Essen-Möller, E.: Individual traits and morbidity in a Swedish rural population, Acta Psychiat. Scand., supp. 100, p. 1, 1956.

Freedman, N., Rosen, B., Engelhardt, D. M., and Margolis, R.: Prediction of psychiatric hospitalization. I. Measurement of hospitalization proneness, J. Abnorm. Psychol. 72:468, 1967.

Hall, J. C., Smith, K., and Bradley, A. K.: Delivering mental health services to the urban poor, Social Work, No. 2, April, p. 35, 1970.

Hanlon, J. J.: Principles of public health administration, ed. 5, St. Louis, 1969, The C. V. Mosby Co., chaps. 5, 28, and 32.

Hollingshead, A. B., and Redlich, F. C.: Social class and mental illness, New York, 1958, John Wiley & Sons, Inc.

Kramer, M.: Epidemiology, biostatistics and mental health planning, Psychiat. Res. Rep. Amer. Psychiat. Ass. no. 22, Apr., 1967.

Mental health in the metropolis, the midtown Manhattan study, New York, 1962, The Blakiston Division of the McGraw-Hill Book Co.

More for the mind, a study of psychiatric services in Canada, Toronto, 1963, Canadian Mental Health Association.

Murphy, J. M., and Leighton, A. H., editors: Approaches to cross-cultural psychiatry, Ithaca, N. Y., 1965, Cornell University Press.

Querido, A.: The Amsterdam psychiatric first aid scheme and some proposals for new legislation, Proc. Roy. Soc. Med. 48:741, 1955.

Reid, D. D.: Epidemiological methods in the study of mental disorders, Public Health Papers no. 2, Geneva, 1960, World Health Organization.

Rosen, B. M., Bahn, A. K., and Kramer, M.: Demographic and psychiatric characteristics of psychiatric clinic outpatients in the United States, 1961, Amer. J. Orthopsychiat. 34:455, 1964.

Services for children with emotional disturbances, New York, 1961, American Public Health Association.

Sletten, I. W., Ulett, G. A., Wood, M. J., and Thompson, W. A.: Standard system of psychiatry, Jefferson City, Mo., 1972 (abbreviated edition), Missouri Division of Mental Health.

Squire, M. B.: Current administrative practices for psychiatric service, Springfield, Ill., 1970, Charles C Thomas, Publisher.

Srole, L., et al.: Mental health in the metropolis, New York, 1962, McGraw-Hill Book Co.

Ulett, G. A., Schnibbe, H., Ganser, L. J., and Thompson, W. A.: Mental health director—bird of passage, Amer. J. Psychiat. 127:126, 1971.

Ulett, G. A., and Sletten, I. W.: Computers and psychiatric case records—state of the art, Brit. J. Hosp. Med. 6:291, 1971.

United States Public Health Service: Fact sheet: the Comprehensive Community Mental Health Center Program, Washington, D. C., 1965, U. S. Department of Health, Education, and Welfare.

Index

Grandeur, delusions of, definition
of, 80
Griesinger, Wilhelm, 5-6
Grimaces, 82
Group therapy, 276-281
flexible, 280
history of, 276-277
psychoanalytic, 279
psychodrama in, 280
social group work, 279-280
Guardianship proceedings, 337-339
Guilford-Martin Temperament Profile, 55
Gyrectomy, 297

H

Habitual excessive drinking, 184
Habituation, definition of, 187
Hall, G. Stanley, 9
Hallucination
definition of, 77
types of, 77-78
Hallucinogens
addiction to, 194
in chemotherapy, 304
Hallucinosis, alcoholic, 104
Harlow, 10
Hashish addiction, 193
Headache, tension, 203
Healy, William, 220
Hearing, hallucinations of, 77
Heart action, disturbances of, 205
Heautoscopy, definition of, 77
Hebephrenic schizophrenia, 147
Heinroth, Johann, 6
Hematophobia, 171
Hemic psychophysiological disorder, 207-208
Hippocrates, 5
History taking and diagnostic procedures, 13-82
examination
for agnosia, 32
for aphasia, 28, 31, 32, 33-34
for apraxia, 33
physical and neurological, 23-27
of psychiatric patient, 15-22
psychological, 44-63

History taking and diagnostic procedures—cont'd
psychiatric disorder symptoms, 76-82
psychodynamic concepts of personality development, 64-75
Histrionic personality disorder, 179
Homosexuality, 182
Horney, Karen, 9
psychotherapy theory of, 263-264
Hull, Clark, 269
drive reduction theory of, 271
Huntington's chorea, 232
psychosis associated with, 110
Hydrophobia, 171
Hydrotherapy, 293
Hyperkinetic reaction, 222
Hypermnesia, definition of, 78-79
Hypertension, essential, 205-206
Hyperthyroidism, 212
Hyperventilation syndrome, 204
Hypnopompic hallucinations, definition of, 77
Hypnotherapy, 268-271
Hypnotics, addiction to, 193
Hypnotizability, definition of, 269
Hypochondriacal neurosis, 175-176
Hypomania, 81
Hypothalamic seizures in epilepsy, 124
Hysteria
definition of, 167
seizures in, 121
Hysterical neurosis, 163, 167-169
Hysterical personality, 179
Hysterical pseudostupidity, 196

I

Id, definition of, 256
Ideas of reference, definition of, 80
Idiocy, amaurotic, 233
Illusion, definition of, 77
Impulse (s)
instinctual, 256
irresistible, definition of, 334
Impulse neurosis, 179
Inadequate personality, 180-181
Incompetency, mental, forensic psychiatry and, 337